LGBTQ Cultures:

What Health Care Professionals Need to Know About Sexual and Gender Diversity

3rd Edition

Michele J. Eliason, PhD
Peggy L. Chinn, RN, PhD, FAAN

D0862709

. Wolters Kluwer

Philadelphia • Baltimore • New York • London
Buenos Aires • Hong Kong • Sydney • Tokyo

Acquisitions Editor: Nicole Dernoski
Editorial Coordinator: Jeremiah Kiely
Production Project Manager: Kim Cox
Marketing Manager: Linda Wetmore
Manufacturing Manager: Kathleen Brown
Design Coordinator: Larry Pezzato
Vendor: Aptara, Inc.

9 8 7 6 5 4 3 2 1

Printed in China

Library of Congress Cataloging-in-Publication Data

Names: Eliason, Michele J., author. | Chinn, Peggy L., author.
Title: LGBTQ cultures : what health care professionals need to know about
    sexual and gender diversity / Michele J. Eliason, Peggy L. Chinn.
Description: 3rd edition. | Philadelphia : Wolters Kluwer, [2018] | Includes
    bibliographical references and index.
Identifiers: LCCN 2017038782 | ISBN 9781496394606
Subjects: | MESH: Sexual Minorities | Gender Identity | Attitude of Health
    Personnel | Health Services Accessibility | Culturally Competent Care
Classification: LCC RA564.9.H65 | NLM WA 300.1 | DDC 362.1086/6–dc23
LC record available at https://lccn.loc.gov/2017038782

DISCLAIMER
Care has been taken to confirm the accuracy of the information present and to describe generally accepted practices. However, the authors, editors, and publisher are not responsible for errors or omissions or for any consequences from application of the information in this book and make no warranty, expressed or implied, with respect to the currency, completeness, or accuracy of the contents of the publication. Application of this information in a particular situation remains the professional responsibility of the practitioner.

To purchase additional copies of this book, please visit Lippincott's NursingCenter.com or call our customer service department at (800) 638-3030 or fax orders to (301) 223-2320. International customers should call (301) 223-2300.

Visit Lippincott Williams & Wilkins on the Internet: http:/www.lww.com. Lippincott Williams & Wilkins customer service representatives are available from 8:30 am to 7:00 pm, EST.

Dedication

We started this book as a group of four White nurses who had spent many years in educational institutions. We said goodbye to Jeanne DeJoseph and Sue Dibble after the first edition when they retired. Mickey and Peggy updated the content for the second edition, but retained most of the information from the first edition. We dedicate this work to Sue and Jeanne who were pivotal in getting the project up and running in the first place.

We also dedicate this book to the LGBTQ nurses and other health professionals and the allies who helped us see the need for this book, and the LGBTQ people who need to have culturally sensitive healthcare providers to feel safe and included when they seek out health services.

Michele J. Eliason, PhD
Peggy L. Chinn, RN, PhD, FAAN

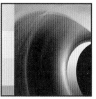

Preface

When we wrote the first edition of this book, published in 2007, we felt that there was a dire need for an introductory level book on sexual and gender identities for healthcare provider audiences. There were a few books focused on medical care or specific health issues such as substance abuse and lots of books on HIV/AIDS, but in our own experience, students in healthcare-related educational programs, whether medicine, nursing, physical therapy, psychology, social work, or other majors, often lacked the basics. In that first edition, we found little research on specific physical health problems other than HIV/AIDS and other sexually transmitted infections, and not that much information about the experiences of LGBTQ people in hospitals or clinics either. The only area where research was fairly robust was about substance abuse and mental health problems.

When we updated the book in 2016, there was much more information available about physical health and links between minority stress and chronic illnesses. Along with health information, there was a virtual explosion of writing about gender identities, and much more study of nonbinary identities that expanded the possible identities for people beyond male, female, or transgender. There was an expansion of sexual identities as well. We appreciated how fast the field has evolved.

Now, in 2017 as the ebook becomes available in a physical book format, we are in an almost unimaginable time in the United States when hard-won LGBTQ rights are being threatened at local, state, and especially national levels once again. Religious freedom bills are proliferating, workplace protections for government workers have been rolled back, there are movements to limit adoptions by same-sex couples, and so much more. Repeal of the Affordable Care Act would remove health insurance from thousands of LGBTQ people who were finally covered by health insurance for the first time. Transgender, gender variant, genderqueer, and gender nonbinary folks are the targets of anti-LGBTQ hatred, with much of the emphasis in the media focused on access to bathrooms. At the same time, transgender women of color are being murdered on a regular basis. There is a resurgence of anti-LGBTQ sentiment across the world, from death threats and detention and torture camps for gay men in Chechnya to extremist Islamic groups murdering gay men. White supremacists have gained power and influence in the United States, and they threaten the lives of people of color, women, and LGBTQ people (and some people embody all of these oppressed minority identities in one body).

The only way we can ensure continued progress in civil rights for all people is through thorough and accurate education about human variations and differences, without labeling them as disorders. We hope that having this book available in hardcopy will encourage its use in classrooms across the world as an introductory text that will benefit all students, who will encounter LGBTQ people not only in their work in healthcare settings, but also in their daily lives; in their families, their neighborhoods, their congregations and schools and elsewhere. Education is one part of a larger strategy to ensure human rights, and until healthcare curricula consistently address LGBTQ issues, myths and stereotypes are perpetuated.

Michele J. Eliason, PhD
Peggy L. Chinn, RN, PhD, FAAN

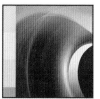

Table of Contents

Chapter 3: The Deadly Effects of Stigma

Chapter 4: Myths and Facts about Sexual Orientation and Gender Identity

Chapter 5: LGBTQ Families

Chapter 1

Overview and Theoretical Framework

"I have come to believe over and over again that what is most important to me must be spoken, made verbal and shared, even at the risk of having it bruised or misunderstood...My silences had not protected me. Your silence will not protect you...What are the words you do not yet have? What do you need to say? What are the tyrannies you swallow day by day and attempt to make your own, until you will sicken and die of them, still in silence?" —African American lesbian poet, Audre Lorde (1980, pp. 19–20)

This first chapter is offered in the spirit of the opening quote—breaking the silence about LGBTQ health care. We believe that open dialogue about sexual and gender diversity is healthy and will benefit all people. That dialogue has raged in recent years primarily over same-sex marriage, and a telling sign of the times is that at this writing (July 2015), Ireland just approved same-sex marriage by popular vote, and the U.S. Supreme Court ruled in favor of legalized same-sex marriage in all 50 states (Masci, Posts, & Bio, 2015). This is a good start, but it means that conversations about equitable and quality healthcare services need to ramp up. In many states in the United States, a person might now be able to marry, but could be fired from a job for that marriage, or evicted from their home. Employment and housing discrimination protection is not uniform in state laws yet.

Changes in law do not automatically erase years of bias and stigma. We know that 50 years after civil rights legislation based on race/ethnicity, that our nation is still torn by constant racial incidents and both blatant and subtle racism. We expect the same will be true of civil rights based on sexual orientation and gender identity. Some of the issues we raise in this book are controversial and have no easy resolution, and indeed, we struggle with many of the thorny issues ourselves. We raise them in order to challenge healthcare professionals to begin conversations about these issues and start identifying the steps that are needed to change the healthcare climate to one that is open, welcoming, and inclusive to all the people it serves.

Medical, nursing, and other healthcare professional schools have historically ignored the needs of lesbian, gay, bisexual, transgender, and queer (LGBTQ) patients/clients. In recent years, however, with growing recognition of health disparities based on race/ethnicity, class, gender, and sexual orientation, the health professions have increasingly acknowledged the need for culturally sensitive care. We believe that providing generic care means that many people receive inadequate or culturally inappropriate care. Failing to address health disparities means that some patients/clients do not enter healthcare institution doors until their illnesses are far advanced, because they fear poor treatment, because they do not have insurance, or on occasion, because a healthcare professional has refused to care for them.

This book introduces basic concepts and terminology related to sexual orientation and gender identity, and addresses such diverse topics as myths and stereotypes about LGBTQ people, developmental issues, diversity, LGBTQ families, the effects of stigma on health, and individual provider level and structural changes that need to occur to create culturally sensitive healthcare services. In this first chapter, we introduce some of the most basic terminology and present our assumptions and theoretical perspectives that will set the tone for the rest of the book.

This third edition has been challenging to write, since there has been an explosion of new research on LGBTQ populations since we completed the first edition. We have updated the entire book, added new chapters, but decided to stay with our focus on the issues that are shared by each of the subgroups in the alphabet soup of LGBTQ. We wanted this book to stay at the level of an introduction to the broad issues that affect LGBTQ cultures, and not try to be comprehensive or all inclusive. Readers who wish for subgroup specific information will be given resources in later chapters to access that information.

Terminology

A lot of space is devoted in this book to the definition and critique of words and concepts used to describe people and behaviors. Language both reflects and creates deepseated cultural biases and anxieties, and the terminology we use sets the climate for social interactions and the parameters for research on LGBTQ populations (Eliason, 2014). Chapters 2 and 3 focus on the definitions related to the concepts of sex/gender, sexuality, and stigma, but some terms are used throughout the book and need to be defined before we proceed any further. We have chosen to be as inclusive as possible in our language, but any terms we select have some limitations. We provide a rationale for our choice of those core terms now.

LGBTQ

We have chosen to use the shorthand LGBTQ when talking about the shared influences of stigma among lesbian, gay, bisexual, transgender, and queer-identified people, and other terms if we are talking about a specific group or groups. The Q could also stand for questioning, and represents those people who are at particular risk for health disparities as they struggle internally about coming out as LGBTQ. Some of the previous books have focused only on gay men and lesbians, or on men who have sex with men, or on transgender individuals, or on lesbian, gay, and bisexual people, or LGBT populations (Institute of Medicine, 2011). We wanted to be as broadly inclusive as possible in this book, and chose to include another "Q," or "queer" in our list of identities because a growing number of youth, and a fair number of adults, use this term to refer to their identities. Some use it as a way to reclaim a term previously used as an insult. If you call yourself "queer," it no longer has the power to intimidate or degrade. Others use queer as a more inclusive identity that encompasses a wide diversity of sexual and gender expression, and some people use it for political reasons to point out the unique experiences of many LGBT people, who are *not* just like everyone else. Some use it in order to avoid the traditional male/female binary that has been imposed on gender, wishing to break free of gender stereotypes. We also recognize that the term offends some people, and that there is no one satisfactory umbrella term for all the diversity contained within categories of sexuality, gender, class, race/ethnicity, age groups, trans-nationality, and geographic locations, to name just a few.

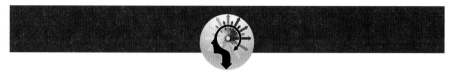

There Are No Dumb Questions 1.1

Question: I just cannot warm up to the term "queer"—it is hard enough to begin to accept many of these things that I never before knew existed, and to add a word that is so negative is too much. Why do you have to use it?

Answer: Indeed this is not a dumb question at all, and it is important to consider why this term has "caught on" for many LGBTQ people. Not all LGBTQ people like or use the term, in fact some folks feel exactly as you do! However, for many, it is now the preferred term for self-identity because it does not box them in to a strict male or female or gay or straight identity. Using the term defies and overcomes gender "opposites" (binaries) and instead creates a culture where people are free to just express themselves as they wish. In academic circles, the term "queer studies" refers to the study of cultural, linguistic, and social factors that create gender, sexual, and heteronormative stereotypes. Another reason it is gaining popularity is that using a negative or derogatory term in a new way—as a positive term of pride—eventually defies and deflates the negative connotations that it once carried. It is true that many derogatory and negative terms are so offensive that they can never acquire a positive image in the larger culture. But at this point in time, the term "queer" is widely acknowledged, and has gained standing as a term that can be used to shift values and attitudes by breaking down gender and sexual stereotypes and assumptions. You certainly do not have to use it yourself, and it may not be possible for you to overcome how you feel about it at this point. As a healthcare provider, you are quite likely to encounter individuals, either as colleagues or as patients, who use this term comfortably, and your acceptance of their choice of terms will open the way for a positive relationship.

Language is always a limitation, but it is a necessary evil when communicating with each other. On one hand, it lets us share information with others, but on the other hand, it is often the source of misunderstandings and confusion. In various literature sources and in social service agencies, you may see different terms used, or a different order of the terms, such as GLBT, LGBTAIQQ (lesbian, gay, bisexual, transgender, allies, intersex, queer, and questioning), or LGBTQFF (the FF standing for friends and family), LGBTQ2S (the 2S standing for two spirit), same-gender loving, and so on. Recently the great diversity within trans communities has given rise to using an asterisk, as in trans*, to indicate the intention to be inclusive of any term that a person might use in connection with a "trans" identity. A telling sign of the times is that Facebook went from having two options for gender (male or female) to 58 categories.

Sexual and Gender Minorities

In some contexts we use this phrase to indicate inclusion of all people who identify in a way that is not heterosexual male or female. This phrase has the advantage of words that are inclusive and generally understood without the mystifying use of a set of alphabet letters. It also is capable of including a large proportion of the population who identify as "mostly heterosexual" or "not entirely heterosexual" (Vrangalova & Savin-Williams, 2012). But the term has the disadvantage of being so general that it obscures meanings that are unique to each of the many groups who might be included. This term also runs the risk of "sanitizing" the powerful connotations conveyed by the terms represented by LGBT and Q, so in some contexts we use specific terms deliberately to draw attention to the feelings, attitudes, and stereotypes that need to be challenged and overcome.

Healthcare Professional

We wanted a book that could be used in all types of healthcare settings and situations, from professional schools (medicine, nursing, dentistry, pharmacy, physician assistant, health and clinical psychology, chiropractic, medical social work, physical therapy, osteopath schools, occupational therapy, and so on) to clinical settings (hospitals, clinics, residential programs, and private practices) to health policy settings (departments of public health, elected officials). The individuals who might find this book useful include, but are not limited to, clinicians of every sort, student services personnel and educators in health training programs, human resource and continuing education specialists in health fields, community health workers and policy-makers. There is no one term that encompasses them all, so we chose what we thought was the broadest term, healthcare professional.

Patient/Client/Consumer

Similarly, we wanted to discuss the needs of all LGBTQ people who access healthcare services. In various settings, they are called patients, clients, residents, or consumers. We have decided to alternate between the use of patient and client, since those are the most commonly used terms. People who fall into those categories may be interested in the content of this book, but we have written it primarily to address a healthcare professional audience.

Culturally Appropriate Care

There are a multitude of terms in the literature to denote some level of knowledge, skills, and attitudes about people who are different from the healthcare professional. These terms include cultural diversity, multiculturalism, cultural competency, cultural sensitivity, cultural awareness, culturally specific care, cultural humility, cross-cultural care, and so on. We believe that no one can fully achieve cultural competency for all the types of people they will encounter in healthcare settings, and recognizing the limitations of all the terms, have chosen to use "culturally appropriate." A process to becoming culturally appropriate that is gaining momentum in health fields is the concept of cultural humility (Tervalon & Murray-García, 1998). This lifelong process of self-reflection and discovery posits that everyone is a unique blend of qualities and cannot be reduced to any one group membership. Healthcare professionals practice cultural humility by learning about other cultures as well as examining their own beliefs and considering how their own identities might affect patients (Yeager & Bauer-Wu, 2013).

Why a Book on LGBTQ Cultures?

Why do we need a book on LGBTQ people for healthcare professionals? Haven't we come a long way toward acceptance and adequately addressed the negative stereotypes? Indeed, considerable progress has been made, but a substantial segment of the population continues to hold negative attitudes about LGBTQ people based on lack of information, misinformation, and/or deeply ingrained belief systems about the nature of gender and sexuality. Sometimes those belief systems are rooted in religious or moral value systems, and sometimes they stem from beliefs about the way things are or are supposed to be (what is "natural" or "normal"). A portion of those people with negative attitudes treat LGBTQ people differently. When those people are healthcare professionals, the results can be poor quality of care, inappropriate care, or even refusal of care, and whether the violence is subtle or blatant, LGBTQ people suffer. Figure 1.1 shows data on healthcare experiences of LGBT people, and people living with HIV (Lambda Legal, 2010). When more than one in four trans* individuals and one in five people living with HIV are refused health services, we still have a problem. Many respondents reported that healthcare professionals had refused to touch them or used excessive precautions when making physical contact, and many felt that healthcare professionals had blamed them for the presenting health concern. The author of the opening quote, Audre Lorde, died of breast cancer in 1992, and throughout her life, experienced health disparities related to the totality of her experience, including her race/ethnicity, gender, and sexuality. She was a champion for "breaking the silence" and we owe her a great debt for paving the way.

The negative attitudes have receded somewhat in recent years. A survey by the Pew Research Center (2013a) found that 51% of the U.S. general population favored same-sex marriage, but yet 45% considered homosexuality to be a sin and significant numbers of LGBTQ people still experience discrimination and social rejection (Pew Research Center, 2013b). Sheldon and colleagues (2007) conducted phone interviews about the "causes" of homosexuality with randomly selected respondents from the

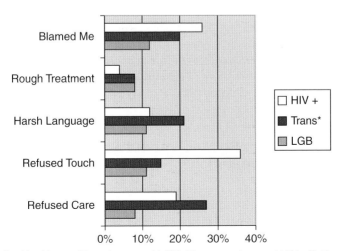

Figure 1.1 – Healthcare Experiences of LGB, Transgender, and HIV+ Patients (Based on **Lambda Legal, 2010**).

United States, and the stereotypes and misinformation elicited were staggering. Here are a few examples of respondent comments:

> "It's a female brain inside of a male body, and vice versa with a lesbian." (p. 124)
>
> "It's something wrong with them—a brain defect or something." (p. 124)
>
> "Part of their genitals are outside and they have to make a decision whether they're gonna be a boy or a girl at birth, so they did surgery and sometimes they didn't always make the right decision." (p. 125)
>
> "He wasn't accepted by his father and that had a lot to do with him being a homosexual." (p. 126)
>
> "The reason they started going with each other—because of the bad experiences that they had had with men." (p. 127)
>
> "I think a lot of time when people revert over to the same sex it's because they done been raped by a man or a woman." (p. 127)
>
> "It might be someone at a young age was approached by someone or introduced to it." (p. 127)
>
> "It's Satan's work." (p. 129)

These statements highlight the confusion that some people in the general population have regarding the overlapping concepts of gender and sexuality. Some respondents did not know the difference between lesbian, gay, bisexual, transgender, and intersex identities (also called disorders of sexual development, see Chapter 2). The comments also highlight lack of understanding of the research on the relative influences of nature and nurture on development. Surely people in the healthcare professions are more knowledgeable about these issues? Historically, healthcare training programs have been notoriously poor at including accurate, research-based information about LGBTQ issues, or sexuality in general, for that matter. A recent survey of medical school curricula showed that one-third had no LGBT-related content at all, and the rest had a median of 5 hours, but 44% of medical school deans thought their coverage of LGBT issues was only fair (Obedin-Maliver et al., 2011). Nursing schools are similarly thin on LGBTQ content, with a median of just over 2 hours of LGBT content across the nursing curriculum, and with 17% reporting no LGBTQ content at all (Lim, Johnson, & Eliason, 2015). These findings mean that the majority of healthcare professionals go into clinical settings with little or no more information than people in the general population. There are few or no sources of factual information in the textbooks of their discipline or the lectures/discussions in their classes or clinical rotations to counteract the stereotypes learned in childhood and adolescence, so they persist among many healthcare providers today.

Why Should I Learn So Much About Such a Small Segment of the Population?

Healthcare professionals have so much to learn about health, disease states, treatment options, and technical skills and procedures. Why should they spend time learning about subsets of the clinical population? Isn't that a bad use of limited time in healthcare training programs? We give you four reasons here why it is important to learn the content in this book—there may be several other reasons, but these will resonate with at least some readers.

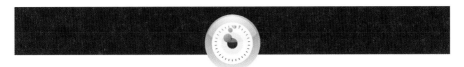

Watch This 1.1

Watch this video summarizing the experiences of Chris Tanner and Lisa Chickadonz, both lesbian nurses who are prominent nurse leaders in nursing and the LGBTQ community in Oregon, and who have carried on a legal struggle to gain basic healthcare benefits for their family for over 15 years.
https://goo.gl/dXtzRq

First, LGBTQ people make up a larger portion of the population than many people think. Surveys of the LGBTQ population are flawed and unreliable for a number of reasons, including how one asks the questions (e.g., many more people have engaged in same-sex activities than will adopt an LGBQ identity; many transgender people consider themselves male or female, thus are not counted). Stigma plays a major role in responding to questions about sexuality and gender and LGBTQ populations are suspicious of people who ask for this information and may not reveal their identities or behaviors to researchers or healthcare providers they do not yet trust. Stigma leads to an under-reporting of LGBTQ identities. No one knows what the actual number is, but it is likely to be close to the one in ten figure that is so often quoted (that is, about 10% of people are not entirely heterosexual or have a gender identity consistent with the sex assigned at birth). There are more LGBTQ people than there are people of the Jewish faith (about 2%), people in the world with green eyes (about 2%), and about the same number as left-handers (10%). LGBTQ patients will be found in every type of healthcare setting, from dermatology clinics to birthing suites; from pediatrics to geriatrics; from substance abuse residential programs to community-based free clinics. Professionals from every discipline and specialty will encounter some LGBTQ clients and coworkers. In addition, LGBTQ people contain every other form of diversity, including race/ethnicity, gender, social class, educational levels, and national origins.

Second, everyone has gender and sexuality identities and expresses them in various ways. The information in this book will help healthcare professionals be more aware of and sensitive to the needs of all patients/clients and more comfortable asking them about these issues. Many patients/clients of any sex/gender or sexuality want their primary healthcare providers to be more knowledgeable and approachable about topics related to sexuality and gender.

Third, the information may be personally relevant. Everyone has LGBTQ friends, relatives, children, coworkers, neighbors, and so on. Being more comfortable talking about these issues will open the individual up to the possibility of deeper, richer relationships with others, and allow some readers to explore how their own sex/gender and sexuality have impacted their lives as healthcare professionals.

Finally, the ethical standards of most healthcare professionals demand quality healthcare services to all patients. It is the ethical responsibility of healthcare professionals to educate themselves in areas where they have knowledge gaps. It is not acceptable to wait for patients to educate healthcare professionals about their needs, because they are in a highly vulnerable state when entering healthcare systems. Laws and policies do not always support the best ethical actions, and it is important to examine your own ethical responsibilities and know where you stand from both an ethical and a legal perspective. Fortunately, as LGBTQ rights are increasingly recognized as valid human rights, laws and policies are beginning to change to be consistent with ethical responsibilities of healthcare providers.

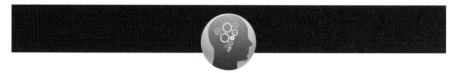

Think About It 1.1

To underscore the importance of understanding LGBTQ healthcare issues, here is one story. In 2007, Janice Langbehn, her partner of 18 years Lisa Pond, and three of their four children arrived in Miami for a family cruise, when Lisa collapsed and was taken to the hospital. Janice was denied any access to her partner or information about her condition even though she presented legal documents (power of attorney for health care) and was told by the social worker that she was in an anti-gay city and state. Janice was allowed just one 5-minute visit, while last rites were administered. Later she was denied access to the death certificate. She filed a lawsuit against the hospital and the publicity ultimately resulted in a presidential memo in 2010 requiring hospitals to allow same-sex visits.

How do you think you might have responded to this situation, or to another similar situation? What are the local laws and policies where you live, and how might these influence your decision in a case like this?

Our Philosophy and Basic Assumptions

Most authors have agendas, often hidden. The messages they give in their writing may be obvious or subtle. We choose to state our agenda directly in the form of a mission statement and underlying assumptions that we have about LGBTQ identities and healthcare professionals. Our mission for this book can be expressed as follows: To positively change the culture of healthcare for LGBTQ individuals.

More specifically, we believe that:
- When healthcare professionals know more about LGBTQ populations they can provide better care, make better decisions, and make better referrals.
- Each healthcare professional is responsible to learn about the populations for whom they provide care or develop policies.
- Background knowledge about LBGTQ health issues can assist both healthcare recipients and their direct care providers to better understand one another and to focus their questions for each other.
- Dialogue from a position of mutual understanding is necessary to bring about social justice within healthcare.

Underlying Assumptions Within this Book

- Sexual orientation and gender identity are not risk factors for health problems: stigma associated with those identities creates the risk.

- The world, including healthcare settings, can be unsafe for LGBTQ people.
- There is a lack of knowledge among the majority of healthcare professionals about LGBTQ cultures and people.
- There are many different communities and cultures within LGBTQ populations; each letter in the alphabet soup represents groups with different needs, but as a collective, the issue is one of dealing with stigma.
- Even members of LGBTQ communities have misunderstandings about health needs of other members of their own communities and may have biases and prejudices about others, because few of us have received adequate or accurate education about sexual orientation and gender identity in school, at home, or in the media. Just because a healthcare professional identifies as LGBTQ does not mean that they are knowledgeable about the health issues of the community.
- Clarity about definitions can facilitate understandings, but we recognize that language is in constant evolution so some of these definitions will change over time.
- Education can facilitate awareness which can improve sensitivity and build a knowledge base that facilitates social justice. This education is essential in all healthcare profession training programs.
- Most healthcare professionals are good people with good intentions, but lack knowledge about ways to communicate their acceptance of their LGBTQ clients.
- All people are experts on their own health, body, and experiences. It is the responsibility of the healthcare provider to "tune in" to that expertise of their patients.

Theoretical Framework for the Book

The ASK™ model (Lipson & Dibble, 2005) serves as the framework for this book (see Figure 1.2). The three components of the model are Awareness (A), Sensitivity (S), and Knowledge (K), and apply to learning about any new cultural group. We can never be totally culturally competent about every group of people we may care for, but the ASK model allows us a framework for approaching new learning.

We come to each patient encounter bringing along all of our beliefs, stereotypes, and morals/values. We do not practice in a vacuum away from the lifelong influences

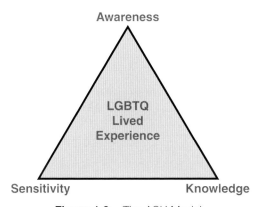

Figure 1.2 – The ASK Model.

of our cultural socialization from the media, friends, family, and religious leaders. It is critical that each person identify and take the time to reflect on potential internal barriers to quality care that have been produced by our environment. This reflection will facilitate AWARENESS of our biases about specific groups of people and the impact these biases might have on providing quality care (both overtly and covertly). This awareness allows us to avoid verbal and nonverbal social gaffes that potentially might offend our clients and their families. We hope that all of the chapters in this book will facilitate a greater awareness of LGBTQ cultures in healthcare settings.

The second part of the model teaches us to be SENSITIVE in our approach to similarities as well as differences in cultures. For example, we can examine the art, magazines, questionnaires, and forms in various healthcare setting from multiple perspectives. Have we unconsciously created a space that conveys a message that everyone is heterosexual by our choice of language in the intake forms, brochures, and the posters on the walls? Do the materials we use reflect the cultures we serve in terms of language and visual images? Are we aware of gender diversity and have we set a climate that will allow patients to discuss their real lives with us? We address the issue of a welcoming environment further in Chapter 13. Sensitivity necessitates approaching each new patient with an open mind and heart, no expectations or assumptions, as a unique human being.

KNOWLEDGE is the final component of the ASK™ model and the purpose of this book is to provide the reader with some basic information about LGBTQ cultures to build the individual healthcare professionals' knowledge base. Notice we use the plural term; the cultures within and among each LGBTQ community vary by race/ethnicity, age, gender, socioeconomic status, educational preparation, social class, and disability status, among others. Sexual orientation and gender identity are other threads in the tapestry of being human. All "facts" especially those that we use to make decisions about patients' needs must be checked out with the individual, not just assumed to be true.

Conclusion

We have explained our use of basic terminology, laid out the rationale for this book, and made transparent our assumptions and philosophy about sex/gender and sexuality in healthcare settings. Finally, we have introduced a framework, ASK™ that is useful for understanding a wide variety of cultural differences. In the next chapter, we deal with definitions of terms and concepts related to sex/gender and sexuality; concepts that are fascinating and complex manifestations of human diversity.

References

Eliason, M. J. (2014a). An exploration of terminology related to sexuality and gender: Arguments for standardizing the language. *Social Work in Public Health, 29,* 62–175. Retrieved from http://doi.org/10.1080/19371918.2013.775887

Eliason, M. J. (2014b). Chronic physical health problems in sexual minority women: A review of the literature. *LGBT Health, 1,* 259–268.

Institute of Medicine. (2011). *The health of lesbian, gay, bisexual, and transgender people: Building a foundation for better understanding.* Washington, DC: National Academies Press. Retrieved from http://www.iom.edu/Reports/2011/The-Health-of-Lesbian-Gay-Bisexual-and-Transgender-People.aspx

Lambda Legal. (2010). When health care isn't caring: Lambda Legal's survey of discrimination against LGBT people and people with HIV. Retrieved May 29, 2015, from http://www. lambdalegal.org/publications/when-health-care-isnt-caring

Lim, F., Johnson, M., & Eliason, M. J. (2015). A national survey of faculty knowledge, experience, and readiness for teaching lesbian, gay, bisexual, and transgender health in baccalaureate nursing programs. *Nursing Education Perspectives, 36*(3), 144–152. Retrieved from http://doi.org/10.5480/14–1355

Lipson, J., & Dibble, S. L. (Eds.) (2005). Providing culturally appropriate health care. In *Culture and critical care.* San Francisco, CA: UCSF Nursing Press.

Lorde, A. (1980). *The cancer journals.* Argyle, NY: Spinsters, Ink.

Masci, D., & Posts, & Bio. (2015). 5 facts about same-sex marriage. Retrieved May 30, 2015, from http://www.pewresearch.org/fact-tank/2015/04/27/same-sex-marriage/

Obedin-Maliver, J., Goldsmith, E. S., Stewart, L., White, W., Tran, E., Brenman, S., … Lunn, M. R. (2011). Lesbian, gay, bisexual, and transgender-related content in undergraduate medical education. *JAMA: The Journal of the American Medical Association, 306*(9), 971–977. Retrieved from http://doi.org/10.1001/jama.2011.1255

Pew Research Center. (2013a). A survey of LGBT Americans: attitudes, experiences and values in changing times. Retrieved July 20, 2015, from http://www.pewsocialtrends. org/2013/06/13/a-survey-of-lgbt-americans/

Pew Research Center. (2013b). In gay marriage debate, both supporters and opponents see legal recognition as 'inevitable.' Retrieved May 30, 2015, from http://www.people-press. org/2013/06/06/in-gay-marriage-debate-both-supporters-and-opponents-see-legal-recognition-as-inevitable/

Sheldon, J. P., Pfeffer, C. A., Jayaratne, T. E., Feldbaum, M., & Petty, E. M. (2007). Beliefs about the etiology of homosexuality and about the ramifications of discovering its possible genetic origin. *Journal of Homosexuality, 52*(3–4), 111–150. Retrieved from http://doi.org/10.1300/J082v52n03_06

Tervalon, M., & Murray-García, J. (1998). Cultural humility versus cultural competence: A critical distinction in defining physician training outcomes in multicultural education. *Journal of Health Care for the Poor and Underserved, 9*(2), 117–125.

Vrangalova, Z., & Savin-Williams, R. C. (2012). Mostly heterosexual and mostly gay/lesbian: Evidence for new sexual orientation identities. *Archives of Sexual Behavior, 41*(1), 85–101. Retrieved from http://doi.org/10.1007/s10508–012–9921-y

Yeager, K. A., & Bauer-Wu, S. (2013). Cultural humility: Essential foundation for clinical researchers. *Applied Nursing Research: ANR, 26*(4), 251–256. Retrieved from http://doi. org/10.1016/j.apnr.2013.06.008

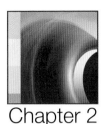

Chapter 2

What's in a Word? Concepts Related to Sex/Gender and Sexuality

"Silence is a knife—it cuts both ways" (Hemphill, 1989)

Chapter 2 contains an introduction to important concepts and terminology related to sex/gender and sexuality in order to ensure that all readers are on the same page before focusing on health care. Language/terminology, styles, and fashions change over time, and are highly contextual and culturally bound, and this is particularly the case with terminology related to matters of sex and gender. Non-Western cultures and even some subsets of westernized regions of the world have very different understandings of the same concepts, and slang terms in particular are often specific to specific age groups and/or geographical regions. For the purposes of this book, we rely on dominant U.S. cultural construction of sex/gender and sexuality that define sexuality and gender.

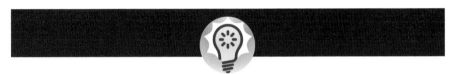

Imagine This 2.1

You are meeting your new supervisor for the first time, a person named Chris Chinn. What do you assume about Chris? If you do not know Chris' gender, does that cause any anxiety about the first meeting? How about Chris' ethnicity? Why do those things matter?

Part of the reason that many people are confused about issues related to sex/gender and sexuality is that usually we are not taught a language as children about these topics in school or in our homes. They are still considered "controversial" topics and families may not discuss them openly. Peers may use slang terms or use words inappropriately or in derogatory ways, and most schools shy away from comprehensive sexuality education. Taboo topics are imbued with secrecy, guilt, and a titillating anxiety for many people. No wonder our language is imprecise and laden with emotionality. This chapter provides some discussion of the words sex, sexual orientation, gender identity, intersex, gender expression or presentation, and the diversity of the definitions for these terms. The chapter ends with a brief discussion on disclosure of gender and sexuality.

Sex

This term has two meanings. The first definition refers to the physical/biological characteristics thought to distinguish men and women, such as

- Chromosomes: women have an XX pattern; men have an XY pattern;
- Genitals: men have a penis and testicles; women have a clitoris, vulva, and vagina;
- Reproductive organs: men have a prostate and testes; women have a uterus and ovaries; and
- Hormones: women have estrogen and men have testosterone.

We will address the reality of these distinctions between women and men in a later section, but for now, will just point out that they are not as simple and straightforward as they appear.

The second meaning of the word sex has to do with those behaviors or internal desires that are related to pleasure and/or reproduction. We will discuss those issues in a section labeled "sexual expression." Sometimes you will hear people refer to "gay sex." This term has little meaning, as any persons can engage in a wide variety of behaviors that result in arousal—these behaviors are not limited by one's sexual orientation or identity. The only fairly consistent difference between same-sex encounters and other-sex encounters is the likelihood of pregnancy, and even this is not a reliable difference. Neither of the two meanings of the word "sex" is universal, completely straightforward, or consistent, as we shall see as we proceed through this book.

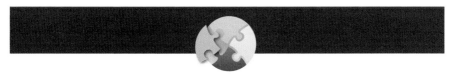

Try This 2.1

Write a definition for the word, "sex." Was it an easy task? Is your definition clear and unambiguous? Does it reveal underlying assumptions about sex (there are only two sexes and they are "opposites," sex is an activity between a man and a woman, sex is for reproduction, and so on). We have not been taught to talk about sexuality openly, which means that every individual learns about sexuality in quite different ways, and there is no one universally accepted definition of sex.

Gender

Usually one of the first things we notice about people is their gender. Not their sex, because that would require asking the person to undress so we could observe their genitals, or take a blood test so we could check their chromosomes. We rarely, if ever, use the biological sex markers to categorize people; we use the gender markers, such as hair style, clothing, amount or type of adornment, posture, voice, and communication styles. On written form and surveys, we rely on self-report—a person is typically asked to respond to an either-or, male or female question. Sometimes we rely on names to give us clues about a person's gender and sometimes their race/ethnicity as well. All of these "markers" that we use to label and categorize people by gender are socially constructed, unlike sex, which is based on a set of biological characteristics (but that are given social meaning).

There are many characteristics that a particular culture determines are the appropriate appearance and behavior for someone who is male-bodied or female-bodied. This means that sex and gender are conflated (interdependent), and that the use of the term sex/gender is more accurate when we are talking about issues of maleness/femaleness or their cultural expressions as masculinity/femininity.

Sexual Orientation

Sexual orientation is the umbrella term used to refer to all the factors related to objects of sexual attraction, and with whom we form sexual and romantic relationships. The American Psychological Association defines it this way:

> *Sexual orientation is an enduring emotional, romantic, sexual, or affectional attraction toward others. It is easily distinguished from other components of sexuality including biological sex, gender identity (the psychological sense of being male or female), and the social gender role (adherence to cultural norms for feminine and masculine behavior). Sexual orientation exists along a continuum that ranges from exclusive heterosexuality to exclusive homosexuality and includes various forms of bisexuality. Bisexual persons can experience sexual, emotional, and affectional attraction to both their own sex and the opposite sex.* (American Psychological Association, 2015)

There are three terms that are sometimes used interchangeably in the literature: sexual orientation, sexual preference, and sexual identity. Each has a distinct underlying assumption about sexuality, as expressed below:

- Sexual orientation: refers to biological or early childhood experiences that determine sexuality. Some think of it as biologically "hard-wired," innate attractions that cannot be altered. This term is mostly used by scientists who believe sexuality to be biological, and LGBTQ rights activists who are fighting for civil rights based on the idea that sexuality is immutable like sex or race (although the concepts of sex and race are equally contested and complex social terms, not as rooted in biology as most of us were raised to believe).
- Sexual preference: the choices we make regarding sexuality; a preference can be changed or another object can be substituted fairly easily for the "preferred" choice. This term is mostly used by opponents of LGBTQ rights, who claim that people could change if they wanted to, and that sexual attraction is a learned behavior. This term is the most politicized of the three.
- Sexual identity: our internal schemas about our sexuality; the way we think about or label our sexuality. Sexual identity is one of the many components of our self-concept, working in interactions with other social identities related to our sex/gender, race/ethnicity, social class, occupation, and family roles.

Since we do not really know the differential role of biology or environment in the development of sexualities, the term sexual identity is the most neutral choice. Orientation, identity, and preference all refer to our attractions to others—what characteristics of individuals we find sexually attractive. They do not provide any information about the specific sexual behaviors a person enjoys or practices. That topic is dealt with in the next section.

In the academic literature, the first four sexual orientations or identities are often presented. There is growing consensus that there is a fifth sexual orientation: asexuality.

1. Gay—men whose primary sexual attractions are to men.
2. Lesbian—women whose primary sexual attractions are to women.
3. Bisexual—men or women who are sexually attracted to people on the basis of characteristics other than their sex/gender. Bisexuality can be threatening to heterosexuals and gays and lesbians who base their identities on the sex/gender of the people to whom they are attracted.
4. Heterosexual—men or women who are sexually attracted to people of the other sex/gender.
5. Asexual—an individual who is not sexually attracted to people of either sex/gender.

Both men and women are often referred to as gay or homosexual. Many LGB individuals consider the word "homosexual" to be an insult, because it was a term imposed upon the community by a largely negative medical establishment. The terms homosexual and homosexuality are slowly dropping out of the English language.

The sexual identity categories break down when talking about the sexuality of transgender individuals. How would one label a postoperative transgender woman (born biological male) who is attracted to women? How about a preoperative transgender man who likes athletic blonds regardless of their sex/gender? Gender identity and sexual identity are relatively independent of each other, but our language has conflated the two, and discussion of same-sex and different-sex couples is still based on the idea of a binary of sex (male and female, same or different).

The term "queer," despite long-standing negative connotations, has become more common among some people, particularly younger individuals, as a way to defy the labels and stereotypes of "male" and "female." "Queer" is also used as a badge of pride in defiance of the hate and disdain that has been perpetrated toward sexual/gender minority individuals or communities. The term "queer" is the only term that does not imply a gender binary or opposite, and can be used to convey the intent to overcome culturally imposed "norms" based on gender. There is also a growing academic literature about queer identity, and the potential of gender-free social constructions.

Asexual is a relatively new term for an old concept. Throughout time, some people (estimates of about 1% of the population) report a lack of sexual attraction to anyone. In some contexts, this has been defined as a sexual dysfunction, as in the DSM's hypoactive sexual desire disorder. On the other hand, if the low sexual desire does not produce any distress for the person, it is better described as a sexual orientation (Bogaert, 2015; Yule, Brotto, & Gorzalka, 2015).

The idea that people can be defined by their sexual orientation or identity is a relatively new one, stemming back to the rise of sexology a little over 100 years ago. Prior to that time, in all cultures and all studied time periods, some people engaged in same-sex behaviors and deviated from social norms related to sex/gender, however, they were not thought to be a different type of person because of it. The term "homosexual" was first coined in the 1860s, and the labeling of same-sex behavior in the medical literature allowed people to recognize that others shared their differences and were able to form communities based on the label (Katz, 2007). In some other cultures, less influenced by western medical ideas than the United States, same-sex behavior is something you do, not who you are.

Given the lack of clarity about the terminology of sexual orientations and identities, it is safest for healthcare professionals to use the words that patients use to describe themselves, or use the more neutral "sexual identity." In general, avoid terms like "sexual preference" and do not refer to individuals as "queer" or "homosexual' unless they expressly ask you to. Sexual identities are the public facts about who people are attracted to and say nothing about a person's private sexual behaviors. Behaviors may not be congruent with sexual identity—that is, a woman who identifies as a lesbian may have recent or past sexual experiences with men, a self-identified heterosexual man may have considerable same-sex experience, and a bisexual woman may never have had a sexual relationship with a woman. Many people use the terms MSM (men who have sex with men) and WSW (women who have sex with women) or WPW (women who partner with women) to reflect the disconnection between sexual identities and sexual behaviors. If the purpose is only to identify people who are engaging in same-sex sexual activities (keep in mind that sex/gender of the partner is not a risk factor—only actual behaviors are risky or not risky), then MSM and WSW are adequate terms, although bisexual health advocates have pointed out that it would be more accurate to say "men who have sex with men and women" (MSMW) and "women who have sex with women and men" (WSWM) (Miller, Andre, Ebin, & Bessonova, 2007). However, some people feel that to use any of these behavioral terms too broadly is an erasure of LGBTQ culture, identity, and community (Young & Meyer, 2005). After all, knowing about communities is essential to developing environmental prevention strategies to improve the health of any subpopulation, and to reduce people merely to their behavior does not reflect their whole being. Healthcare professionals need to address both behavior and identities.

Because it gets cumbersome to write or say LGBTQ all the time, the field has often used shortcuts or umbrella terms, although none have been accepted as the standard. Examples of language found in health research include sexual and gender minority (SGM), gender and sexual diversity (GSD), and nonheterosexual populations. Some use LGBT; others add more letters to the alphabet soup: LGBTQQAI for example.

Think About It 2.1

When were you first aware of, or begin to question, your own sexual identity? What do you think "caused" your sexual attraction patterns? These are relatively easy questions for openly LGBTQ individuals, because the coming out process requires thinking about these issues, but heterosexual people often must think long and hard about this. Heterosexuality is taken-for-granted, but if people take this question seriously, they will see that many expectations and pressures were put upon them from family, religion, popular culture, education, and peers, to be heterosexual (Eliason, 1995).

Sexual Expression

Sexual expression refers to how we act out our sexual desires, including what we like or do not like sexually and what arouses us or turns us off. Some of this comes from our biology, but probably most of it comes from our conditioning, societal taboos or norms, personal experiences, personality styles (thrill-seekers vs. don't rock the boat), and our partners' characteristics and wishes. People engage in a wide variety of sexual behaviors for a wide variety of reasons, ranging from solitary activities (looking at sexually explicit materials on the computer, fantasizing, or masturbating) to behaviors with one or more other people; and from motives of curiosity, seeking pleasure, wanting to get pregnant, or other less lofty motives such as revenge, boredom, wanting to please a partner, rebellion, or wanting to hurt someone. These motives are not attached to particular sexual identities.

There are huge cultural variations in what is considered sexual (and sexy), and those cultural norms are often contradictory. What is pronounced as "normal" or "conventional" by some forms of popular culture varies considerably from what is "normal" by conservative religious standards. What one person labels as sex, another does not (think about the controversy over whether or not former U.S. president Bill Clinton had sex with Monica Lewinsky—the debate about whether oral sex is "real" sex persists today in some ways). In contemporary U.S. culture, behaviors that are portrayed in the media as "sex" might include kissing, fondling, masturbation, mutual masturbation, rubbing genitals against each other, oral sex, vaginal sex, and anal sex. Other things that may or may not be considered sex might be bondage, role-playing, wearing fetish clothing (e.g., leather), watching sexually explicit images, watching others have sex, etc. None of these behaviors are linked tightly with one's sexual orientation or identity. There are infinite combinations of sex, gender, sexual orientations, sexual expressions, and gender expressions, testimony to the diversity of the human experience and imagination.

Gender Identity

Gender identity refers to one's self-concept as male or female, masculine or feminine, or as a continuum with many points between the extremes. Gender identity is established quite early in life, with most children being able to identify their own gender by age 3, and categorizing others on the basis of gender stereotypes (called gender schema in the developmental psychology literature) soon after that. Most women and men, regardless of their sexual identities, have a gender concept that is fairly consistent with their physical bodies. People who do not have a consistent gender identity and physical body gender presentation are referred to as trans*. This relatively new way to designate the broad category of gender difference from the norm comes from the way internet search terms can be configured with a stem and asterisk to search all terms with that stem. In this case, the stem "trans" can be followed by many other phrases (transgender, transsexual, transmasculine, trans man, trans woman, etc.). Some of the terms that make up the trans* community include:

Transgender is probably the most common term used to describe people whose gender identity is not congruent with their sex as assigned at their birth.

Coined in the late 1980s, the term transgender caught on in a big way in the 1990s following the publication of a pamphlet by Leslie Feinberg entitled, Transgender Liberation (Stryker, 2006). People who use the term to describe themselves are quite diverse.

Transsexual is the term first used by the medical profession to define those individuals who seek interventions to change their bodies to align with their psychological gender. Some activists use the term "transexual" (one "s") instead of transsexual (Wilchins, 1997). Some people object to this term because of its origins in medical disciplines that have often been obstacles in receiving transition services.

Other trans* terminology includes:

- A male-to-female (also written as MTF, MtF, or M2F) transgender individual is a transgender woman ("trans woman" or "trans female"). Some simply identify as women.
- A female-to-male transgender (FTM, FtM, or F2M) individual is a transgender man ("trans man"). Some simply identify as men.
- Some individuals in the transgender community do not identify as either male or female, but "genderqueer" or gender crosser (McCloskey, 1999) or some other term such as transmasculine, boi, nonbinary, or gender nonconformer.

It is important to be aware that the term "transvestite" is sometimes mistakenly taken to refer to people who are trans*. As explained in the next section, "transvestite" refers exclusively to people who sometimes cross-dress for limited occasions not associated with gender identity, and it should not be used in a discussion about sexual and gender identities. Neither should it be used to designate men who perform publicly as "drag queens."

Transitioning is the process that some trans* people undergo to bring their outward gender expression into alignment with their internal gender identity. Transitioning can involve medical treatments such as hormonal therapy, cosmetic procedures, chest surgery ("top surgery") and genital surgery ("bottom surgery") as well as behavioral/psychological interventions such as speech coaching, electrolysis, counseling, and learning how to dress/present like the other sex (Israel & Tarver, 1997; Lawrence, 2007; Lombardi, 2007). The World Professional Association of Transgender Health (WPATH) has guidelines for helping trans* people with transition-related care (see http://www.wpath.org/).

Some gender nonconforming people do not identify as trans* and may express their individuality in dress, in behaviors, and/or speech (Skidmore, Linsenmeier, & Bailey, 2006). Some of these individuals identify as "genderqueer," "butch," or other terms. Cross-dressers, who are often called "transvestites" in the medical literature, are predominantly heterosexual men who like to dress in women's clothing on occasion, but do not wish to permanently become women. They may or may not identify with a community or call themselves trans*. The organization Tri-Ess (The Society for the Second Self: http://www.tri-ess.org/) addresses common issues of heterosexual cross-dressers. Finally, some people "play" with gender for political or theatrical reasons; this is typically called "drag" and people born into male bodies who cross dress are called "drag queens," whereas those born into female bodies dressing and acting as men are called "drag kings."

Intersex/Differences in Sexual Development

"Intersex" is an identity term used by some people who have a number of biological conditions or physical variations in which a person has reproductive or sexual anatomy that does not fit the typical parameters of female or male bodies. Increasingly the term "disorders of sex development" or DSD is used in the medical community to denote the wide range of conditions that are associated with genital anatomical, chromosomal, or hormonal variations. Because of the stigma attached to the term "disorder," some choose to say "differences in sexual development" instead (Association of American Medical Colleges [AAMC], 2014). The outdated term "hermaphrodites" is no longer used because it is both inaccurate and offensive, and was dropped by the medical establishment in 2006 and replaced by DSD. A person might be born appearing to be female on the outside, but having mostly male-typical anatomy on the inside, or with genitals that seem to be in-between the usual male and female types—for example, a girl with a noticeably large clitoris, or lacking a vaginal opening, or a boy with a notably small penis, or with a scrotum that is divided like a labia. Some people who appear to have completely female bodies are found to have XY chromosome patterns. Many of these conditions are not noticed at birth, and only manifest later in childhood or around puberty, yet others are not identified unless the person seeks assessment for infertility or on autopsy. Some of the conditions require medical or surgical interventions, but many others do not. Some authors suggest that as many as 1 in 100 individuals has some form of intersex variation (Blackless et al., 2000). The most common of these include congenital adrenal hyperplasia, androgen insensitivity, and hypospadias. Keep in mind that biomedical fields may use DSD as the major term, but some individuals will still choose to identify with the term intersex.

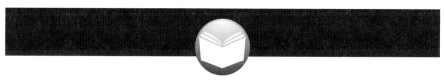

Read This 2.1

Alliance Accord provides information for parents and healthcare professionals about disorders of sexual development. This link leads to their site where you can download for free and read "Clinical Guidelines" for providers, and "Handbook for Parents." https://goo.gl/FwLEpN

People with DSD may have lesbian, gay, bisexual, heterosexual, or asexual orientations and identities, and they vary as much as any other group on gender identity and gender expression. In the past 20 years, some people with intersex conditions who were subjected to invasive procedures as children before they could be consulted about their wishes, have formed social and political organizations to campaign for more humane treatment. Some people who identify with the intersex label also align with the LGBTQ communities, because of the similarities of experiences of stigma, shame, and secrecy.

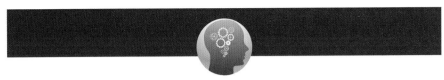

Think About It 2.2

A well-publicized case that was reported in many news venues in 1997 told the story of one of the twin brothers who was mutilated during circumcision at the age of 8 months. A decision was made to raise this biological boy as a girl, renamed as Brenda. Famous sexologist, John Money, followed the case and reported successful adaptation to a female role. However, years later researcher Milton Diamond encountered this individual who wanted the story to go public. Diamond found that Brenda never felt comfortable in a female role. When he found out at age 14 what had happened in infancy, he reverted back to a male role and started living as David. David committed suicide at age 38. In this tragic case, nature seemed to trump nurture (see Colapinto, 2001 for whole story.). What do you think is needed to change a scenario like this from unfolding as it did?

Gender Expression

As noted above, sex/gender can include biological components such as genitalia, but mainly we recognize gender by the way people express themselves through choices in clothing, hair styles, accessories, body postures, communication styles and voice, and other behaviors. A person with XX chromosomes, a vagina and uterus may be comfortable being a woman, regardless of sexual identity, but may choose more "masculine" attire (defined by the culture) and body postures and may self-identify or be called, "butch." Other biological women may choose more traditionally feminine gender expression and use a label or be recognized as "femme," "girly," or "feminine." Yet others are androgynous in their appearance and behaviors. The same is true of people with typically biological male bodies, although the terms may differ. For example, the term "effeminate" has sometimes been applied to boys or adult gay men who have feminine interests or behaviors rather than the term "femme." Because "effeminate" is not a word of the LGBTQ communities' choosing, it may be considered offensive by many. Some gay and bisexual men may call each other "girl" or "girlfriend" in a jesting play on gender, but it does not mean that they identify as trans* or think of themselves as female in any way.

Trans* individuals may express a disconnection between their physical bodies and the gender they perceive themselves to be, and they may strive to match their physical appearance with their internal gender concepts. Some individuals "play" with gender expression, such as cross-dressing for fun or political reasons on occasion, whereas others live more permanently within one part of the gender continuum and would be offended by any suggestion that they are playing with gender. Gender expression is an ever-changing cultural construct, determined by fashion trends, religious beliefs, family socialization, developmental phase, and many other factors. Because sex and gender are so overlapping, some theorists use the terms together "sex/gender" to refer to gender expression.

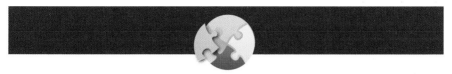

Try This 2.2

How did you express your gender today? Did you make a conscious choice to appear more masculine, feminine, or androgynous in your appearance? How much variation is there in your own gender expression from day to day? If you have access to childhood pictures, what clues are there in those pictures about your gender expression? Were these signs of gender of your own choosing?

Sexuality, Gender, and Cultural Diversity

Definitions of sex/gender and sexuality in the academic literature developed out of White European, middle class values and belief systems, and people from other cultural groups may use different terms (e.g., mahu in French Polynesia; hijras in India and Pakistan; fa'afafine in Samoa; or tomboy in the Philippines) and have different understandings about sex/gender and sexuality (Eliason, 2014; Herdt, 1996; Roscoe, 1998). As an example, the term "two spirit" is used by some people who are indigenous to the Americas to describe sexuality and gender. The term does not equate exactly to lesbian, gay, bisexual, transgender, or intersex, but denotes a greater level of sexual and gender fluidity that is common to many American-Indian groups (Fieland, Walters, & Simoni, 2007; Tafoya & Rowell, 1988). Some African-American people who are not heterosexual use the term "same-gender loving." Similarly, the slang terms used to refer to gender expression vary by geographical region and community, and terms like "bull-dyke," "fairy," "stud," and "bulldagger" might be used to describe a person's gender expression. Many researchers use the term "sexual minority" rather than lesbian, gay, or bisexual, as an umbrella term that encompasses same-sex attraction, behavior, and identity, since there is considerable fluidity and flux among these different ways of viewing one's sexuality, particularly in many adolescents (Diamond, 2006; Russell, 2006), regardless of whether or not the youth attach a label to their sexualities. We will discuss diversity in sexual and gender expression and identities in more detail in Chapter 7.

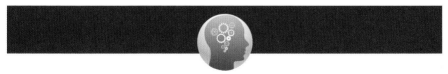

Think About It 2.3

Youth often reject labels (and a growing number of adults do as well) as people recognize that sexual desire does not need to be attached to gender. As one respondent in a study said: "Labels don't really matter because when I'm falling in love or whatever, I'm falling in love with the person's soul and packaging is incidental" (Diamond, 2006, p. 84). What labels do you use that you might discard? What purposes do the labels you use serve?

Another issue related to "cultural diversity" is the criticism some people make about including LGBTQ issues in larger diversity training programs or curriculum. They often argue that sexual or gender identities do not constitute "culture." It is certainly true that there are differences between ethnic minority cultures and LGBTQ cultures (see Chapter 7 for a longer discussion of this issue). Most LGBTQ people are not born into a sexual/gender minority culture where they are socialized for their role in the culture during childhood. Instead, most LGBTQ people consciously adopt the culture later in life. Reasons that LGBTQ may be considered a cultural community include the following:

1. LGBTQ people often organize around a common identity—most express that they are part of a community that has some shared beliefs. For example, the majority of LGBTQ people believe that homophobia, biphobia, and transphobia need to be eradicated; that LGBTQ people deserve full rights and benefits; and that same-sex relationships are normal and healthy.

2. There is a long and extensive LGBTQ history. Same-sex behaviors and gender crossings have been noted through-out recorded history, although the trend to label these behaviors as identities only has a history of about 150 years. The contemporary LGBTQ movement often dates itself from two major events: January 1, 1965 when police raided a San Francisco drag ball, and June 27, 1969, the day that a police raid on a gay bar in New York City called the Stonewall Inn erupted into a riot that lasted several days and spawned gay liberation groups to emerge across the country. Of course it was not as simple as one or two events creating a movement. Rather, the entire climate of the 1950s and 60s civil rights, anti-war, and women's liberation movements set the stage for a gay liberation movement as well.

3. LGBTQ communities have developed a unique language. Terms like coming out, passing, the closet, transitioning, stealth, top/bottom, butch/femme, queen, MTF and FTM, are commonly understood by people in LGBTQ communities.

4. There are well-organized social and political organizations within LGBTQ communities, including restaurants, book stores, social service agencies, choirs and bands, clubs, informal online chats and message boards, bars, music festivals, cruises, and local, state, and national political organizations. There are even "gay holidays" such as pride festivals, National Coming Out Day, and National Day of Silence.

5. There are almost universal rituals and rites of passage in LGBTQ communities, including individual rites such as coming out to self, coming out to others, and the experience of rejection and discrimination; and group rituals such as gay pride rallies and parades, and the experience of the first time attending a gay bar or social group.

6. There is clear evidence of cultural productions. LGBTQ people have created music, poetry, literature, and art that reflect their experiences as oppressed minorities and as part of a unique cultural group. For example, the AIDS quilt reflects grief over loss of so many LGBTQ people to AIDS, but is also a form of artistic and social expression about community. Another example is the rainbow flag that represents the vast diversity of LGBTQ communities.

Just because LGBTQ communities might be considered a "culture" or community does not mean that all LGBTQ people agree on everything. On the contrary, there are vast differences in opinion about marriage, monogamy, sexual values, how to go about getting equality, politics, religion, gay pride parades, and everything else you can think of. This is true of any social identity: put a group of people who call themselves "feminists" or "democrats" in a room and see if they agree on all the important issues!

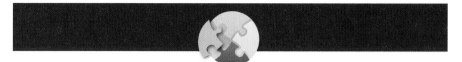

Try This 2.3

Find an event or a place where people who have a different sexual orientation or gender identity than you do gather. For example, if you identify as heterosexual, find a place in your community where people who identify as gay, lesbian, or bisexual tend to gather (a community center, bar, or event). Spend some time there and strike up a conversation with some of the people who are there. How did you feel being part of the minority in this group? How did others react to you?

Disclosure

Most of the time sexual and gender identities are not visible differences, and most LGBTQ people cannot be reliably identified by their appearance. The majority must proclaim their identities in some way if they want others to know. Disclosure is both a process and an outcome. Research on disclosure of sexual/gender identity has taken two forms: most of the literature has focused on the processes that LGBTQ people undergo to adopt an LGBTQ identity, often referred to in the lay literature as "coming out." A smaller body of research has examined the effects of revealing one's sexual or gender identity to others, including healthcare professionals, an outcome called disclosure. Both sexuality and gender identities are important factors for healthcare professionals to know to provide the highest quality and most relevant care.

Coming Out

Levitt and Ippolito (2014) described coming out as the process of "balancing a desire for authenticity with demands of necessity" (p. 1727). Older models of sexual identity formation described it as a linear process progressing from recognizing a same-sex attraction to engaging in same-sex behavior, exploring an identity, and culminating in adopting a stable and consistent gay or lesbian sexual identity (Cass, 1979; Eliason, 1996; Troiden, 1988). The studies that informed these early models were generally based on retrospective memories of adults (mostly men who identified as gay). Prospective studies, and those with more diverse samples have indicated that the processes are much more complex than a simple set of stages, and involve a great deal of fluidity, periodic re-evaluations of the identity, differing circumstance of a particular context, and changes in the labels used for one's sexuality or gender (Diamond, 2006; Eliason & Schope, 2007). Some people never adopt a label of lesbian, gay, or bisexual in spite of considerable same-sex experience, and some explore various forms of gender expression without adopting a trans* identity.

There has been little research on sexual identity formation processes for bisexual and transgender individuals (Devor, 2004; Exceptions include Fox, 1995; Rust,

1996), but it does appear that identity formation is even more complex for people who fall between the binary positions of society, such as man/woman and gay/straight. For example, Devor (2004) noted 14 distinct stages in the process of a trans* identity. Levitt and Ippolito (2014) identified seven clusters of experiences in the process of coming out as trans*. The overriding category was one of "developing color vision in a mono-chromatic world" (p. 1736). This included finding labels or concepts for one's gender, finding ways to communicate about gender in order to be seen by others, and balancing identity needs with safety in a discriminatory and hostile world.

Another alternative way to view identity formation is to examine whether the person considers their sexuality or gender as fixed and stable, or fluid (Ross, Daneback, & Månsson, 2012). A growing number of youth prefer not to label their sexuality and experience it as flexible and ever-changing (see also Farr, Diamond, & Boker, 2014). Ultimately, though, "fluid" is also a sexual identity on the nonheterosexual continuum.

Whether or not coming out is a linear process with identifiable steps or stages, or a more cyclical, fluid, or free-flowing process, all people who have a sexual identity (whether LGBTQ or heterosexual) have experienced some sort of process that informs their self-identities (Eliason & Schope, 2007). Common experiences of that process include confusion and questioning, experimenting, feeling alienated, feeling different from others, fearing rejection from others if they reveal their identity, but also feeling inauthentic or fraudulent for not disclosing, preferring to be around other people of the same identity (isolating oneself in LGBTQ communities), integrating the sexual or gender identity into the larger self-concept or becoming an activist, and celebrating the difference. For hetero-sexual people, the processes may be taken-for-granted and not involve alienation or fears of rejection, or they may include confusion, anxiety, and experimenting.

There is some evidence that the process of questioning one's sexual or gender identity is the most stressful point of the process, because thoughts of having a nonnor-mative gender or sexuality raise fears of rejection by loved ones and by peers (Meyer, 2007). The stress of the questioning phase may be associated with increased frequency of depression/anxiety, suicide thoughts or attempts, and other health risk behaviors such as substance use and misuse, and unsafe sexual experiences. These will be explored in more detail in a later chapter.

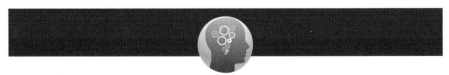

Think About It 2.4

George is a 32-year-old middle school teacher in a small city with only one hospital. Following a nasty cold, he develops pneumonia and goes to the emergency room. He informs the doctor that he is gay, but not out in the community. He is tested for HIV and is negative, and is also treated for the pneumonia. The next week when he returns to school, there is a derogatory message written on the blackboard of his home room. He eventually discovers that the husband of one of his coworkers was employed as a nurse in the ER and told his wife the details of George's ER visit, and the wife then told other teachers and students that he is gay. George's faith in confidentiality has been destroyed and he now faces harassment and potential discrimination in his workplace. What needs to change in the hospital to prevent this situation in the future?

Disclosure to Healthcare Professionals

Since sexual and gender identities are usually not visible differences, they generally require disclosure to others, including healthcare professionals. The majority of healthcare professionals do not ask about sex/gender identities, instead making the assumption that all patients are heterosexual. This puts the onus on the client to disclose, creating undue burden on the one who is in the most vulnerable position. Therefore, deciding whether to disclose one's identity to a healthcare professional can be a very stressful event. In a study of lesbians in Oregon, 90% had disclosed to a healthcare professional, and 92% of those had to raise the issue themselves (White & Dull, 1997). In another study, 61% of lesbians and gay men reported that a healthcare professional had never asked them about their sexuality (Stein & Bonuck, 2001), and a national survey of lesbians found that 37% had delayed health care in the past year because of fear of discrimination (van Dam, Koh, & Dibble, 2001). In one of the few studies to compare gay mens' and lesbians' experiences with disclosure (Eliason & Schope, 2001), lesbians were more likely to have disclosed their sexuality to a healthcare provider, and were also more likely to report that they were hypervigilant in healthcare settings than were gay men. Whereas many gay men and lesbians had actively told their healthcare professionals about their sexual identities (37%), a subset had relied on "passive disclosure" (15%) and assumed that their providers knew even though they had not actually told them, and others reported that the healthcare professional did not ask, so they did not tell (38%). Patients with bisexual identities are less likely to disclose to healthcare professionals than are gay or lesbian patients (Durso & Meyer, 2013).

There are many reasons that LGBTQ people may not disclose, including fear of homophobic reactions, being early in the coming out process, being single, holding a belief that one's sexual orientation is private, or simply, because no one asked (Austin, 2013; Boehmer & Case, 2004; Eliason & Schope, 2001; Hitchcock & Wilson, 1992; Metcalfe, Laird, & Nandwani, 2014; Schatz & O'Hanlan, 1994; Stevens, 1994). LGBTQ people who disclose often do so because the environment seems safe and/or they had done preparatory work in researching the healthcare professional before scheduling an appointment. And there appear to be advantages to disclosure: in one study, patients who disclosed were more likely to receive regular preventative healthcare services than patients who did not disclose (Steele, Tinmouth, & Lu, 2006).

Talk About It 2.1

A woman in treatment for breast cancer remarked about her decision whether or not to disclose to the surgeon that she worried that finding out she was a lesbian might cause the surgeon to "… take another snip out that she is not supposed to?" (Boehmer & Case, 2004, p. 1885). Discuss this dilemma with your colleagues and brainstorm what needs to change to address this kind of concern.

LGBTQ people of color may be even less likely than White LGBTQ people to disclose their sexuality to a healthcare professional because of cultural norms about the privacy of sexuality (Chng, Wong, Park, Edberg, & Lai, 2003; Diaz, 1998; Dowd, 1994; Gómez & Marín, 1996), religious beliefs (Woodyard, Peterson, & Stokes, 2000), not relating to the White gay culture (Wolitski, Jones, Wasserman, & Smith, 2006), or family obligations related to marriage and family (Morales, 1990). There may be even greater mistrust of healthcare professionals and systems among LGBTQ people of color than White LGBTQ people because of historical abuses (Battle & Crum, 2007; Greene, 1997; Wilson & Yoshikawa, 2007).

Disclosure decisions may vary by generation, gender, ethnicity, couple status, immigration status, and reason for seeking care. Several studies have indicated that many LGB patients would prefer that healthcare professionals ask them directly about their sexuality, either in written or oral assessments. Lucas (1992) reported that 64% of lesbians wanted healthcare professionals to ask directly about sexual identities, and in a study of LGBT youth, 64% also indicated that they wanted their healthcare professionals to ask (Meckler, Elliott, Kanouse, Beals, & Schuster, 2006). As a note of caution, though, some authors have raised an ethical dilemma resulting from the frequent recommendations in the literature that healthcare systems and providers start asking questions about sexual orientation and gender identity (Wahlert & Fiester, 2014). If an individual healthcare provider has not been adequately trained to deal with such disclosure, and the healthcare systems do not have appropriate policies and procedures in place to humanely deal with LGBTQ patients, asking these questions may cause more harm than good and further marginalize LGBTQ people.

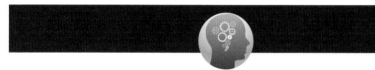

Think About It 2.5

Some LGBTQ people seem to believe that just the fact that a written form includes questions about sexual orientation means that the provider is probably more sensitive. One research respondent said: "On the questionnaire, optional information was 'Were you heterosexual, lesbian, or gay or bisexual?' And that was wonderful. I could just tell him and they wouldn't be asking if they weren't open and aware" (Barbara, Quandt, & Anderson, 2001, p. 56). What do you think? Does having a question on a written form guarantee awareness and openness?

Situations where disclosure might be unlikely could include:
- Older LGBTQs who grew up in a more restrictive, homophobic environment than today;
- LGBTQs of color who have more to lose by disclosing, for example, losing the support of family within a racist society;
- LGBTQ people from working class backgrounds who might not feel as empowered or privileged as middle or upper class LGBTQ people;

- LGBTQs in the military for whom "don't tell" was a mandate until recently. Ingrained fears about negative treatment may still affect active service members and people seeking services at VA hospitals;
- LGBTQ people who receive support and comfort from religious institutions that would potentially reject them if they came out;
- Situations where sexuality is not considered to be relevant, such as being treated in an ER for a minor injury;
- LGBTQ people who fear loss of custody of children if they disclose;
- Others who are early in the coming out process themselves and not ready to talk to anyone about it;
- LGBTQ healthcare professionals who fear gossip about them will spread, or fear that their confidentiality will be compromised;
- LGBTQ teachers and childcare workers for whom "don't tell" is an understood but unspoken rule;
- Those who fear loss of insurance benefits; and
- Those who are not heterosexual, but consider themselves fluid, flexible, or another term that is often not widely known to healthcare professionals.

Of course, some individuals in all of these situations may disclose their sexuality/ gender identities to a healthcare professional because they feel they will receive more appropriate care that way or they have developed a level of trust in the healthcare professional so they feel safe. Disclosure decisions are highly individual, and only the individual can determine if conditions are "safe" enough for disclosure.

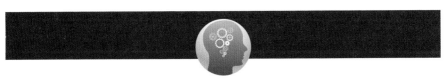

Think About It 2.6

Jamie is a 24-year-old bisexual woman who came out to her gynecologist after the question, "Are you sexually active?" She told her doctor that she was currently in a monogamous relationship with a woman, but 8 months ago, had ended a relationship with a man. Her doctor scribbled something on her tablet, then moved on to another question. Jamie left feeling unsettled. Was her doctor OK with her disclosure or not? She couldn't tell, and that worried her. What should have been different in this situation?

Conclusions

Concepts related to sex/gender and sexuality are under constant transformation in our rapidly changing world. Our understandings of the role of biology, social environment, and societal norms and expectations influence the language we use. However, all language is ultimately limiting and too often becomes a barrier to communication. For healthcare professionals, the best way to work with LGBTQ clients is to put aside all assumptions and expectations, and treat each person as a unique individual.

References

American Psychological Association. (2015). Sexual orientation and homosexuality: Answers to your questions for a better understanding. Retrieved June 20, 2015, from http://www.apa. org/topics/lgbt/orientation.aspx

Association of American Medical Colleges (AAMC). (2014). Implementing curricular and institutional climate changes to improve health care for individuals who are LGBT, gender non-conforming or born with DSD. Retrieved July 25, 2015, from https://www.aamc.org/ download/414172/data/lgbt.pdf

Austin, E. L. (2013). Sexual orientation disclosure to health care providers among urban and non-urban southern lesbians. *Women & Health, 53*(1), 41–55. Retrieved from http://doi.org/ 10.1080/03630242.2012.743497

Barbara, A. M., Quandt, S. A., & Anderson, R. (2001). Experiences of lesbians in the health care environment. *Women and Health, 34*, 45–61.

Battle, J., & Crum, M. (2007). Black LGB health and wellbeing. In I. H. Meyer & M. E. Northridge. (Eds.), *The health of sexual minorities: Public health perspectives on lesbian, gay, bisexual, and transgender populations* (pp. 320–352). New York: Springer Publishing.

Blackless, M., Charuvastra, A., Derryck, A., Fausto-Sterling, A., Lauzanne, K., & Lee, E. (2000). How sexually dimorphic are we? Review and synthesis. *American Journal of Human Biology: The Official Journal of the Human Biology Council, 12*(2), 151–166.

Boehmer, U., & Case, P. (2004). Physicians don't ask, sometimes patients tell. *Cancer, 101*(8), 1882–1889. Retrieved from http://doi.org/10.1002/cncr.20563

Bogaert, A. F. (2015). Asexuality: What it is and why it matters. *Journal of Sex Research, 52*(4), 362–379. Retrieved from http://doi.org/10.1080/00224499.2015.1015713

Cass, V. C. (1979). Homosexual identity formation: A theoretical model. *Journal of Homosexuality, 4*(3), 219–235. Retrieved from http://doi.org/10.1300/J082v04n03_01

Colapinto, J. (2001). *As nature made him: The boy who was raised as a girl*. New York: HarperCollins

Chng, C. L., Wong, F. Y., Park, R. J., Edberg, M. C., & Lai, D. S. (2003). A model for understanding sexual health among Asian American/Pacific Islander MSM in the U.S. *AIDS Education and Prevention: Official Publication of the International Society for AIDS Education, 15*(Suppl 1), 21–38.

Devor, A. H. (2004). Witnessing and mirroring: A fourteen stage model of transsexual identity formation. *Journal of Gay & Lesbian Psychotherapy, 8*(1–2), 41–67. Retrieved from http:// doi.org/10.1300/J236v08n01_05

Diamond, L. (2006). What we got wrong about sexual identity development: Unexpected findings from a longitudinal study of young women. In A. Omoto & H. Kurtzmann (Eds.), *Sexual orientation and mental health: Examining identity and development in LGB people* (pp. 73–94). Washington, DC: APA Press.

Diaz, R. M. (1998). *Latino gay men and HIV: Culture, sexuality, and risk behavior*. New York: Routledge.

Dowd, S. A. (1994). African American gay men and HIV and AIDS. In S. Caldwell, R. Burnham, & M. Forstein (Eds.), *Therapists on the frontline: psychotherapy with gay men in the age of AIDS* (pp. 319–338). Washington, DC: American Psychiatric Press.

Durso, L. E., & Meyer, I. H. (2013). Patterns and predictors of disclosure of sexual orientation to healthcare providers among lesbians, gay men, and bisexuals. *Sexuality Research & Social Policy: Journal of NSRC: SR & SP, 10*(1), 35–42. Retrieved from http://doi.org/10.1007/ s13178–012–0105–2

Eliason, M. J. (1995). Accounts of sexual identity formation in heterosexual students. *Sex Roles, 32*, 821–834.

Eliason, M. J. (1996). Identity formation for lesbian, bisexual, and gay persons: Beyond a "minoritizing" view. *Journal of Homosexuality*, *30*, 31–58. Retrieved from http://doi.org/10.1300/J082v30n03_03

Eliason, M. J. (2014). An exploration of terminology related to sexuality and gender: Arguments for standardizing the language. *Social Work in Public Health*, *29*, 162–175. Retrieved from http://doi.org/10.1080/19371918.2013.775887

Eliason, M. J., & Schope, R. (2001). Does "Don't Ask, Don't Tell" apply to health care? Lesbian, gay, and bisexual people's disclosure to health care providers. *Journal of the Gay and Lesbian Medical Association*, *5*, 125–134.

Eliason, M. J., & Schope, R. (2007). Shifting sands or solid foundation: Lesbian, gay, bisexual, and transgender identity formation. In I. H. Meyer & M. E. Northridge (Eds.), *The health of sexual minorities* (pp. 3–26). New York: Springer Science.

Farr, R. H., Diamond, L. M., & Boker, S. M. (2014). Female same-sex sexuality from a dynamical systems perspective: Sexual desire, motivation, and behavior. *Archives of Sexual Behavior*, *43*(8), 1477–1490. Retrieved from http://doi.org/10.1007/s10508–014–0378-z

Fieland, K., Walters, K., & Simoni, J. (2007). Determinants of health among two-spirit American Indians and Alaska Natives. In I. H. Meyer & M. Northridge (Eds.), *The health of sexual minorities: Public health perspectives on lesbian, gay, bisexual, and transgender populations* (pp. 268–300). New York: Springer Publishing.

Fox, R. C. (1995). Bisexual identities. In A. R. D'augelli & C. J. Patterson (Eds.), *Lesbian, gay, and bisexual identities over the lifespan: Psychological perspectives* (pp. 48–86). Columbia University Press.

Gómez, C. A., & Marín, B. V. (1996). Gender, culture, and power: Barriers to HIV-prevention strategies for women. *Journal of Sex Research*, *33*(4), 355–362. Retrieved from http://doi.org/10.1080/00224499609551853

Greene, B. (1997). Ethnic minority lesbians and gay men: Mental health and treatment issues. In B. Greene (Ed.), *Ethnic and cultural diversity among lesbians and gay men*. Thousand Oaks, CA: Sage Publications, Inc.

Hemphill, E. (1989). Excerpt from the documentary, Tongues Untied by Marlon Riggs, MTR Production.

Herdt, G. H. (1996). *Third sex, third gender: Beyond sexual dimorphism in culture and history*. New York: Zone Books.

Hitchcock, J. M., & Wilson, H. S. (1992). Personal risking: Lesbian self-disclosure of sexual orientation to professional health care providers. *Nursing Research*, *41*(3), 178–183.

Israel, G. E., & Tarver, D. E. (1997). *Transgender care: Recommended guidelines, practical information, and personal accounts*. Philadelphia, PA: Temple University Press.

Katz, J. (2007). *The invention of heterosexuality*. Chicago, IL: University of Chicago Press.

Lawrence, A. A. (2007). Transgender health concerns. In I. H. Meyer & M. E. Northridge (Eds.), *The Health of Sexual Minorities: Public health perspectives on lesbian, gay, bisexual, and transgender populations* (pp. 473–505). New York: Springer. Retrieved from http://doi.org/10.1007/978–0–387–31334–4_19

Levitt, H. M., & Ippolito, M. R. (2014). Being transgender: The experience of transgender identity development. *Journal of Homosexuality*, *61*(12), 1727–1758. Retrieved from http://doi.org/10.1080/00918369.2014.951262

Lombardi, E. (2007). Public health and trans-people: Barriers to care and strategies to improve treatment. In I. H. Meyer & M. E Northridge (Eds.), *The Health of Sexual Minorities: Public health perspectives on lesbian, gay, bisexual, and transgender populations* (pp. 638–652). New York: Springer. Retrieved from http://doi.org/10.1007/978–0–387–31334–4_26

Lucas, V. A. (1992). An investigation of the health care preferences of the lesbian population. *Health Care for Women International*, *13*(2), 221–228. Retrieved from http://doi.org/10.1080/07399339209515994

McCloskey, D. N. (1999). *Crossing: A memoir*. Chicago, IL: University of Chicago Press.

Meckler, G. D., Elliott, M. N., Kanouse, D. E., Beals, K. P., & Schuster, M. A. (2006). Nondisclosure of sexual orientation to a physician among a sample of gay, lesbian, and bisexual youth. *Archives of Pediatrics & Adolescent Medicine*, *160*(12), 1248–1254. Retrieved from http://doi.org/10.1001/archpedi.160.12.1248

Metcalfe, R., Laird, G., & Nandwani, R. (2014). Don't ask, sometimes tell. A survey of men who have sex with men sexual orientation disclosure in general practice. *International Journal of STD & AIDS*. Retrieved from http://doi.org/10.1177/0956462414565404

Meyer, I. H. (2007). Prejudice and discrimination as social stressors. In I. H. Meyer & M. E. Northridge (Eds.), *The health of sexual minorities: Public health perspectives on lesbian, gay, bisexual, and transgender populations* (pp. 242–267). New York: Springer. Retrieved from http://doi.org/10.1007/978–0–387–31334–4_10

Miller, M., Andre, A., Ebin, J., & Bessonova, L. (2007). *Bisexual health: An introduction and model practices for HIV/STI prevention programming*. New York: National Gay & Lesbian Task Force Policy Institute, Fenway Institute, and BiNetUSA.

Morales, E. S. (1990). HIV infection and Hispanic gay and bisexual men. *Hispanic Journal of Behavioral Sciences*, *12*(2), 212–222. Retrieved from http://doi.org/10.1177/07399863900122009

Roscoe, W. (1998). *Changing ones: Third and fourth genders in Native North America*. New York: St. Martin's Press.

Ross, M. W., Daneback, K., & Månsson, S.-A. (2012). Fluid versus fixed: A new perspective on bisexuality as a fluid sexual orientation beyond gender. *Journal of Bisexuality*, *12*(4), 449–460. Retrieved from http://doi.org/10.1080/15299716.2012.702609

Russell, S. T. (2006). Substance use and abuse and mental health among sexual-minority youths: evidence from add health. In A. Omoto & H. Kurtzmann (Eds.), *Sexual orientation and mental health: Examining identity and development in LGB people* (pp. 13–36). American Psychological Association. Retrieved from http://doi.org/10.1037/11261–001

Rust, P. C. (1996). Sexual identity and bisexual identities: The struggle for self-description in a changing sexual landscape. In B. Beemyn & M. Eliason (Eds.), *Queer studies: A lesbian, gay, bisexual, and transgender anthology* (pp. 64–86). New York: New York University Press.

Schatz, B., & O'Hanlan, K. A. (1994). *Anti-gay discrimination in medicine: Results of a national survey of lesbian, gay, and bisexual physicians*. San Francisco, CA: American Association for Human Rights.

Skidmore, W. C., Linsenmeier, J. A., & Bailey, J. M. (2006). Gender nonconformity and psychological distress in lesbians and gay men. *Archives of Sexual Behavior*, *35*(6), 685–697. Retrieved from http://doi.org/10.1007/s10508–006–9108–5

Steele, L. S., Tinmouth, J. M., & Lu, A. (2006). Regular health care use by lesbians: A path analysis of predictive factors. *Family Practice*, *23*(6), 631–636. Retrieved from http://doi.org/10.1093/fampra/cml030

Stein, G. L., & Bonuck, K. A. (2001). Attitudes on end-of-life care and advance care planning in the lesbian and gay community. *Journal of Palliative Medicine*, *4*(2), 173–190.

Stevens, P. E. (1994). Protective strategies of lesbian clients in health care environments. *Research in Nursing & Health*, *17*(3), 217–229.

Stryker, S. (2006). (De) Subjugated knowledges: An introduction to transgender studies. In S. Stryker & S. Whittle (Eds.), *The transgender studies reader* (pp. 1–18). New York: Routledge.

Tafoya, T., & Rowell, R. (1988). Counseling gay and lesbian Native Americans. In M. Shernoff & W. Scott (Eds.), *The sourcebook on lesbian/gay health care*. Washington, DC: National Lesbian and Gay Health Foundation.

Troiden, R. R. (1988). *Gay and lesbian identity: A sociological analysis*. Lanham, MD: Rowman & Littlefield.

Van Dam, M. A. A., Koh, A. S., & Dibble, S. L. (2001). Lesbian disclosure to health care providers and delay of care. *Journal of the Gay and Lesbian Medical Association*, *5*(1), 11–19. Retrieved from http://doi.org/10.1023/A:1009534015823

Wahlert, L., & Fiester, A. (2014). Repaving the road of good intentions: LGBT health care and the queer bioethical lens. *The Hastings Center Report*, *44* Suppl 4, S56–S65. Retrieved from http://doi.org/10.1002/hast.373

White, J. C., & Dull, V. T. (1997). Health risk factors and health-seeking behavior in lesbians. *Journal of Women's Health/The Official Publication of the Society for the Advancement of Women's Health Research*, *6*(1), 103–112.

Wilchins, R. (1997). *Read my lips: Sexual subversion and the end of gender*. Ithaca, NY: Firebrand Books.

Wilson, P. A., & Yoshikawa, H. (2007). Improving access to health care among African-American, Asian and Pacific Islander, and Latino lesbian, gay, and bisexual populations. In I. H. Meyer & M. E. Northridge (Eds.), *The health of sexual minorities: Public health perspectives on lesbian, gay, bisexual, and transgender populations* (pp. 607–637). New York: Springer. Retrieved from http://doi.org/10.1007/978–0–387–31334–4_25

Wolitski, R. J., Jones, K. T., Wasserman, J. L., & Smith, J. C. (2006). Self-identification as "down low" among men who have sex with men (MSM) from 12 US cities. *AIDS and Behavior*, *10*(5), 519–529. Retrieved from http://doi.org/10.1007/s10461–006–9095–5

Woodyard, J. L., Peterson, J. L., & Stokes, J. P. (2000). "Let us go into the house of the Lord": Participation in African American Churches among Young African American men who have sex with men. *The Journal of Pastoral Care & Counseling: JPCC*, *54*(4), 451–460. Retrieved from http://doi.org/10.1177/002234090005400408

Young, R. M., & Meyer, I. H. (2005). The trouble with "MSM" and "WSW": Erasure of the sexual-minority person in public health discourse. *American Journal of Public Health*, *95*(7), 1144–1149. Retrieved from http://doi.org/10.2105/AJPH.2004.046714

Yule, M. A., Brotto, L. A., & Gorzalka, B. B. (2015). A validated measure of no sexual attraction: The Asexuality Identification Scale. *Psychological Assessment*, *27*(1), 148–160. Retrieved from http://doi.org/10.1037/a0038196

Chapter 3

The Deadly Effects of Stigma

"The healthcare system is so imposing and it is so daunting. It is not me looking in someone's eyes and having them understand that I have a problem that they have the expertise to help me, but it is in fact me out here off to the side terrified that the first person that I see is going to do something to shame me or embarrass me or cause me to be ridiculed in front of other people." (Hussey, 2006, p. 137)

In Chapter 2, we introduced terms related to sexuality and gender. The question remains: why have variations in the development of sex and gender been considered as forms of deviance? We do not have an easy answer to this "why" question, but it is without doubt that viewing variations in sexual and gender identities as deviant is prevalent, damaging, and unfounded in fact. This process of making some groups deviant is commonly known as stigmatization. This chapter defines and critiques the terminology used to describe the effects of stigma. From the Greek, *stigma* is derived from the term "tattoo" referring to marks placed on the body of a person labeled as criminal or deviant. Stigma operates through a process of separating oneself from people who are "not like me," a practice often called "othering." This process of rendering some people as "others" can lead to de-humanizing of the other group. People learn to stigmatize some human differences such as skin color or minority sexual identifications, whereas other differences are not stigmatized, such as left handedness or eye color. As you will see, there are many terms and concepts used to describe stigma, leading to some confusion. Language is constantly evolving, and terms used in psychology or sociology may differ from terms used in the health sciences. We will try to include as many of the terms used for each concept as possible, but recognize that we will miss some of them, and define other terms differently from some other authors in this field. That is an occupational hazard of being in a newly emerging field of study. But it can also be a benefit, since different meanings and understandings can contribute to a more complete understanding of human experience. In the first section of this chapter we examine the concepts and terms related to stigma, and the second section addresses the effects of stigma.

Goffman (1963) first applied the term stigma to sexuality, likening minority sexual identification to a "spoiled identity," leading to a sense of inferiority and isolation from the mainstream. We will explore the far-reaching effects of gender and sexual stigma on health and well-being in Chapters 8, 9, and 10, but it is becoming abundantly clear that the stress of being LGBTQ arises from stigma, not from the sexual or gender identities in and of themselves. Stigma is the umbrella concept under which the other terms in this chapter fall. Stigma results in inordinate stress that increases the chance of physical and mental health problems in LGBTQ people. The rest of this chapter explores the terminology used to describe the effects of stigma based on minority sexual or gender identifications, but the concept of stigma is also useful when exploring health disparities for women, racial/ethnic minority individuals, people with disabilities, and many other vulnerable populations.

Stigma-related terms pertaining to LGBTQ people include homophobia, biphobia, transphobia, AIDS-related stigma, heterosexism and heteronormativity, gender normativity, "lifestyle," and internalized oppression. Similar processes of stigmatization underlie racism, sexism, classism, and other systems of oppression that intersect with gender and sexual identities for many LGBTQ people. Near the end of this chapter, we discuss some of the similarities and differences among the various forms of oppression that are common today. All forms of oppression are related because they involve power and privilege. In our use of the word, privilege refers to the unearned rewards that are granted solely on the basis of belonging to a certain class of people and is based on a belief that one class of people is superior to others. Men, regardless of other identities, have male privilege; White people have white privilege; heterosexual people have heterosexual privilege. These privileges are largely invisible and taken-for-granted by those who have them, but painfully obvious to those people who do not. People with privilege are the ones who have the power to set the "norms" of society, and those norms often exclude or marginalize those without privilege. The terms described in the next section help to demonstrate how privilege is maintained.

Terms/Concepts Related to Stigma

Homophobia

Coined by a psychologist in the 1970s (Weinberg, 1972), homophobia originally was defined as an irrational fear of lesbian and gay persons. The term has been widely criticized in the research literature, as often it is not based in irrational fear and it is not similar to other kinds of phobias, but the term caught on despite its shortcomings. Sometimes homophobia is based on fear, but sometimes on deliberate hatred or ignorance, or it stems from internalized self-hatred. Sometimes it comes from an unexamined belief that one's religion condemns LGBTQ people or behaviors. The term homophobia is now understood to refer to any negative attitudes about LGBTQ persons. One good thing about the term is that it puts the blame for stigma on the person who holds the negative attitudes, not the LGBTQ person. Some authors suggest that the term "sexual prejudice" (Herek & McLemore, 2013) is more appropriate and more inclusive. Another term that is used in some of the literature is "homonegativity."

Considerable research has examined the predictors or correlates of homophobia or sexual prejudice (Eliason, 1998; Eliason & Raheim, 2000; Herek, Chopp, & Strohl, 2007). In general, this research shows that sexual prejudice is more common among:

- men than women,
- youth and older adults than young and midlife adults,
- people from evangelical and fundamentalist religions than less conservative religions, or people without formal religious affiliations,
- people who are racist and sexist versus those who are not,
- people who have conservative views about sexuality, such as negative attitudes about masturbation and premarital sex,
- in the United States, people from the south and Midwestern regions rather than other regions,
- people with unacknowledged or unaccepted same-sex desires in themselves.

Homophobia or sexual prejudice is seldom an "all or none" phenomenon. It is best described as a continuum of attitudes that range from very mild discomfort to very negative reactions. The varieties of homophobia may also be qualitatively different from one another, and require different interventions to address them. Table 3.1 shows one attempt to categorize some of the varieties of attitudes about LGBTQ people (Eliason & Raheim, 1996) and suggests what interventions might work best to move individuals with negative attitudes to more positive positions along the continuum.

Biphobia

This term has similar conceptual problems to homophobia, but is commonly used to refer to negative attitudes about bisexual persons. There is sufficient evidence that homophobia and biphobia have considerable overlap and many of the same factors (such as conservative religious affiliation and sexist beliefs) predict both, but there are also unique differences (Eliason, 1997). Some gay men and lesbians are biphobic, sometimes for different reasons than heterosexual people may be biphobic. Those reasons may be related to a sense of betrayal. Some gay men and lesbians have been heard to wonder "If there is a revolution, whose side will you take?" In reality, many people have dual or multiple identities that are experienced as part of their whole. We often have situations where one part of our identity is in conflict with another and we must choose. For example, when a child is sick or in trouble, many people choose to express their parental role over the expectations of their work role. LGBTQ people of color may experience racism more acutely than sexual prejudice and choose to belong to political organizations that combat racism rather than LGBTQ organizations. That does not mean that they reject their sexual identities, but prioritize where to put their energies at any given time.

For heterosexual as well as gay and lesbian persons, sexual orientation is defined by the sex/gender of the partner or potential partner. Bisexuality challenges the centrality of sex/gender to a person's core identity by proposing that characteristics other than sex/gender are more critical in sexual desire and relationships. In general, there is more stigma attached to male bisexuality whereas female bisexuality is sometimes glorified, particularly in heterosexual male-oriented pornography (Eliason, 1997; Mohr & Rochlen, 1999). Bisexual men have been accused of spreading HIV and other sexually transmitted infections to their heterosexual female partners, and have been labeled as deceitful and deviant. There is a big difference between cheating on one's partner or spouse with a person of a different gender, and adopting a bisexual identity. People of any gender or sexual identity can be deceitful and unfaithful—bisexual people are no more likely to cheat on their partners than anyone else. Anyone who is having unsafe sex behind a partner's back is putting the partner at risk. Later in the book, we will discuss the phenomenon called "the down-low," a concept that unfairly links Black gay and bisexual men to the HIV/AIDS epidemic among African-American women.

In one study, a woman who had identified as lesbian reported that she unexpectedly fell in love with a male friend and shared, "Overall, people have been supportive, but I've definitely seen some nastiness because of it. One lesbian I know, she said it was just a phase, that I was misguided, that she didn't want him in her house. It made me angry, it made me cry, it made me question—I mean these were the same types of things I heard from straight people when I first came out about having relationships with women" (Diamond, 2006, p. 82).

Table 3.1 – Continuum of Attitudes About LGBTQ People and Proposed Interventions (Eliason & Raheim, 1996)		
Label	**Description. A Person Who:**	**Possible Responses**
Celebration	Believes that having people in the community with a variety of sexual and gender identities and expressions is good and benefits society.	Encourage and publicize. Be a role model for others at your workplace to celebrate the contributions of LGBTQ people.
Acceptance	Believes that all people should be treated fairly and that no one should be discriminated against on the basis of personal characteristics such as race/ethnicity, religion, sexuality, gender, socioeconomic class, etc.	May intellectually believe in civil rights for all people but harbor some emotional baggage about LGBTQ people. Education to counteract stereotypes may be helpful.
Tolerance	Does not actively discriminate against LGBTQ people, but believes that heterosexuals are superior and that LGBTQ people should not "flaunt" their sexuality or be too visible in society. A "don't ask, don't tell" philosophy.	Point out the invisibility of heterosexual privilege and focus on the ways that LGBTQ people are similar to heterosexual people rather than focusing on the differences. Help the person to develop one-on-one relationships with LGBTQ people.
Disapproval	Disapproves of LGBTQ people and/or behaviors on the basis of religious or moral/ethical beliefs about the nature of gender and sexuality (that the only options are two sexes that are fixed and unchangeable; and that other-sex couples are the only normal option for relationships because they are the only ones who can reproduce). Carries a strong sense of superiority. May espouse the belief of "loving the sinner, hating the sin."	Religion: if amenable, have discussions about the context of passages in the Bible that are supposedly about same-sex conduct. Use Bible scholars like Daniel Helminiak (2000) to critique these passages. Unnaturalness: Discuss how sex and reproduction have become unlinked in the past 50 years, and that the majority of sexual encounters even among heterosexuals are not for reproduction, but for intimacy. Discuss the diversity of sex/gender and sexuality throughout the world and in nearly every animal species.
Disgust	Involves strong emotional reactions to LGBTQ people and/or behaviors, such as revulsion and disgust. May involve a physiological reaction like other phobias that cause the person to avoid LGBTQ people or discussion of LGBTQ issues.	This type of reaction might be related to some deep-seated traumas or unacknowledged same-sex desires and may require psychotherapy. Widespread cultural change in the direction of acceptance may eventually change this attitude.
Hatred	A strong disliking and belief that LGBTQ people should be punished for their behaviors or their very existence. Operates through an extreme form of de-humanizing of LGBTQ people.	Victim empathy approaches may be helpful with those who have perpetrated violence, but if they repeatedly show this behavior, they need to be prosecuted, fired, expelled, etc. Discrimination and violence cannot be tolerated.

Biphobia arises from the stereotypes about bisexuality, such as:
- it does not exist; people are either gay or straight,
- it is a phase,
- it is "trendy,"
- it means that monogamy is not possible,
- bisexuals are confused,
- bisexuals are fence-sitters (unable to commit to gay or straight), and,
- bisexuals are responsible for introducing HIV/AIDS to heterosexual communities.

Gay men and lesbians may hold these stereotypes about bisexual people, as well as believe that bisexuals can exercise heterosexual privilege. These untrue stereotypes are addressed in Chapter 4.

Transphobia

Negative attitudes about transgender people often stem from deeply ingrained cultural beliefs that there are two and only two sexes, therefore a person must be male or female, and that gender is derived from biological sex. For example, if you have a male body, you are a man (forever) and your gender expression must be stereotypically male and masculine. We are only recently beginning to comprehend that these are stereotypes, not as rooted in biology as we once thought. But gender stereotypes run deep and hate crimes against transgender individuals are often even more horrific and violent than those reported for other groups. Sometimes the terms transmisogyny (negative attitudes about trans women) or transmisia (negative attitudes about transgender people in general) are used in the literature.

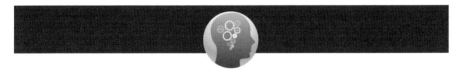

Think About It 3.1

"On the night of October 3, 2002, four young men found out that their friend, Gwen Araujo, was biologically male. They kneed her in the face, slapped, kicked, and choked her, beat her with a can and a metal skillet, wrestled her to the ground, tied her wrists and ankles, strangled her with a rope, and hit her over the head with a shovel. She begged for mercy, offered money in a desperate attempt to buy her freedom, and said her last words, 'Please don't. I have a family.' Her killers buried her in a shallow grave and went to McDonalds for breakfast." (Steinberg, 2005, pp. 499–500). This and many other similar accounts of brutal hate crimes against people who are transgender remind us of the urgency to do everything possible to end social stigma based on sexual and gender identities. Think about your own personal experiences as you read things in this book that may change how you think about these issues.

Notably, whereas homosexuality was removed from the Diagnostic and Statistical Manual of Mental Disorders (DSM) in 1973, gender identity disorder, defined as a strong and persistent cross-gender identification combined with discomfort with anatomical sex, and transsexualism, were added to the DSM in 1980. In the next version of the DSM in 1994, transsexualism was collapsed into the gender identity disorder

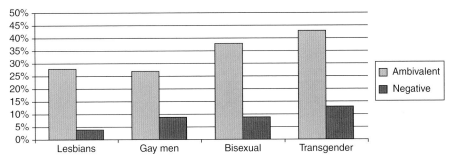

Figure 3.1 – Percent of Substance Abuse Counselors with Ambivalent or Overtly Negative Attitudes About Lesbians, Gay Men, Bisexuals, and Transgender Individuals (Based on **Eliason, 2000**).

category (Stryker, 2006). At the time when sexual orientation was de-pathologized, gender identity disorder became a psychiatric diagnosis. In the 2013 DSM-5 publication, this term was replaced with the term "Gender Dysphoria" along with this explanation:

> *Part of removing stigma is about choosing the right words. Replacing "disorder" with "dysphoria" in the diagnostic label is not only more appropriate and consistent with familiar clinical sexology terminology, it also removes the connotation that the patient is "disordered."* (American Psychiatric Association [APA], 2013).

However, the DSM is still the manual of "mental disorder" so the term still refers to pathology, and many argue the change in words has not reduced the stigma (Lev, 2013).

Even people with fairly positive attitudes about lesbians and gay men may have more negative attitudes about transgender people. For example, in one of the few studies that examined attitudes toward LGB and T people separately, there were more reports of feeling uncomfortable and carrying negative attitudes about transgender clients among a large sample of substance abuse counselors from urban and rural communities (Eliason, 2000; Eliason & Hughes, 2004). Figure 3.1 shows these data.

HIV/AIDS-Related Stigma

HIV/AIDS is also a stigmatized condition, related to its potential "contagion," the fact that it is often terminal, and the fact that it can be transmitted through sexual activities. HIV/AIDS-related stigma represents the intersections among homophobia/biphobia/transphobia, racism, and classism. Assigning a label of "diseased" or "contagious" has been one way that stigma has formed the boundaries between the acceptable and the unacceptable. HIV/AIDS is still considered by some people to be a "gay" disease and contributes to shunning LGBTQ people whether or not they are HIV positive (Padilla, del Aguila, & Parker, 2007). The high prevalence of HIV/AIDS among IV drug users, poor people, and people of color as well as gay, bisexual, and MSMW contributes to the idea of HIV positive people as "throw-away" populations, who got what they deserved from engaging in deviant behavior. No one deserves death and disability, and HIV risk is associated with specific behaviors, not classes of people, yet the perception that HIV is common or isolated within certain populations (gay men, people of color, IV drug users) persists.

Heterosexism/Heteronormativity

Homophobia, biphobia, and transphobia are generally used to refer to individual belief systems or attitudes (prejudice) and behaviors that stem from those attitudes. However, there are larger societal and institutional level influences that support and give power to the individual attitudes and behaviors. The terms heterosexism and heteronormativity are used more widely in the academic literature than in lay usage, and refer to institutionalized belief systems found in most or all of the dominant discourses of a society, such as the media, education, medicine and healthcare literatures, legal systems, and religion (Morin, 1977). These are the systems that set laws and the unspoken "norms," establish how people who deviate from the laws and customs will be dealt with, and often, how they will be punished. Heterosexist belief systems state that only heterosexual relationships between one man and one woman are "normal." This belief system was solidified into federal law by the Defense of Marriage Act (DOMA), passed in 1996, struck down in part by the US Supreme Court on June 26, 2013, and finally dismantled by the U.S. Supreme Court in June 2015. The first Supreme Court ruling did not completely overturn DOMA but found the part that denied federal benefits to same-sex couples legally married in states that permit same-sex marriage was unconstitutional. Until the U.S. Supreme Court ruled that bans on same-sex marriage were unconstitutional in June of 2015, it was still up to each state to decide whether to legalize same-sex marriage or not. Similarly, the "Don't Ask, Don't Tell" policy in the U.S. military, instituted by the Clinton administration in 1994 and struck down by the Obama administration in 2011 was also grounded in the belief that any sexual identity other than heterosexuality is abnormal and not tolerable. The fact that these US policies were struck down represented the "evolving" attitudes toward diverse sexual identities, but changes in laws do not translate to widespread acceptance or understanding of the range of human sexuality and gender expression that actually exists in human experience. In reality, no one knows what "causes" a person to be LGBTQ, or heterosexual for that matter—there is virtually no good research on this. Freud was one of the first theorists to challenge the belief that heterosexuality is biological, by proposing that family and environmental circumstances in early childhood determined sexual orientation. Most research takes for granted that people are born male or female and straight or gay, but as we have seen, there is considerable diversity within the categories of gender and sexuality.

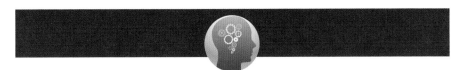

Think About It 3.2

Think about your elementary school days. Did any of the storybooks that your teachers or parents read to you have children from households with two dads? Did the Dick and Jane readers or their equivalent have any transgender boys and girls? If your family went to church, synagogue, temple, or mosque, what did you hear about LGBTQ people there? In the media? From your family? Until fairly recently, LGBTQ people were absent from most discourses, or if present, were discussed in the most negative light. What effect does that have on adult attitudes about LGBTQ people?

One example of heteronormativity can be found in the forms that people are asked to fill out in healthcare settings. Most standardized forms are based on the assumption that everyone is heterosexual and there are no other options for same-sex identities or relationships. Some people consider heteronormativity to be the source of heterosexual privilege. Privilege plays out in everyday activities as well; people who are heterosexual in the United States, can, among other things, take a date to the prom without raising an eyebrow, get engaged and married with family and community support and be legally recognized as a couple/family, profit from the multiple financial benefits given to legally married couples, not feel afraid that they may be beaten because of their sexual identity, not worry that their children will be discriminated against or taken away from them, and not feel they were passed over for promotion because of their sexual orientation. The power of heteronormativity can be seen when some LGBTQ people mimic heterosexual relationship patterns, because that is all they have been exposed to. This concept is sometimes called "hetero-relational," and refers to thinking that relationships need a male figure and a female figure to be viable or acceptable.

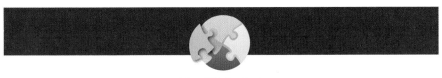

Try This 3.1

Imagine that tomorrow morning you wake up in the body of the other sex. You are still the same person in every other way, except for your physical body. How do you think your life would change?

Gender Normativity

Similar to the concept of heteronormativity, gender normativity refers to institutionalized belief systems about sex/gender: that there are only two sexes (and therefore, genders), the sexes are "opposite," and that everyone must be one or the other. This is sometimes called the "binary" system of sex and gender because there are only two choices. Gender normativity is more strictly enforced for boys than girls in childhood. Being a tomboy is often tolerated, but being a "sissy" is usually punished by parents, teachers, religious leaders, peers, and even strangers. Some authors think that this strict enforcing of gender and the linking of gender nonconformity in boys with same-sex orientation is what makes adolescent and adult men more likely to have negative attitudes about LGBTQ people than women generally have (Herek, 2000).

Homophobia is often part of masculine identity formation in a way that is not found in feminine identity formation. Girls are not as severely or as consistently punished for deviations in gender as are boys, and are allowed more freedom in clothing, interests, behaviors, and the ability to form emotional attachments and show physical affection for their same-sex friends. Boys on the other hand, are socialized that masculinity equals heterosexuality and being gay means not being a man. As Pascoe (2007) noted, "boys lay claim to masculine identities by lobbing homophobic epithets at one another" (p. 5). Boys who deviate from masculine gender activities are punished by their peers by taunts and beatings on the playground, and sometimes are taken to psychologists for "gender identity" therapy because of parents' and teachers' anxiety about boys who are not masculine enough by societal standards. Girls may also be taken to therapists for gender identity therapy, but not as often as are boys. For a biological male to want to transition to a female gender identity in our society is considered "crazy." Why would a man want to give up his male privilege for the inferior class status of a woman? And how dare a woman try to deceive society and assume the power position of male? The documentary, *The Brandon Teena Story*, and Hollywood version of that story, *Boys Don't Cry*, illustrated how one community reacted to what they perceived as a monumental betrayal when Brandon attempted to pass as male. He was brutally raped and murdered when his biological sex was revealed.

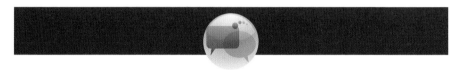

Talk About It 3.1

Find a group of friends and colleagues to explore and discuss the "Gwen Araujo Justice for Victims Act (AB1160)," the nation's first bill to address use of panic strategies. The Act was signed into law September 28, 2006 by California Governor Arnold Schwarzenegger. The bill states that a defendant may not use societal bias against their victim to decrease their own culpability for a crime. "This is a victory for fairness in our criminal justice system and a tribute to the courage of Gwen Araujo," said Assemblywoman Sally Lieber of her bill that also mandates the creation of practice materials for District Attorney's offices. "Too many Californians live with the very real fear that they will be victimized simply because of who they are. Making sure that our court system treats every one fairly, regardless of individual differences, is essential." (**https://goo.gl/R5zkdG**) Gwen's mother, Sylvia Guerrero, supported Gwen's transition as a teenager, and has continued the work for social change ever since her daughter's murder. Read about the 2012 update related to activism based on this case here: **https://goo.gl/S3t7Kq**.

For your discussion, focus on your feelings about this case, and what you as individuals and as a group can do to contribute to creating the changes needed to end this kind of hate crime and serve justice when it does happen.

As a basis for your discussion, you can watch the movie at **https://goo.gl/ef2xMF**. You can also read more about Gwen: **https://goo.gl/voeUBD**

Microaggressions

In recent years, there has been a slight decrease in the occurrence of many overt forms of discrimination and the most negative attitudes. However, LGBTQ people still experience many negative effects that are more subtle, and these are often called microaggressions (Nadal, 2013). On a personal and emotional level, a very damaging consequence of stigma is rejection by family and friends. Many families and friends are not prepared and do not know how to react when they learn one of their loved ones is lesbian, gay, bisexual, or transgender and they sometimes react in hurtful ways. These reactions can range from mildly harmful to extremely harmful. Some LGBTQ youth have been ejected from their homes; some LGBTQ adults have been treated as if they never existed. Research by Caitlin Ryan and colleagues found that young LGB adults from rejecting families had much higher rates of suicide attempts, depression, substance abuse, and unsafe sexual behavior than young adults from accepting families (Ryan, Huebner, Diaz, & Sanchez, 2009). Some find support and a path toward ultimate acceptance, but the hurt and damage is devastating for everyone involved, especially when initial negative responses cannot be overcome or healed. Many LGBTQ people remain closeted to their families and friends because of the fear, and the probable reality, of rejection. Rejection can occur in any setting, including schools, religious institutions, neighborhoods, and workplaces. People who are visibly identifiable as LGBTQ are also likely to experience social rejection from strangers in public places.

Another form of microaggression is when people dismiss the experiences of LGBTQ people as being "too sensitive" or less important than other forms of oppression. Statements such as "Now that same-sex couples can marry in this state, there is no reason for LGBTQ people to complain" trivialize the importance of other issues besides marriage. Another example is when people dismiss horrific murders of LGBTQ people as "just an isolated case," refusing to acknowledge that violence is institutionalized and is a pattern, not a random act.

Another way that microaggressions harm LGBTQ people is the seemingly innocuous comments such as "That's so gay." Serious consequences of stigma, such as losing a job because of one's gender or sexual identity are devastating. However, microaggressions happen every day and can be equally damaging. The study of microaggressions is a promising new line of investigation into the effects of stigma on people's daily lives and overall stress levels (Balsam, Molina, Beadnell, Simoni, & Walters, 2011; Bostwick & Hequembourg, 2014; Nadal, Davidoff, Davis, & Wong, 2014).

Internalized Oppression

When people are stigmatized by negative attitudes or institutionalized belief systems about sex/gender and sexuality, sometimes those negative attitudes are incorporated into their self-concepts, resulting in self-doubt, guilt, shame, depression, and/or self-hatred (Meyer, 2007). Internalized oppression appears to contribute to many of the health risk factors seen in LGBTQ people, such as suicide attempts, mental health disorders, unsafe sexual behaviors, and substance abuse. Other terms that appear in the literature to describe this concept include internalized homophobia (biphobia, transphobia), internalized homonegativity, and internalized heterosexism. Internalized oppression can result in a self-fulfilling prophecy.

For example, if a young man is socialized to believe the stereotype that bisexuals are "promiscuous," and has internalized this view, when he comes out as bisexual, he may think that it is his destiny to engage in many casual sexual encounters. If a young woman who is attracted to women is raised within a conservative religion to believe that all LGBTQ people will go to hell, she may be terrified of coming out, go to great lengths to hide her true identity, and may think that suicide is her only option. The internalization of the negative stereotypes begins very early in life and is rarely contradicted or counteracted by authority figures or role models in the child's life. For example, children hear taunts of "fag," and "lezzie" and "sissy" in school every day and teachers rarely challenge this on the playground when it occurs. Teachers rarely address issues of sexual and gender minorities in the classroom, sending a message that it is okay to make derogatory remarks about LGBTQ people, or use those words to try to control or hurt people. Sex education programs in the climate of abstinence only until marriage programs either do not mention LGBTQ people at all, or discuss them as "abnormal."

Talk About It 3.2

"Sticks and stones may break my bones but names can never hurt me." Discuss this child-hood saying. Did you believe this as a youngster? Do you believe this now? Share your memories of derogatory names that you heard as children, and what it felt like when you heard them. Notice what feelings come up for you now when you remember these inci-dents. What does it feel like to think about it now? What do your friends believe and why?

Lifestyle

Many opponents of LGBTQ civil rights refer to "the gay lifestyle." The term "lifestyle" has virtually no meaning, because it can refer to so many different things, such as the pace of our lives, where we live, our diet and exercise patterns, how fashionable we are, the amount of stress in our lives, whether we are single or partnered, and so on. LGBTQ people have diverse lives, not one universal lifestyle. Using the term "lifestyle" only to refer to one's choice of sexual partners is a form of stigmatization. A similar notion to this idea of a gay lifestyle is the idea that LGBTQ people are asking for "special rights." Most LGBTQ people merely want what heterosexual people can take for granted—lives free of discrimination, harassment, and violence based on their sexuality or gender—and the ability to form relationships and families that are recognized and respected.

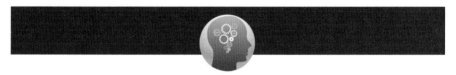

Think About It 3.3

In recent years, there have been bills introduced in many state legislatures proposing that healthcare workers can refuse to treat certain individuals if they feel those individuals violate their moral, ethical, or religious beliefs. Most of these bills were primarily focused on addressing healthcare professionals like pharmacists who did not want to administer emergency contraception, but the wording of these bills paints a broad stroke. Healthcare professionals of all sorts could refuse to treat LGBTQ people (as well as women who are seeking abortions, illegal immigrants, people with HIV/AIDS or other sexually transmitted infections) on the basis of beliefs that LGBTQ people are unnatural or immoral. Do you think that healthcare professionals have an obligation to provide quality care to all people, or can they choose not to care for some patients? These bills were mostly about individual worker's rights to refuse care.

In early 2014, the Supreme Court decided in favor of Hobby Lobby, a craft store chain owned by conservative Christians, that they could not be forced to do anything that goes against their religion, such as offer contraception to female employees in their health plan. The bill has potentially far-reaching effects, such as allowing businesses to discriminate against LGBTQ people in hiring as well. Can for-profit corporations be considered to have "religious beliefs?"

Other Forms of Stigma

Stigma stems from the stereotypes that pervade the institutional belief systems of a culture (the power structures) and affect individual attitudes (prejudice). Oppression results from the combination of power and prejudice. Look at the characteristics of the people with wealth and power in the United States and around the world—who are the senators, judges, CEOs of Fortune 500 companies, presidents of the TV channels and newspapers? Who are the administrators at hospitals, the deans of medical schools, and the makers of healthcare policies? They are still overwhelmingly wealthy, White, and (presumably) heterosexual men. Maintaining the status quo means not letting any other groups gain power and recognition. If the group in control is in charge of the legal system, medicine and healthcare systems, the media, and education, they can consciously or unconsciously maintain the stereotypes and reinforce the barriers to true equality. That is why stigma is so hard to address. It is not in the best interests of the people in power to share or give up their power. People who do not have the power of the "movers and shakers" of society try to hang on to whatever power (or privilege) they do have and often oppress people who are perceived to be lower than they are in the hierarchy. Even well-intentioned White people may stand quietly and not challenge racism for fear of the repercussions on their own lives, and some moral and ethical men do not question sexist jokes or object to violence against women for fear of being shunned by their peer group. White LGBTQ people may ignore racism in their communities, maintaining their white privilege. Finally, heterosexuals may not challenge sexual and gender prejudices for fear of being labeled as LGBTQ or "too sensitive." It takes great courage to be an ally to LGBTQ communities and other stigmatized groups.

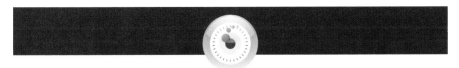

Watch This 3.1

It is rare to see someone with privilege acknowledge their privilege and explain how important it is to do this. Here are two videos that serve as excellent examples!
Privilege Checklist: https://goo.gl/hJzR6i
What is white male privilege? https://goo.gl/QXCUQh

Stigma operates through stereotypes, the topic of Chapter 4. Eliason (1996) proposed a model for understanding how oppression works. Dominant discourses (controlled by those people in power) bestow privilege on people who are white, male, heterosexual, able-bodied, and with some degree of wealth. These are the primary privileges in U.S. society as in most of the world, and those who do not have those privileges are marked by stigma. We call the various forms of stigma or oppression racism, sexism, heterosexism, ageism, ableism, sizism, and classism. The dominant discourses create and maintain stereotypes for each of these forms of stigma. This is where the different oppressed groups diverge somewhat, because the stereotypes differ in many ways, although they do overlap as well. The common basis of stereotypes

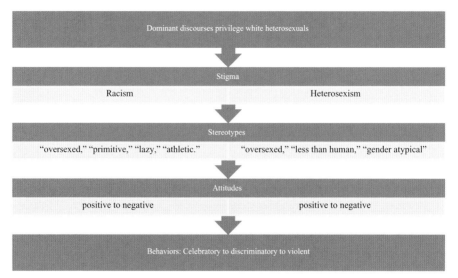

Figure 3.2 – The Processes of Oppression Based on Intersections Between Race and Sexuality (Based on **Eliason, 1996**).

is that they render the "other" group as inferior to the dominant groups. Stereotypes lead to attitudes, ranging from positive to negative, and when they are negative we call them homophobia/transphobia, biphobia, or sexual prejudice. These attitudes also influence behavior. It is possible to have a negative attitude about some group of people or some behaviors, and not express it in one's outward behavior, but in general, the more negative the attitude, the more likely that it will be expressed in behavior.

Figure 3.2 shows a simplified model of oppression, based on two common forms of oppression in contemporary society: race/ethnicity and sexuality. In the United States, society certainly privileges other statuses as well, such as male gender, upper and middle class, Christian, able-bodied, U.S.-born, and English-speaking. Stereotypes about most stigmatized groups involve some element of sexual deviance (such as myths that African-American people are "over-sexed," Latina women are "hot," Asian women are sexual slaves, working class women are "sluts," Asian men are "asexual," and so on). Labeling someone as a "sexual deviant" is one of the major ways of stigmatizing or dehumanizing another person. For many people, these stereotypes are compounded because the person has multiple stigmatizing identities. How might an American-Indian bisexual man be perceived? A disabled Asian-American transgender woman? People often respond to others first on the basis of their visible cues—race/ethnicity signifiers like skin color and facial characteristics or gender markers, not seeing the whole person.

Returning to the model, individual stereotypes and discriminatory and even violent behavior toward people in the oppressed minority classes are encouraged by those who create the dominant discourses that establish the laws, enforce laws, and police the unspoken norms. For example, if the state or country where one lives does not include gender identity in its human rights codes, transgender people could be fired for their gender expression and have no legal recourse. If a bisexual person of color is denied medical care, there are few legal organizations that will take on the case.

Table 3.2 – Experiences of Discrimination in Midlife Adults in the United States (Based on Mays & Cochran, 2001)

Lifetime Experiences	Lesbians	Heterosexual Women	Gay Men	Heterosexual Men
Not hired for a job	39%	17%	23%	19%
Denied or given poor medical care	7%	3%	3%	4%
Hassled by the police	5%	3%	18%	12%
Poor service at restaurants or stores	27%	11%	5%	9%
Called names or insulted	20%	6%	16%	6%
Threatened or harassed	15%	3%	11%	4%
Any experience of discrimination	58%	36%	51%	34%

The next section outlines the consequences of stigma on the lives and livelihoods of LGBTQ persons. The effects can be far-reaching, particularly for LGBTQ people with multiple stigmatized identities. Table 3.2 shows some examples of how LGBTQ people perceive the effects of stigma on their lives. Imagine how you would feel if you experienced these events just by being who you really are. The next section reviews some of the more common non–health-related effects of stigma on LGBTQ individuals, families, and communities and later chapters deal with the health-related effects.

Social Effects of Stigma

The rest of this chapter deals with the effects of stigma on the lives of LGBTQ people, their families, and communities. These effects set the stage for a potentially chronically stressful life, and that stress can affect one's health and well-being.

Lack of Recognition of Relationships and Family

The most apparent social and legal discrimination against same-sex couples is the fact that, historically, and currently in some locations, they are not afforded the same rights to marriage as those who are in heterosexual relationships. While many countries, provinces, and states have recently passed legislation to allow either marriage equality or a form of civil union or domestic partnership, the issue remains deeply divisive with highly charged negative feelings toward same-sex couples who seek the right to marry. This lack of legal recognition of relationships can have significant impact on access to more than one thousand federal rights and benefits, and hundreds of state benefits, including healthcare coverage (NCLR, 2015). Lack of recognition of close emotional ties and bonds of commitment directly influences access to healthcare benefits for LGBTQ people and their families, and can be especially devastating as the cost of healthcare soars in the United States. The recent Supreme Court ruling upholds the right to marry, but in the first few months, has been inconsistently implemented. Some clerks of court still refuse to issue marriage licenses, and politicians still speak forcefully about defying the Court's decision. This political climate is stressful for many LGBTQ people, who worry that the new rights will soon be taken away.

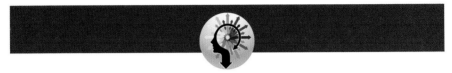

There Are No Dumb Questions 3.1

Question: Things related to same-sex marriage are happening so fast, and they are so complicated, how can I possibly keep up?

Answer: You are right, and by the time this book is published many changes will have happened from the time we finished writing it! The big events are broadcasted widely by news outlets, but there are many important changes that are easy to miss. Here are the Web sites that we recommend to check regularly for current information:

- The interactive map from Pew Research shows the dramatic change in laws affecting marriage equality in the United States since 1995, and it is a resource that is reliably updated in real time. **https://goo.gl/HXxkKf**
- "Freedom to Marry" project has an excellent summary of marriage laws around the world. **https://goo.gl/Wn3zvv**
- The Human Rights Campaign (HRC) provides a selection of maps that show laws in all of the U.S. states: **https://goo.gl/WPfbZH**

Transgender individuals have a more complicated relationship to marriage. If one of a couple in a same-sex relationship legally change their sex, they were now allowed to marry. If they were in heterosexual marriages/relationships prior to a legal sex change, their relationships were sometimes considered null and void. Trans people challenge the very definitions of same-sex and other-sex.

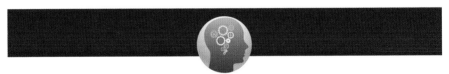

Think About It 3.4

As soon as the California Supreme Court ruled that same-sex couples could marry (June 2008), opponents organized a petition that put an initiative to ban same-sex marriage on the November ballot (Prop 8), which passed with 52% of the vote. Why do you think there was so much opposition to same-sex marriage in one of the most liberal states in the United States? Ultimately, Prop 8 was struck down by the Supreme Court.

The Right to Adopt

A related legal right that has been denied LGBT people is that of the adoption of children. Adoption is sometimes the best option for LGBTQ people who wish to have children, and denial of this right can be a severe and painful form of discrimination. LGBTQ people are often denied the right to second-parent adoptions as well, which can significantly impair the ability of the nonlegal parent if a child becomes ill or injured in their presence. Adoption rights should not be granted only to married couples, as many families differ from the two married adult and children model that is considered "normal."

Hate Crimes and Violence

Another devastating consequence of stigma is expressed in hate crimes against LGBTQ people (see Table 3.3). Lombardi, Wilchins, Priesing, and Malouf (2001) found that

Table 3.3 – Summary of Hate Crime Laws in the United States as of July 2015 (for Details see "Hate Crime Laws," 2015, "Maps of State Laws and Policies: State Hate Crimes," 2015, "State Hate Crime Laws," 2013, "State Religious Freedom Restoration Acts," 2015)	
Type of Protection	**States**
No laws that address hate crimes	5 states: Arkansas, Georgia, Indiana, South Carolina, and Wyoming
Laws that address hate crime but do not address sexual orientation or gender identity	15 states: Alabama, Alaska, Idaho, Michigan, Mississippi, Montana, North Carolina, North Dakota, Ohio, Oklahoma, Pennsylvania, South Dakota, Utah (no categories listed), Virginia, and West Virginia.
Laws address hate or bias crimes based on sexual orientation only	15 states: Arizona (2003), Florida (2001), Illinois (2001), Iowa (2002), Kansas (2002), Kentucky (2001), Louisiana (2002), Maine (2001), Nebraska (2002), New Hampshire (2002), New York (2002), Rhode Island (2012), Tennessee (2001), Texas (2002), and Wisconsin (2002).
Laws address hate or bias crimes based on sexual orientation and gender identity	15 states and District of Columbia: California (1999), Colorado (2005), Connecticut (2004), Delaware (2001/2013), District of Columbia (1989), Hawaii (2003), Maryland (2005), Massachusetts (2002/2011), Minnesota (1993), Missouri (2001), Nevada (2001/2013), New Jersey (2002/2008), New Mexico (2003), Oregon (2001/2008), Washington (1993/2009) and Vermont (2001).
Laws that grant businesses the right to honor their "religious beliefs" by potentially discriminating against LGBTQ people: Religious Freedom Restoration Acts (RFRAs) plus Supreme Court Hobby Lobby decision.	21 states: Arkansas, Alabama, Arizona, Arkansas, Connecticut, Florida, Idaho, Illinois, Indiana, Kansas, Kentucky, Louisiana, Mississippi, Missouri, New Mexico, Oklahoma, Pennsylvania, Rhode Island, South Carolina, Tennessee, Texas, and Virginia.

27% of transgender individuals in their survey had been victims of violence in their lifetime; studies of gays and lesbians find similar rates (20% to 25%; Herek, 2009). All too often these crimes result in death, with inadequate law enforcement to apprehend or justly prosecute the perpetrators. Hate crime legislation is beginning to be enacted to protect LGBTQ people, but the fact remains that people of minority sexual and gender identities experience great danger and fear that is simply nonexistent for people who are not LGBTQ. Non-LGBTQ people also do not have to worry about being re-traumatized by the people who are supposed to help them after a violent attack— police, hospital ER staff, social workers, ambulance attendants, etc.

In 2001, the Fenway Community Health Center distributed a handout that summarized the common reactions that people have to hate crimes based on sexual or gender identity:

1. Even if the event was random, the victim may feel personally targeted.
2. Victims may question their own identity and self-worth.
3. Victims may feel shame, guilt, and self-blame.
4. They may lose trust in law enforcement and service providers.
5. They may have an increased perception that the world is a dangerous place.
6. They may experience an increase in mental health symptoms.

Historically, perpetrators of violence against LGBTQ people have received light sentences, or no legal punishments, for their crimes. Since the national publicity about the murder of gay college student, Matthew Shepard, this has begun to change, as noted in the news release below.

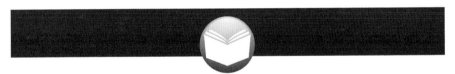

Read This 3.1

September 27, 2007

WASHINGTON, Sept. 27—The National Gay and Lesbian Task Force, Inc., hails today's landmark passage of a gay and transgender-inclusive federal hate crimes measure, included as an amendment to the Department of Defense reauthorization bill. The amendment, introduced by Sens. Edward Kennedy (D-Mass.) and Gordon Smith (R-Ore.), passed by a 60–39 cloture vote, which ended debate and sent the bill to the floor where it was approved by a voice vote.

Statement by Matt Foreman, Executive Director
National Gay and Lesbian Task Force, Inc.

"At long last, Congress is putting a bill on the president's desk to condemn and respond to violent crimes based on hatred of a person's sexual orientation, gender, gender identity, or disability. Laws ultimately reflect a nation's values and today's vote says that America rejects all forms of hate violence, including bias-motivated crimes against lesbian, gay, bisexual, and transgender people. This victory is all the more sweet given the right wing's hysterical, defamatory and lying campaign against it."

"We are deeply disappointed by President Bush's past statements that he would veto hate crimes legislation. The president has also threatened to veto the larger Department of Defense reauthorization bill to which this measure is attached. We call upon the president to work with—rather than oppose—the Congress, the overwhelming majority of the public and national and local law enforcement leaders in enacting this important legislation."

(continued)

"Violence against lesbian, gay, bisexual, and transgender people has escalated over the past 25 years. Since establishing our groundbreaking Anti-Violence Project in 1982, we have been working to get the federal government to take a stand against this epidemic. Until today, sadly, little progress has been made in the 17 years since Congress passed the Hate Crimes Statistics Act, because right-wing forces would rather see hate crimes against lesbian, gay, bisexual, and transgender people ignored than have the words 'sexual orientation' or 'gender identity' appear alongside other protected classes in federal law."

Background

The Local Law Enforcement Hate Crimes Prevention Act of 2007 (LLEHCPA) extends federal authority for investigation and prosecution of hate violence to crimes based on the victim's actual or perceived sexual orientation, gender, gender identity, or disability. Current federal hate crimes law covers crimes motivated by race, religion, and national origin. LLEHCPA also removes the existing limitation on federal involvement that a victim of a bias-motivated crime must have been attacked because the victim was engaged in a specific federally protected activity such as serving on a jury or attending public school. The Department of Justice will now have the authority to provide assistance to local law enforcement agencies in addressing all forms of hate violence.

Lesbian, gay, bisexual, and transgender people are disproportionately affected by hate violence. In fact, lesbian, gay, and bisexual people are more likely to be victims of hate-motivated physical assaults than other minorities, including African Americans, Jews, and Muslims. According to the FBI, 14% of hate crime victims in 2005 were victims of crimes motivated by hatred of lesbian, gay, or bisexual people. Moreover, reports produced by the National Gay and Lesbian Task Force (1984–1993) and the National Coalition of Anti-Violence Programs (1994–present) have documented more than 35,000 anti-LGBT crimes over the last 22 years. It is important to note that these statistics are based on reports from only a handful of local LGBT crime victim assistance agencies.

The version of the hate crimes bill passed today includes crimes based on a victim's actual or perceived gender identity. The clear inclusion of transgender people in hate crimes laws is especially important because violence against transgender people is widespread, largely underreported, and disproportionately greater than the number of transgender people in society. In 2011, the Matthew Shepard and James Byrd Hate Crimes Prevention Bill forced the FBI to add gender identity to the definition of hate crimes and they began to collect statistics on targeted violence against the transgender population of the United States. However, these statistics may not reflect the actual rates of hate crimes because transgender victims of hate crimes may be afraid to report them to the police.

Imagine This 3.1

Imagine how would you feel if this happened to you?

"The women's room is a war zone for my girlfriend and me, as well as for countless other butch lesbians across the United States. Dressed in leather jackets, jeans, button-down men's shirts, and boots, with our haircuts barely brushing the tops of our ears, we strike fear into many women's hearts, as they glance pointedly from the sign on the door to us … Not uncommonly, a braver woman will walk up and tap one of us on the shoulder and say, 'This is the *ladies* room.' This happens with such frequency that I enter a public restroom with trepidation. I smile and try to appear nonthreatening, attempting to diffuse any hostility or

(continued)

confusion. Yet I am still stared at" (Inness, 1997, p. 233). In October of 2007, a 28-year old African-American lesbian, Khadijah Farmer, filed a lawsuit against a New York City restaurant after a bouncer kicked her out of the restroom because he thought she was a man, and he refused to look at her identification.

Imagine how you would feel if you had this experience nearly every time you used public facilities? How would you react?

Discrimination in Employment and Education

Many LGBTQ people remain in the closet in their public lives because of the fear or the reality of stigma and discrimination that they would face if they revealed their sexual or gender identity. They fear job discrimination, and loss or lack of access to educational opportunities. In schools, many LGBTQ children and teens are often afraid to come out to peers, and if they do, often suffer extreme bullying in school, with negative consequences on their grades, mental health, and intentions to continue their education (Markow & Fein, 2005).

There is a stereotype that lesbian and gay people have higher incomes than heterosexuals—an argument often used by the religious right to deny any legal protections to LGBTQ people. The reality is much more complicated. Badgett (1997) found that between one-fourth and two-thirds of LGB people reported that they had lost a job or a promotion because of their sexuality, even in "tolerant" professions such as academics, law, and medicine. When she studied LGB and heterosexual workers with the same qualifications, the LGB workers earned less. Transgender individuals are at even higher risk for employment discrimination. One survey in San Francisco found nearly half had experienced employment discrimination (Minter & Daley, 2003), and the rates of unemployment are much higher among transgender individuals than any other group. Even those who are postoperative and employed may not be able to get health benefits, or stand to lose their benefits if their gender identity is revealed to insurers (National Coalition for LGBT Health, 2004). A recent Gallup Poll (August 2014) assessed well-being of LGBTQ people (www.gallup.com/poll/175418/lgbt-americans-report-lower.aspx). In terms of financial well being, a measure that included questions about standard of living, ability to pay for basic necessities, and degree of financial worries, LGBT people were less likely to be "thriving" financially than heterosexual people. For men, 32% of LGBT and 40% of heterosexual men were thriving; for women, 27% of LGBT and 39% of heterosexual women were thriving.

The U.S. military epitomized the sentiment of contemporary culture, with the "don't ask, don't tell" policy, and even though the policy was struck down in 2011, the effect of cultural endorsement of stigma that the policy perpetrated remains today. Under this policy, military recruiters could not ask about a person's sexuality, and LGBTQ people could only enlist in the service if they did not reveal their sexuality. What constituted the "don't tell" part of the policy once a person enlisted was never clear. LGBTQ people were dismissed for belonging to an LGBTQ chat room on the internet or receiving LGBTQ literature in the mail. Instituted in 1993, the policy was intended to be an improvement over the former armed services view that "homosexuality is incompatible with military service," and was supposed to reduce the rates of harassment and expulsion from the service. However, the policy's implementation actually resulted in an increase in the number of discharges based on sexual orientation. According to the Servicemembers Legal Defense Network (SLDN), more than 9000 service members were discharged under the "don't ask, don't tell" policy at a cost of more than a quarter billion U.S. dollars to taxpayers. A Defense Department inspector general survey (Mancuso, 2000) showed that:

- 80% of service members had heard offensive speech, derogatory names, jokes or remarks about gays in the previous year;
- 85% believed such comments were tolerated by authorities; and
- 37% reported that they had witnessed or experienced direct, targeted forms of harassment, including verbal and physical assaults and property damage. Overwhelmingly, service members did not report the harassment for fear of retaliation.

Women were disproportionately affected by the policy, according to SLDN. Whereas women made up 15% of the armed forces in 2002, they accounted for 31% of those discharged under the policy. Women were affected in part due to a phenomenon known as "lesbian baiting." Lesbian baiting occurs, for example, when a woman superior is accused of being a lesbian in retaliation for receiving a poor performance review, after refusing a man's sexual advances, or after reporting a man for sexual harassment. Many heterosexual women were discharged, or left the military, because of lesbian baiting as well.

A year after the repeal of DADT, researchers surveyed 553 generals and admirals who had predicted negative effects as a result of the repeal, interviewed major activists and organizations opposed to the repeal, and interviewed scholars and active duty LGBT service people from every branch of the service. Their conclusion was that the repeal had no overall negative impact on military readiness, recruitment, retention, harassment, or morale. Those in units with openly LGB service members reported increased understanding, respect, and acceptance (Belkin et al., 2012). However, change in policy does not always translate to change in individual attitudes and behaviors. Some studies of Veteran's Administration (VA) patients finds that many lived under the fear of disclosure for so long that they still do not trust in the system to treat them fairly if they come out (Sharpe & Uchendu, 2014).

Discrimination in Housing

A study done in 30 cities and suburbs in the state of Michigan, sending out same-sex and other-sex pairs of testers posing as life partners, revealed discrimination in 27% of the cases involving the same-sex testers. In Detroit, one landlord handed the testers a list of "forbidden" activities that included homosexuality along with drug use, prostitution, and one-night stands. A real estate agent in a small town told a lesbian couple that he "kind of liked it" that they were lesbians and told them to call him anytime ("Equality Michigan," n.d.; Fair Housing Center, 2007). Other LGBTQ people have reported harassment from neighbors. In January of 2012, HUD outlawed housing discrimination for LGBT Americans (Federal Register, 2012).

Effects of Living in the "The Closet"

The consequences of living the inauthentic existence of the closet are far-reaching. When LGBTQ people are closeted to their families, they are never able to share openly in family events such as holiday and family celebrations, often having to choose between their lover/partner and their family of origin for these important occasions. On the job, LGBTQ people sometimes are not able to bring their lover or partner to social events where heterosexual partners are welcome. In casual conversations with co-workers who frequently and casually mention "my wife" or "my husband," some LGBTQ people remain silent. Pictures of loved ones are displayed prominently on desks of heterosexual people; closeted LGBTQ people refrain from such displays. To add to the stress, closeted LGBTQ people also experience fear and dread of being "discovered" and to avoid this, they carefully monitor their language, where they go, and with whom.

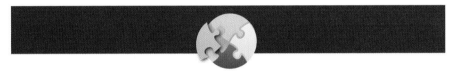

Try This 3.2

Try being "in the closet" for a day by spending a day at work without mentioning your significant other, chosen family, or best friends, or talking about what you did on the weekend or evenings. How would this affect your relationship with coworkers? With your significant other?

Unfortunately, the closet may be a place of necessity for some people where the threat of loss of job, custody of children, or fears for their safety may feel like too high a risk. It is important to keep in mind that most LGBTQ people are on a continuum of being "out"—few people are completely out or completely closeted—and that the closet has a revolving door.

Stigma has a great impact on the LGBTQ person's ability to lead the "normal" life that is taken for granted by heterosexual couples and individuals. The rights that LGBTQ people are requesting are the ability to marry (and receive the financial and legal benefits and protections for their families), adopt and raise children, and live free of discrimination, harassment, and violence. In short, LGBTQ people just want to be themselves and be accepted.

Conclusions

This chapter has tackled the difficult concept of stigma, showing how the invisible privileges conferred in our culture set up the boundaries of what is designated as normal/abnormal and natural/unnatural. Stigma works through the dominant discourses and societal-level power structures that facilitate individual prejudice and allow for discriminatory behaviors, even violence to go unpunished. The negative attitudes toward LGBTQ people can become internalized and result in shame, doubt, and guilt, which are risk factors for unhealthy coping mechanisms. The effects of stigma are potentially profound, from the inability to have "legitimate" relationships and families to employment discrimination and violence. The everyday effects of social rejection and invalidation are pervasive, and the most devastating effect might be the hit they take on socioeconomic status. Later chapters will deal with the consequences of stigma on individual physical and mental health, as well as access to and quality of healthcare services.

References

American Psychiatric Association (APA). (2013). Gender dysphoria. Retrieved July 25, 2014, from http://www.dsm5.org/Documents/Gender%20Dysphoria%20Fact%20Sheet.pdf

Badgett, M. V. L. (1997). Beyond biased samples: Challenging the myths on the economic status of lesbians and gay men. In A. Gluckman & B. Reed (Eds.), *Homo economics: Capitalism, community, and lesbian and gay life* (pp. 65–71). New York: Routledge.

Balsam, K. F., Molina, Y., Beadnell, B., Simoni, J., & Walters, K. (2011). Measuring multiple minority stress: The LGBT People of Color Microaggressions Scale. *Cultural Diversity & Ethnic Minority Psychology*, *17*(2), 163–174. Retrieved from http://doi.org/10.1037/a0023244

Belkin, A., Ender, M., Frank, N., Furia, S., Lucas, G. R., Packard, G., Jr, … Segal, D. R. (2012). One year out: An assessment of DADT repeal's impact on military readiness. DTIC Document. Retrieved from http://www.dtic.mil/cgi-bin/GetTRDoc?AD ADA567893

Bostwick, W. B., & Hequembourg, A. (2014). "Just a little hint": bisexual-specific microaggressions and their connection to epistemic injustices. *Culture, Health & Sexuality*, *16*(5), 488–503. Retrieved from http://doi.org/10.1080/13691058.2014.889754

Diamond, L. (2006). What we got wrong about sexual identity development: Unexpected findings from a longitudinal study of young women. In A. Omoto & H. Kurtzmann (Eds.), *Sexual orientation and mental health: Examining identity and development in LGB people* (pp. 73–94). Washington, DC: APA Press.

Eliason, M. J. (1996). *Who cares: Institutional barriers to health care for lesbian, gay, and bisexual people*. New York: National League for Nursing.

Eliason, M. J. (1997). The prevalence and nature of biphobia in heterosexual undergraduate students. *Archives of Sexual Behavior*, *26*, 317–326.

Eliason, M. J. (1998). Correlates of prejudice in nursing students. *The Journal of Nursing Education*, *37*, 27–29.

Eliason, M. J. (2000). Substance abuse counselor's attitudes regarding lesbian, gay, bisexual, and transgendered clients. *Journal of Substance Abuse*, *12*(4), 311–328. Retrieved from http://doi.org/10.1016/S0899-3289(01)00055-4

Eliason, M. J., & Hughes, T. L. (2004). Substance abuse counselor's attitudes about lesbian, gay, bisexual, and transgender -clients: Urban versus rural counselors. *Substance Use & Misuse*, *39*, 625–644.

Eliason, M. J., & Raheim, S. (1996). Categorical measurement of attitudes toward lesbian, gay, and bisexual people. *Journal of Gay & Lesbian Social Services*, *4*, 51–65.

Eliason, M. J., & Raheim, S. (2000). Experience and level of comfort with culturally diverse groups. *The Journal of Nursing Education*, *39*, 161–165.

Equality Michigan. (n.d.). Equality Michigan. Retrieved June 24, 2015, from https://www.equalitymi.org/issues/discrimination#sthash.VC3RlqEK.dpuf

Fair Housing Center. (2007). Sexual orientation and housing discrimination in Michigan: A report of Michigan's fair housing centers. Retrieved June 24, 2015, from http://www.fhc-michigan.org/images/Arcus_web1.pdf

Federal Register. (2012). *Federal Register*, 77(23), Friday, Feb 3, 2012 (No. 77(23)).

Goffman, E. (1963). *Stigma: Notes on the management of spoiled identity*. Englewood Cliffs, NJ: Prentice-Hall.

Herek, G. M. (2000). Sexual prejudice and gender: Do heterosexuals' attitudes toward lesbians and gay men differ? *The Journal of Social Issues*, 56(2), 251–266. Retrieved from http://doi.org/10.1111/0022–4537.00164

Herek, G. M. (2009). Hate crimes and stigma-related experiences among sexual minority adults in the United States: Prevalence estimates from a national probability sample. *Journal of Interpersonal Violence*, 24(1), 54–74. Retrieved from http://doi.org/10.1177/0886260508316477

Herek, G. M., Chopp, R., & Strohl, D. (2007). Sexual stigma: Putting sexual minority health issues in context. In I. H. Meyer & M. E. Northridge (Eds.), *The health of sexual minorities: Public health perspectives on lesbian, gay, bisexual, and transgender populations* (pp. 171–208). New York: Springer. Retrieved from http://doi.org/10.1007/978–0–387–31334–4_8

Herek, G. M., & McLemore, K. A. (2013). Sexual prejudice. *Annual Review of Psychology*, 64, 309–333. Retrieved from http://doi.org/10.1146/annurev-psych-113011–143826

Hussey, W. (2006). Slivers of the journey: The use of photovoice and storytelling to examine female to male transsexuals' experience of health care access. *Journal of Homosexuality*, 51(1), 129–158. Retrieved from http://doi.org/10.1300/J082v51n01_07

Lev, A. I. (2013). Gender dysphoria: Two steps forward, one step back. *Clinical Social Work Journal*, 41(3), 288–296. Retrieved from http://doi.org/10.1007/s10615–013–0447–0

Lombardi, E. L., Wilchins, R. A., Priesing, D., & Malouf, D. (2001). Gender violence: Transgender experiences with violence and discrimination. *Journal of Homosexuality*, 42(1), 89–101.

Mancuso, D. (2000). Military environment with respect to the homosexual conduct policy. Retrieved July 26, 2015, from http://www.dodig.mil/audit/reports/fy00/00–101.pdf

Markow, D., & Fein, J. (2005). From teasing to torment: School climate in America: a survey of students and teachers. Retrieved June 5, 2015, from http://www.glsen.org/learn/research/national/from-teasing-to-torment

Mays, V. M., & Cochran, S. D. (2001). Mental health correlates of perceived discrimination among lesbian, gay, and bisexual adults in the United States. *American Journal of Public Health*, 91(11), 1869–1876.

Meyer, I. H. (2007). Prejudice and discrimination as social stressors. In I. H. Meyer & M. E. Northridge (Eds.), *The health of sexual minorities: Public health perspectives on lesbian, gay, bisexual, and transgender populations* (pp. 242–267). New York: Springer. Retrieved from http://doi.org/10.1007/978–0–387–31334–4_10

Minter, S., & Daley, C. (2003). Trans realities: A legal needs assessment of San Francisco's transgender communities. Retrieved July 26, 2015, from http://www.hawaii.edu/hivandaids/Trans_Realities__A_Legal_Needs_Assessment_of_SF_s_TG_Communities.pdf

Mohr, J. J., & Rochlen, A. B. (1999). Measuring attitudes regarding bisexuality in lesbian, gay male, and heterosexual populations. *Journal of Counseling Psychology*, 46(3), 353. Retrieved from http://doi.org/10.1037/0022–0167.46.3.353

Morin, S. F. (1977). Heterosexual bias in psychological research on lesbianism and male homosexuality. *The American Psychologist*, 32(8), 629–637.

Nadal, K. L. (2013). *That's so gay! Microaggressions and the lesbian, gay, bisexual, and transgender community*. American Psychological Association. Retrieved from http://doi.org/10.1037/14093–000

Nadal, K. L., Davidoff, K. C., Davis, L. S., & Wong, Y. (2014). Emotional, behavioral, and cognitive reactions to microaggressions: Transgender perspectives. *Psychology of Sexual Orientation and Gender Diversity*, 1(1), 72. Retrieved from http://doi.org/10.1037/sgd0000011

National Coalition for LGBT Health. (2004). An overview of US trans health priorities. Retrieved July 26, 2015, from http://www.seguridadsocial.ccoo.es/comunes/recursos/99922/504930-Transexualidad__US_Trans_Health_Priorities.pdf

NCLR. (2015). Marriage, domestic partnerships, and civil unions: An overview of relationship recognition for same-sex couples within the United States. National Center for Lesbian Rights. Retrieved June 6, 2015, from http://www.nclrights.org/legal-help-resources/resource/marriage-domestic-partnerships-and-civil-unions-an-overview-of-relationship-recognition-for-same-sex-couples-within-the-united-states/

Padilla, M. B., del Aguila, E. V., & Parker, R. G. (2007). Globalization, structural violence, and LGBT health: A cross- cultural perspective. In I. H. Meyer& M. E. Northridge (Eds.), *The health of sexual minorities: Public health perspectives on lesbian, gay, bisexual, and transgender populations* (pp. 209–241). New York: Springer. Retrieved from http://doi.org/10.1007/978–0–387–31334–4_9

Pascoe, C. J. (2007). *Dude, You're a Fag: Masculinity and Sexuality in High School*. Berkeley, CA: University of California Press.

Ryan, C., Huebner, D., Diaz, R. M., & Sanchez, J. (2009). Family rejection as a predictor of negative health outcomes in white and Latino lesbian, gay, and bisexual young adults. *Pediatrics, 123*(1), 346–352. Retrieved from http://doi.org/10.1542/peds.2007–3524

Sharpe, V. A., & Uchendu, U. S. (2014). Ensuring appropriate care for LGBT veterans in the Veterans Health Administration. *The Hastings Center Report, 44* Suppl 4, S53–S55. Retrieved from http://doi.org/10.1002/hast.372

Steinberg, V. L. (2005). A heat of passion offense: Emotions and bias in "Trans Panic" mitigation claims: Hiding from humanity. *Boston College Third World Law Journal, 25*, 499–499.

Stryker, S. (2006). (De) Subjugated knowledges: An introduction to transgender studies. In S. Stryker & S. Whittle (Eds.), *The transgender studies reader* (pp. 1–18). New York: Routledge.

Weinberg, G. H. (1972). *Society and the healthy homosexual*. New York: St. Martins Press.

Chapter 4

Myths and Facts about Sexual Orientation and Gender Identity

"We are on the edge of World War III, and you know what? This time the United States of America does not have divine protection because we've become a nation of homosexuals and atheists and lesbians and God-haters... "What if [God] got out [of America]? What if he left? What are you gonna do, America, if he left, and the Russian nukes show up, if the Russian submarines show up, and you find out God left? Who are you gonna call on, all you atheists, all you homosexuals, all you God-haters, all you Jesus-despising people out there that hate the name of Jesus... what are you going to do when the Russian submarines show up? Who are you going to call upon? Is your gay god going to come and save you?"
—"End Times" U.S. preacher Rick Wiles, Dec 23, 2014

Myths are widely held beliefs that are false; when they are consistently applied to a group of people with a shared identity, they may also be called stereotypes. Many myths prevail in most of the world concerning lesbian, gay, bisexual, transgender, and queer people. Most of the myths begin to enter people's awareness during childhood and adolescence—a time in life when people are the most impressionable and can be easily swayed by the attitudes, feelings, and behaviors of people around them. For many, including LGBTQ people themselves, unlearning myths can take a lifetime. Even when you know on an intellectual level the difference between fact and myth, the feelings associated with the myths can persist on an unconscious level. This can affect an individual's attitudes toward LGBTQ people, including those who identify as LGBTQ. In this chapter, we present some of the most common myths and provide a brief discussion of what is currently known to be a fact.

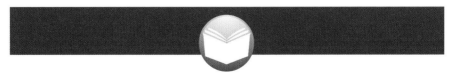

Read This 4.1

Read this: Judge Vaughn R. Walker, U.S. District Chief Judge issued the ruling that struck down Proposition 8 banning same-sex marriage in California. His ruling addresses many facts that dispel myths and stereotypes related to same-sex marriage and is well worth reading! Read the ruling here: https://goo.gl/g8wQ2z

We have divided the myths/facts into two sections. The first section includes those myths/stereotypes associated with sexual orientation and the second section discusses myths based on gender and gender identity, although we recognize that there can be considerable overlap. Many of the stereotypes about LGBQ people are based on perceptions that those individuals violate gender norms, and many of the stereotypes about transgender people are based on the belief that they are really gay people who are trying to be heterosexual by changing their bodies.

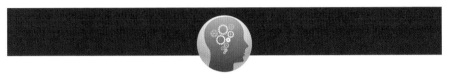

Think About It 4.1

What are your childhood memories? Jorge remembers when he was 5 to 6 years old, hearing a group of boys on the playground taunt a nonathletic boy day after day, calling him "fag" and "sissy." Jorge notes that he did not know the meaning of the words at the time, but he observed the look of fear and humiliation on the face of the taunted boy, and the attitudes of superiority and domination of the pack of popular boys doing the taunting. He still winces whenever he hears the terms as an adult. Do you have similar childhood memories? What words still haunt you from childhood?

Stereotypes are sometimes contradictory (e.g., that lesbians hate men and that lesbians want to be men), some reflect positive characteristics (e.g., that lesbians are strong and gay men are good friends to women). Even positive stereotypes can be bad, because they make assumptions that everyone with the same label has exactly the same characteristics. They dehumanize people. Of course, some LGBTQ people seem to fit some of the stereotypes because they are statements that do fit some people of any identity, and this reinforces the stereotype. When heterosexual people have one of the characteristic traits usually associated with LGBTQ people, they are considered the exception. Keep in mind the discussion from Chapter 3 about how stereotypes work to produce stigma, and how stereotypes or prejudice plus power create oppression. Each myth/stereotype listed in this chapter contributes to the stigma of being LGBTQ.

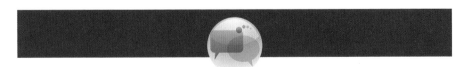

Talk About It 4.1

In a small group of friends/colleagues, brainstorm as many stereotypes as you can about each of following groups: lesbians, gay men, bisexual men, bisexual women, trans women, and trans men. Where/how did you learn these stereotypes? You are likely to find that there are many more stereotypes about gay men and lesbians than there are about bisexual and transgender people. Why do you think that is?

Myths Related to Sexuality

MYTH #1: People could change their sexual orientation if they wanted to.

FACT: Scientific evidence suggests that sexual orientation is something that people are born with or develop fairly early in life. The evidence is sufficiently clear that the American Psychological Association, American Psychiatric Association, American Medical Association, and many other professional organizations have taken the position that therapies designed to change people's sexual orientation (often called reparative or conversion therapy) are unethical (American Psychiatric Association, 1998; Zucker, 2013). For many people awareness of sexual orientation first emerges in childhood or early adolescence prior to any sexual experience (D'Augelli, 2006), and some LGBTQ people report feeling different from a very early age, long before they labeled the difference as related to gender or sexuality. Sexual orientation reflects who or what kind of person one is sexually attracted to, and may or may not be the same as one's sexual identity, the label one attaches to their own sense of sexuality. As of mid 2015, three states—California, New Jersey, and Oregon—Washington, DC—have successfully passed laws banning the use of reparative/conversion therapies with young people under 18 years of age. Legal challenges to these bans have not been successful, with the higher courts citing the scientific evidence that affirms that these therapies are ineffective and unethical (http://news.yahoo.com/jersey-ban-gay-conversion-therapy-upheld-172229347.html).

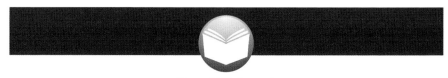

Read This 4.2

Read the full text of the California law that prohibits a mental health provider, from engaging in sexual orientation change efforts, as defined, with a patient under 18 years of age. Senate Bill NO. 1172: An act to add Article 15 (commencing with Section 865) to Chapter 1 of Division 2 of the Business and Professions Code, relating to healing arts. See **https://goo.gl/hqV5Nm**
   Also read the American Psychiatric Association position statements opposing reparative therapies from 2000 to 2013:
   https://goo.gl/qfvLqu

MYTH #2: Minority sexual orientation is caused by sexual trauma in childhood.

FACT: Not all LGBTQ people were abused or experienced traumas as children, although many were, as were many heterosexual people (Balsam, Beauchaine, Mickey, & Rothblum, 2005; Hughes, Johnson, & Wilsnack, 2001; Matthews, Hughes, & Tartaro, 2006; Saewyc et al., 2004; Schneeberger, Dietl, Muenzenmaier, Huber, & Lang, 2014). Heterosexual people and LGBTQ people may have been abused as children, and the abuse can interfere with a person's ability to relate to others in a healthy way or to trust others in intimate relationships. But childhood abuse has not been identified as a cause of sexual orientation. It is a sad fact that some children are abused but there is no single cause or effect of abuse. Some children may have been abused because they were perceived to be gender-noncon-forming, because they were exposed to a perpetrator in their family or community, because they ran away from home and were at risk for abuse on the street, or other reasons related to stigma, not their sexuality (Friedman, Koeske, Silvestre, Korr, & Sites, 2006). To "blame" sexual orientation on child sexual abuse would be anal-ogous to "blaming" left-handedness on child sexual abuse. There may be an asso-ciation between child sexual abuse and later sexual orientation or behaviors, but no research to date has identified a causative link. We take the position that sexual identity is part of normal human variation. There is also no credible evidence that LGBTQ people are more likely to come from broken homes or to have experienced dysfunctional parenting.

MYTH #3: Gay men hate women, and lesbians hate men.

FACT: Gay men and lesbians, like heterosexual people, have dear friends and acquaintances who vary in sex/gender and sexual orientation. Hatred toward any group of people is generally recognized and opposed in the LGBTQ community as prejudice. Like anyone else, LGBTQ people have personal preferences concerning those individuals they like to be around and choose as friends, and most people prefer being together in groups and communities with others who share their own values and identities. But preferring to have certain types of people as friends, or to have an affectionate attraction to a particular type of person does not mean that one hates or even dislikes those who are outside that circle. The majority of heterosexual people also select their friends and potential partners from a pool of people who are similar to them in race/ethnicity, age, sexual identity, religion, education, and other social variables (Laumann, 1994).

MYTH #4: Gay men want to be women; lesbians want to be men.

FACT: This is an interesting stereotype when coupled with the one above—why would you want to be something you hate? Sexual identities are not based on gender—they are two separate (though related) concepts. Most gay men are quite happy being men, they just want the freedom to be whatever kind of man they are. The same is true for lesbians. The stereotype may stem from the fact that some LGBTQ people are drawn to careers or interests that are usually associated with someone of the other sex. For example, because they are less constrained by soci-etal gender norms, gay men may be more likely than heterosexual men to choose nursing, cosmetology, or flight attendant schools, whereas lesbians may be more likely than heterosexual women to choose construction work, law enforcement, and firefighting. But many heterosexual people chose to break from gender stereotypes as well. The stereotypes that relate to beliefs that gay men and lesbians do not fit well with the characteristics of their sex/gender generally do not apply to bisexuals. There are few or no stereotypes about the careers, interests, or physical appearance of bisexual men or women.

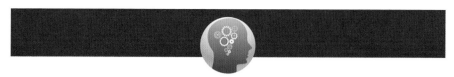

Think About It 4.2

Look back at the list of stereotypes you generated about bisexual people. Why do you think there are fewer stereotypes about bisexuals than there are about gay men and lesbians? Perhaps it is because bisexuality has not been thought to be a "legitimate" identity, or because there are fewer gender-related beliefs associated with bisexuality. How many of the stereotypes about lesbians and gay men that you generated were related to gender?

MYTH #5: Gay men want to look like women, and lesbians want to look like men.

FACT: It is not possible to tell if someone is a gay man or a lesbian from observing how they look. Some gay men and some lesbians do dress or have behaviors that are more typical of the other sex (see the definition of gender expression in Chapter 2). Some heterosexual women or men also dress or behave more typically as the other sex. However, these patterns of dress or behavior do not come from a desire to be or to look like the other sex. Instead, these choices are based on personal preference and refusal to conform to the stereotypes or social expectations for male or female dress and behavior. For lesbians, choice of dress, hairstyle, and whether to wear makeup often has much more to do with comfort and ability to physically navigate than it does with wanting to appear masculine. But many lesbians do dress and act in a manner consistent with social norms for women, and many gay men do dress and act consistent with social norms for men. It is not possible to tell if a person is lesbian, gay, bisexual, transgender, or queer or, for that matter, heterosexual, by the way they dress or act. This stereotype is partly related to people's confusion about the differences between sexual identity and gender identity. Some people erroneously believe that all gay men and lesbians are cross-dressers. The fact is that preferences in clothing, hairstyles, makeup, and accessories change rapidly in our fashion conscious world, and these trends change societal expectations about what men and women are supposed to look like.

MYTH #6: LGB people have uncontrolled sexual urges and try to "hit on" anyone they can.

FACT: The range of sexual drive and variety of sexual practices is similar among LGB people and heterosexual people (Coleman & Rosser, 1996; Matthews, Hughes, & Tartaro, 2006). This myth may come from the fact that LGBQ people are defined by their sexual behavior—the term "homosexual" was coined, it was not characterized as "homo-relational" or "homo-affectional." In fact, LGBQ people do not stalk straight people for casual sex any more frequently than straight people seek out casual sex, nor do they necessarily have sex more often. Like anyone else, there are many factors that influence an LGBQ person's identity besides sex, such as the social groups one belongs to, career or job roles, religious beliefs, etc. This myth of being oversexed particularly affects bisexual men and women who are often perceived to be hypersexual because of the potential to be attracted to people of either sex (Eliason, 1998). Many heterosexual people express considerable distress at the prospect of being "hit on" by someone of the same sex. How does this experience differ from being "hit on" by a member of the other sex when one is not interested?

If you were to analyze this myth by gender, you will find some differences. Men in contemporary society, whether gay, bisexual, or heterosexual, on average, report a higher sex drive and a more frequent desire for engaging in sexual activities than do women (Laumann, 1994). When men have other men for sexual partners, who also seek more frequent sex, it stands to reason that gay and bisexual men, as a group, may have sex more frequently. This myth about the "hypersexuality" of LGBTQ people is related to our cultural anxieties about "promiscuity." How many partners or how much sex is too much? If sexual activity is between adults, consensual, and safe, do the numbers or frequency matter? An older study by Masters and Johnson (1979) compared sexual activity in heterosexual couples, gay male couples, and lesbian couples. One of the main differences they reported was that gay and lesbian couples took more time in love-making, with much more touching, caressing, and focusing on mutuality than heterosexual couples. Perhaps heterosexual couples could learn something about sexual relationships from their gay and lesbian counterparts.

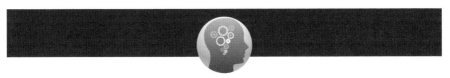

Think About It 4.3

In some murder trials, defense lawyers claimed "gay panic" or "homosexual panic" as the reason for the crime. The defendant is described as having temporary insanity rendered by the spectre of an unwanted sexual advance by someone of the same sex. Should this be considered a legitimate explanation for murder?

MYTH #7: LGBTQ orientation may be "contagious" or stems from close contact.

FACT: Most LGBTQ people were raised by heterosexual parents, but that did not make them heterosexual. Sexual orientation/identity is likely to have genetic components and perhaps other biological influences (Byne, 2007). Therefore, it cannot be "caught." People who are comfortable with a heterosexual identity will not be influenced to become LGBTQ, just as an LGBTQ person will not be influenced to become straight if they spend time with heterosexuals.

MYTH # 8: Children should not be exposed to LGBTQ people nor should adults even discuss LGBTQ issues, as children might be unduly influenced.

FACT: LGBTQ people do not "recruit." This myth is often used as the rationale for keeping LGBTQ people away from children, and affects the ability of some people to be openly LGBTQ daycare workers, teachers, or parents. Evidence of the fallacy of this myth comes from the study of children of same-sex parents—if too much exposure to LGBTQ people makes people become LGBTQ, those children should be mostly LGBTQ as they grow up. In fact, the majority of children of same-sex couples grow up to be heterosexual (Goldberg, Gartrell, & Gates, 2014; Tasker, 2005).

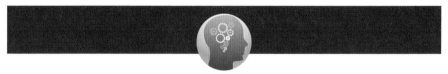

Think About It 4.4

One of the authors was flipping channels one day in June and found a televangelist telling the audience that gay pride parades and rallies were dangerous because "impressionable" children might see them and then grow up to want to be LGBTQ because the parades look fun. She remembered that when she herself was an impressionable child, she was often exposed to Shriner's parades, with grown men driving tiny cars wearing silly hats. She had no desire to be a Shriner when she grew up, despite this overexposure to grown men having fun.

MYTH #9: Gay men are child molesters.

FACT: One of the most damaging stereotypes involves the conflation of child sexual molestation with a gay sexual orientation. They are in fact, entirely different phenomenon. A study published in the *Journal of Pediatrics* (Jenny, Roesler, & Poyer, 1994) reported that a child was 100 times more likely to be abused by a heterosexual man than a gay man (only 1 out of 269 known pedophiles had a gay adult sexual orientation). So where does this myth come from? It is perpetuated by the terminology used in the psychiatric and legal literature to describe child molesters, sometimes called pedophiles. Men who are attracted to prepubescent girls are labeled as heterosexual pedophiles (and make up 60% to 65% of convicted pedophiles) and men who are attracted to prepubescent boys (about 30% of pedophiles) are called homosexual pedophiles. About 20% of pedophiles are attracted to both boys and girls (Cohen & Galynker, 2002). The terms homosexual and heterosexual are misused here, and do not refer to the sexual orientation of the adult relationships of the pedophile.

Although more pedophiles report attraction to girls, there are more male victims than female victims because of circumstances. Boys have much greater social freedom and less supervision by adults than girls, thus pedophiles can have more ready access to boys. In addition, the nature of the sexual acts differs (fondling or exhibitionism occurs more often with boys, activities that are quick and can be done anywhere). Sexual abuse of children is condemned by all LGBTQ social and political organizations, and there is as much concern about child sexual abuse by LGBTQ individuals as there is among heterosexuals. The gray zone in this controversy has to do with age of consent—when is a person old enough to make informed choices about their own sexual behavior?

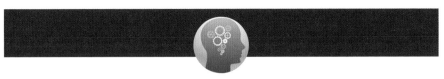

Think About It 4.5

The North American Man Boy Love Association (NAMBLA) was founded in 1978 as a political and educational organization that supports the rights of all people, regardless of age, to participate in consensual sexual activities. They oppose having any age of consent laws and believe that it is best for children to be initiated into sex by experienced adults. Parents and Friends of Lesbians and Gays (PFLAG) released the following statement in 1997: "As a family organization, PFLAG strongly condemns the sexual exploitation of children by any individual, group, or organization, in any form and under any circumstance… NAMBLA is a pedophile organization whose sole purpose is to facilitate sex between adult men and young boys. PFLAG, therefore, repudiates NAMBLA and its aims." Another organization, the Gay and Lesbian Alliance Against Defamation (GLAAD) said this in 1994: "GLAAD deplores NAMBLA's goals, which include advocacy for sex between adult men and boys and the removal of legal protections for children. These goals constitute a form of child abuse and are repugnant to GLAAD … As a group of people who historically have not had legal rights and protections, gay men and lesbians have always worked with and built coalitions with others whose rights are at risk. The true gay and lesbian agenda is ultimately about free human rights for all people."

But what about the first amendment protection of speech? In 2000, the ACLU released a statement about defending the free speech of unpopular organizations, stating that it is not incompatible to support the right of an organization to exist and state their mission, and to oppose that mission, and noted "Those who do wrong are responsible for what they do; those who speak about it are not. The defense of freedom of speech is most critical when the message is one most people find repulsive. That was true when the Nazis marched in Skokie. It remains true today." What do you think?

MYTH #10: Most LGBTQ people are White; homosexuality is rare in other racial/ethnic groups.

FACT: The proportion of people who have same-sex attractions or behaviors, and who are gender-variant is thought to be the same in all racial and ethnic groups, and perhaps in all cultures in the world (Gates & Newport, 2012; Herdt, 1996). However, social and familial acceptance of LGBTQ people varies tremendously among cultures. Because there are wide cultural variations in understandings of the concepts of sexuality and gender, fewer people of color or people from non-Western countries may adopt an open sexual identity as LGBTQ because that is a western concept (Dykes, 2000). In some cultures, revealing one's self as LGBTQ can be very costly personally and socially, even dangerous. Canada, Australia, New Zealand, many European countries, and the United States (all predominantly White populations) have experienced several decades of growing acceptance, which has made it more possible for LGBTQ people of all ethnicities to acknowledge who they are. But even if they are able (or want) to come out publicly, LGBTQ people of color often encounter racism from White LGBTQ communities. Therefore LGBTQ people of color may be less likely to be involved in predominantly White social and political organizations and also less visible in the LGBTQ communities (Battle & Crum, 2007; Fieland, Walters, & Simoni, 2007; Ramirez-Valles, 2007). We discuss this issue in more detail in Chapter 7.

MYTH #11: LGBTQ people are not capable of long-term, stable, or monogamous relationships.

FACT: Despite the fact that LGBTQ people did not have the same legal and social support for their relationships that heterosexual people have until very recently, many LGBTQ people form long-term, monogamous, committed relationships, and consider themselves as much a family as any heterosexual married couple (Kurdek, 2004; Kurdek & Schmitt, 1986; Peplau & Fingerhut, 2007). Many heterosexual people have trouble forming and maintaining stable long-term relationships as do some LGBTQ people. The myth that LGBTQ people are incapable of long-term relationships may stem partly from the historical inability to marry. The lack of social and legal recognition of partner relationships and families in LGBTQ communities may have led to more creative relationship and family formations that do not get validated as authentic. This issue is explored in more depth in Chapter 5.

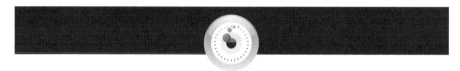

Watch This 4.1

Del Martin and Phyllis Lyon, who were together for over 50 years, were the first couple to legally marry in the state of California when marriage first becomes legal in that state. Watch the ceremony, officiated by Major Gavin Newsom here:
https://www.youtube.com/watch?v=8HksGMTXRxA

MYTH #12: Homophobia, biphobia, and transphobia only exist among heterosexual people.

FACT: Everyone, regardless of sexual identity/orientation, can experience negative attitudes based on fear, shame, guilt, or hatred about LGBTQ people or same-sex feelings in themselves. Lesbians and gay men can harbor negative attitudes toward bisexual or transgender people, older LGBT people can have negative attitudes toward younger people who self-identify as queer. Bottom line—people of any group can and do acquire stereotypes and negative attitudes toward others who are not like themselves. But even more damaging, many LGBTQ people have internalized beliefs about themselves as LGBT or Q, and as a result often have feelings of self-hatred and lack of self-acceptance at some point in the lifespan (Herek, 2009; Meyer, 1995; Szymanski & Chung, 2003). For many young people who are beginning to be aware of their LGBTQ identities, this can lead to devastating consequences—depression, suicide, and self-destructive behaviors. They need as much support as possible from everyone around them to overcome the fear and self-hatred. As they "come out" and learn more about themselves and others in the LGBTQ community, their internalized oppression will begin to decrease. For this reason, it is imperative that issues related to sexuality and gender be discussed in schools, healthcare settings, homes, and as many other places as possible so that youth do not internalize the negative stereotypes and the self-hatred that put them at risk for significant health problems (Elia & Eliason, 2010).

Homophobia operates differently when it occurs among heterosexual people, because they have the power of the dominant institutions supporting their prejudicial beliefs, thus, they have the ability to discriminate against LGBTQ people. When an LGBTQ person has homophobia, it often becomes internalized. This internalization can result in enough self-hate to cause or sustain major depression, anxiety, and suicide, or they avoid, verbally denigrate, or abuse other LGBTQ people. An LGBTQ person can have negative stereotypes about heterosexuals, but since they have no significant societal power to support them, the beliefs lack the strength of homophobia/biphobia that is sustained by heterosexual privilege.

MYTH #13: A person is not lesbian or gay if they have ever had sex with the other sex.

FACT: Many lesbian, gay, and bisexual people have had sex with someone of the other sex, even when they know they are not heterosexual. Sometimes this occurs in an effort on the individual's part to hide or overcome what they know to be their lesbian or gay identity, or for a host of other reasons such as love or attraction for a specific person, curiosity, or peer pressure. In fact, one study identified 237 reasons why people have sex (Meston & Buss, 2007). Diamond (2003) pointed out that sexual desire and romantic love can be two separate things; heterosexual people may have sex with a person of the same sex at some point in their lives, but this behavior does not necessarily affect their identity. Sexual orientation, identity, and sexual behavior are not always consistent. Sometimes concerned parents or friends ask, "How do you know that you are gay, lesbian, or bisexual if you have never had sex with a person of the other sex?" No one asks, "How do you know you are heterosexual if you have never had sex with a person of the same sex?" Human beings explore a variety of behaviors that may or may not affect their core social or sexual identities. Gender and sexuality are not discrete, binary concepts, but each are on a continuum. Kinsey, Pomeroy, & Martin (1948) were among the first to operationalize a sexual behavior continuum. He used a 7-point scale where 0 = exclusively heterosexual and 6 = exclusively homosexual. The points between these extremes included bisexual behavior. Other theorists have expanded on Kinsey's work to develop continua not only of sexual behavior, but of sexual attractions, preferences for romantic partners, preferences for social relationships, and other dimensions of sexuality (e.g., Klein, Sepekoff, & Wolf, 1985).

MYTH #14: LGBTQ people are too blatant: they flaunt their sexuality.

FACT: What is labeled as "flaunting" in the LGBTQ person is considered normal among heterosexual couples: holding hands in public, kissing goodbye or hello, having a picture of a significant other on their desk at work, and so on. Heterosexual relationships are celebrated in many ways; however, even the mere mention of a same-sex partner or relationship can make some people uncomfortable. Some LGBTQ activists may deliberately engage in public behaviors to challenge heterosexual norms, but the typical same-sex couple does not "flaunt" their relationship any more than does a heterosexual couple. In fact, many refrain from any public displays of affection for fear of retaliation.

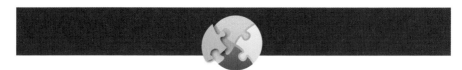

Try This 4.1

List all of the ways that heterosexual people "flaunt" their sexuality. You may be stumped at first, but as the list grows, you may notice many ways that heterosexual people are allowed to express their sexual orientation in public—ways that are considered "normal" for heterosexuals and "flaunting" for LGBT people. For example, heterosexual people can put pictures of significant others and family on their desks at work, they can hold hands in public, kiss goodbye when one drops off the other for work, have their picture printed in the newspaper when they have relationship milestones (engagement, wedding, anniversary, even divorce). Some people have even argued that the tradition of decorating the bride and groom's car and driving around town honking their horns is a "heterosexual pride parade."

Gay pride parades and rallies are often mentioned as examples of flaunting behavior, but similar kinds of celebrations in other communities are rarely scrutinized this way. There are many community celebrations of ethnic pride, cultural diversity, or religious pride that serve similar purposes of community building as gay pride celebrations.

MYTH #15: LGBTQ people are mentally ill.

FACT: Many LGBTQ people do suffer from oppressive, discriminatory, and stressful social circumstances that cause a great deal of suffering (Gilman et al., 2001) and sometimes become diagnosed mental illnesses. But at the same time, many individuals also find a rich source of support and joy in social groups within LGBTQ communities. Hollywood portrayals of lesbian, gay, and bisexual people seldom provide accurate depictions, and reinforce the stereotypes of LGBTQ people as unhappy, or engaging in bizarre, outlandish behaviors (think of the character of Jack on Will & Grace and the exaggerated stereotypes of Mitchell and Cam on Modern Family). The American Psychiatric Association (1973, 1998, 2000) and American Psychological Association (Conger, 1975; DeLeon, 1998) have determined that LGBT identities do not represent mental illnesses. Stigma, not sexual identity, creates the risk for mental health problems. This issue is discussed further in Chapter 9.

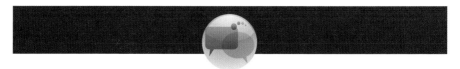

Talk About It 4.2

Consider the story of Evelyn Hooker, an extraordinary ally, and discuss with your colleagues ways that you can also be LGBTQ allies. Evelyn Hooker (1907–1996) was a pioneer in many ways. She was one of the few women psychologists of her day—no easy feat in the male-dominated world of the sciences. In the early 1950s, on the urging of a former student,

(continued)

a gay man, Dr. Hooker received an NIH grant to study the adjustment of a nonclinical sample of gay men compared to a heterosexual comparison group. This was the first nonclinical study of gay men—the earlier studies were done in prisons and mental institutions and did not include adequate comparison groups. It was remarkable that the government funded this study during the highly oppressive McCarthy era, where people with same-sex desires were being routed out of government service as "communists." Dr. Hooker's groundbreaking study published in 1957 showed that experts were unable to distinguish gay men from heterosexual men on the basis of the most widely accepted personality measures of the day, and that there were no reliable differences in ratings of adjustment. Studies by other researchers quickly confirmed her findings, but it took political activists putting pressure on the APA to result in the removal of homosexuality as a mental illness from the Diagnostic and Statistical Manual. This did not occur until 1973. Dr. Hooker is a historical ally—a heterosexual woman with the courage to stand up for LGBTQ rights long before it was safe to do so.

MYTH #16: Religion says it is wrong to be LGBTQ.

FACT: There is considerable variation in religious doctrines and writings about gender and sexuality. We will focus on Christianity in this discussion, since it is the most common religious discourse in the United States. Several Christian churches welcome LGBTQ people and a few ordain openly LGBTQ people to be religious leaders like priests, ministers, or bishops. Many religious denominations are struggling with the best way to deal with issues of sexuality and gender in a changing world, recognizing that the Bible, both the old and the new testaments, was written 2000 years ago. It cannot provide the guidance needed to address all contemporary issues.

In general, both Christian and other fundamentalist and evangelical religions that take the Bible, or some other religious text, as the literal word of God are the most negative about LGBTQ people, because they tend to promote a belief that any same-sex activity is a form of sin. Some religions have programs for converting homosexuals (Exodus International is the largest of these), but research suggests that these programs have been unsuccessful in their goals. In one study, out of 202 people who underwent conversion therapy, only 6 (3%) were "converted" (Schroeder & Shidlo, 2002). The Pew Center report (Pew Research Center, 2013) on LGBT Americans found that 74% of White evangelical protestants and 55% of all Americans with a religious affiliation say that homosexuality conflicts with their religious beliefs. The more often a person attends church services, the more strongly they believe that homosexuality should be discouraged.

An example of an inclusive religious denomination is the United Church of Christ (UCC). In 1973, The *United Church Coalition for Gay, Lesbian, Bisexual, and Transgender Concerns* was formed. In 1975, their General Synod passed a resolution in support of full civil liberties and equal protection under the law to persons of all "affectional or sexual preferences." In 1977, the Church passed a resolution that "deplored the use of scripture to generate hatred, and the violation of civil rights of gay and bisexual persons and called upon individual members, local churches…to continue to work for the enactment of civil rights legislation at the federal, state, and local levels of government." Ordination of openly LGBTQ ministers was formally accepted by the denomination in 1980. UCC clergy are also free to bless same-sex unions. Local associations of UCC congregations have the authority to decide on their own ordination policies. In 1985, the General Synod formally urged local churches to welcome gay and lesbian members and advocate in their behalf against discrimination and persecution. In 2005, the UCC issued a statement in support of same-sex marriage.

MYTH #17: An LGBTQ person cannot be religious.

FACT: The answer depends on the kind of religion. Affiliating with a fundamentalist church is a strong predictor of homophobia (Eagly, Diekman, Johannesen-Schmidt, & Koenig, 2004; Whitley & Kite, 1995), but religious and spiritual beliefs are complex

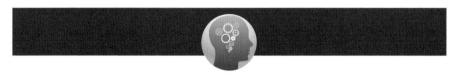

Think About It 4.6

Consider the findings of a survey done by the Pew Research Center (2013). They found that LGBT people are much less religious than the broader American population, with 48%, or more than double the percentage of the general public that says they are not religious. Most LGBT Americans (51%) do have a religion, and for 17%, religion is "very important" in their lives. Of those who are religious, most are Protestant (27%) or Catholic (14%). The survey also reported that one-third of LGBT people felt that there was a conflict between their religious beliefs and their sexual or gender identities. This is echoed in the data from the general population, where 74% of White evangelical Protestants and a majority (55%) of all U.S. adults with a religious affiliation say homosexuality conflicts with their religious beliefs. Among adults in the general public, there is a greater tendency for frequent church attenders to believe that homosexuality is wrong. This chart shows the percentage of LGBT people's religious affiliations compared to the general public.

	LGBT	General Public
Christian	42%	73%
Jewish	2%	2%
Other religions	8%	4%
Atheist/Agnostic	17%	6%
No religion in particular	31%	14%
Total unaffiliated with a religion	48%	20%

Nearly all of those surveyed said at least one of six religious institutions were "unfriendly" to LGBT people: 80% said Islam, Mormonism, and the Catholic Church were unfriendly and 75% said evangelical churches were unfriendly. A substantial number (30%) said they had been made to feel unwelcome at a place of worship. Rejection by religion/religious people is a major source of stress for many LGBTQ people, particularly when it underlies family rejection.

How does your experience compare with these findings? What religious beliefs about LGBTQ people or behaviors did you learn?

and contradictory in the individual (Miller & Stack, 2014; Rodriguez, Lytle, & Vaughan, 2013). Some studies have found that participation in organized religion is detrimental to the mental health of LGBTQ people (Gage-Davidson, 2000; Rodriguez & Ouellette, 2000), but less research has focused on LGBTQ people who belong to welcoming congregations, or churches that specifically serve LGBTQ communities, such as the Metropolitan Community Church. Lease, Horne, and Noffsinger-Frazier (2005) found that belonging to an LGBTQ affirming faith was related to lower levels of internalized homophobia. On the other hand, having a strong, personal spirituality, whether belonging to a formal religion or not, also predicts better health. There is a growing spirituality movement among LGBTQ communities, just as there is in the general population, with people exploring diverse ways to express their spirituality within or outside of formal religious institutions (Helminiak, 2012).

MYTH #18: LGBTQ people want special rights.

FACT: This was a ploy used by anti-gay activists in recent years to imply that LGBTQ people were asking for more than what the general population has. They claim that LGBTQ people are already covered under federal and state laws (as human beings), therefore, do not need or deserve any further legal protections. All LGBTQ activists have ever asked for is to be treated with the same respect and dignity, and to obtain the same legal protections, rights, and benefits that other citizens already have. Theoretically, LGBTQ people are protected under some laws, but as became clear in regards to women's rights and protections and civil rights related to race/ethnicity and religion, sometimes laws are needed to send a clear message to society that harassment, discrimination, and violence against any group of people is not to be tolerated.

MYTH #19: Bisexuals can (and should) choose other sex relationships.

FACT: There is considerable debate in the literature over how much voluntary control anyone has about their sexual attractions—people choose whether to act on them or not, but attraction does not seem to be voluntary. People who are bisexual may be attracted to a person of the other sex, and choose to develop a relationship with that person. Although the relationship may look on the surface like a heterosexual relationship, the person's core identity as bisexual is not changed. One or both partners may be bisexual. Bisexual people can choose whether or not to reveal their sexual identities, as can many gay and lesbian people, but since they face negative attitudes from both heterosexual people and gay and lesbian people, they do not get much "privilege" of any sort, regardless of their relationships. This myth may be expressed differently, depending on who expresses it. For example, a heterosexual man might say, "If you are attracted to both men and women, why not choose to be with someone of the opposite sex and be 'normal?'" A lesbian might say, "That man calls himself bisexual, but by being in a public relationship with a woman, does nothing to further the cause of gay rights." Both viewpoints deny the legitimacy of a bisexual identity.

MYTH #20: Bisexuals are confused about whether they are gay or straight; they are really gay or lesbian, but just cannot commit. In other words, there is no such thing as a true bisexual.

FACT: Nearly everyone is confused about sexuality at some time in life—bisexual people certainly have no corner on the market of confusion. Because there is much less discussion about and less visibility of bisexual people in our culture, it would stand to reason that there may be more confusion about bisexual identity (Balsam & Mohr, 2007), but the majority of bisexual people report a stable sexual identity over time (Diamond, 2005). The sources of confusion come from the culture, not so much from the individual's core sexuality. Because there is little information available to people from their families, churches, schools, and other primary sources of education, and the greater stigma attached to bisexuality than to gay or lesbian identities, the greater fluidity of bisexual experience, and the greater likelihood of questioning when relationships change, it is no wonder that some people feel confused. For example, a man's experience of leaving a relationship with a man and entering one with a woman may represent what Paula Rust (1996) called changes in the "sexual landscape," and being adaptable and more fluid in one's identity is an advantage to healthy adjustment. As to the legitimacy of a bisexual identity, the majority of researchers of sexual orientation have identified a continuum of sexual attraction/behavior rather than a binary, either/or sexuality. This leaves room for a wide variety of identities. For example, some women call themselves "lesbian-identified bisexuals" denoting that they have sexual attractions for men, but tend to prefer women as partners and belong to lesbian social and political organizations. Being confused or adopting a "fluid" identity does not mean that people with these identities can easily change their sexual attraction patterns, and reparative therapy is no more indicated for a "confused" person than it is for someone committed to a sexual identity.

MYTH #21: Bisexuality is just a phase.

FACT: Many well-intentioned persons may tell bisexual people that they are just going through a phase and will eventually find their true identities as gay or lesbian. This stems from the stereotype that bisexuality does not exist and that it is a transitional point on the way to homosexual identity (Mohr & Rochlen, 1999). Some people do indeed label themselves as bisexual early in their coming out process, and then later identify as gay or lesbian, but just as many people first label as gay or lesbian, and then later as bisexual (Rust, 2000). This myth could apply to all LGBTQ people. To tell someone that they are "going through a phase," when they tell you they are LGBT or Q, is to trivialize the very difficult process of sexual and gender identity formation and to deny the reality of their lived experience. There is considerable evidence that many people are bisexual in their sexual behavior, and that some of them adopt a bisexual identity that is stable throughout their lifetimes (Diamond, 2005). Because of cultural pressures, heterosexual identities are the most stable over time, but the majority of lesbian, gay, and bisexual identities were also stable (Mock & Eibach, 2012). There are debates regarding whether one chooses a sexual identity or merely expresses their true nature. There is really no way of knowing if sexuality is predominantly biological, genetic, socially constructed, or some combination of these. Does it matter whether a person chooses their sexuality identity or feels they were born into it? Should their rights and privileges in society differ? Similarly, does it matter if a person with a disability was born with it or acquired it later in life? Does it matter if a person chooses to be a Lutheran, or is one because their family has always been Lutheran?

Myths Related to Gender Identities

"A woman is made, not born" —Monique Wittig

There may be even more strongly held stereotypes about gender than sexuality. A binary gender system is deeply imbedded in contemporary western culture, affecting the way that we perceive people who do not clearly fit into neat categories of male and female. Because language defines two, and only two distinct categories, many people find it difficult to understand a continuum of gender possibilities and jump to the conclusion that anything outside of the binary system must be a matter of choice. Many languages, including English, enforce the idea of two genders by use of two and only two sets of pronouns: she/her and he/his. Most legal institutions also systematize gender, requiring that people must be categorized as male or female on birth certificates, driver's licenses, passports, and marriage certificates. Transgressions from the gender norms are severely punished. Think about how early in life (even before birth) we begin to categorize people by their gender, and start making lists in our heads about the nature of gender. People develop schemas of girls (what girls like, what they do, how they behave, how they look), boys, women, and men based on our interactions with parents, teachers, peers, and what we see in the media. Adults generally recognize these schemas as stereotypes, but they continue to deeply influence our behavior, often on an unconscious level. Have you ever caught yourself saying or thinking something that is totally based on stereotype, like attributing the erratic behavior of the car ahead of you to a "woman driver" or assuming that your nurse would be female? Gender stereotypes hurt us all, but impact LGBTQ people in unique ways. In particular, transgender people are denied existence by strict binary gender stereotypes.

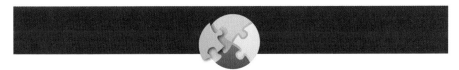

Try This 4.2

List all the stereotypes you can think of about men and women. Check off the stereotypes that fit you personally. Select one, and try changing this for one day. Notice how other people respond to you throughout the day and try to engage at least one person in a conversation about how they respond to you. In what ways have the stereotypes about your own sex/gender affected your life?

MYTH #22: There are two and only two sexes: male and female.

FACT: There is considerable diversity in biological bodies, no matter how sex is defined. We think of sex as determined by chromosomes: people with an XY are male and people with an XX are female. But what about the variations? How about people with XO (Turner syndrome), XXY (Klinefelter syndrome), XXX, XYY, XXYY, and many other variations of sex chromosomes? How about hormones? Both men and women have testosterone and estrogen, just in different proportions at different phases of life. If hormones define sex, then sex can be bought at the local pharmacy. Well, then, what about genitals? Does having a penis make one male and having a vagina make one female? Men can have accidents that result in loss of the penis—are they no longer men? About 1% of infants in the United States are born with a difference of sexual development (DSD) where genitals or internal organs of reproduction are not clearly male or female and about 4% have some form of DSD that may not be apparent at birth (Fausto-Sterling, 1993, 2000).

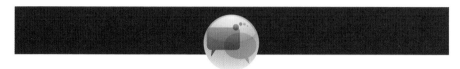

Talk About It 4.3

Get together with a group of colleagues and talk about the ways in which you have learned to think about the world in terms of either/or binaries. Consider this quote: "The world is not divided into sheep and goats. Not all things are Black and White. It is a fundamental of taxonomy that nature rarely deals with discrete categories. Only the human mind invents categories and tries to force facts into separated pigeonholes. The living world is a continuum in each and every one of its aspects. The sooner we learn this concerning human sexual behavior the sooner we shall reach a sounder understanding of the realities of sex" (Kinsey et al., 1948, p. 639). Discuss the ways in which this statement applies equally well to sex/gender.

MYTH #23: Men and women are different mainly because of their biology, not their socialization.

FACT: That is an almost impossible statement to evaluate. How does one go about separating out the effects of biology and environment, when we are born into a culture with stereotypes and beliefs about the nature of men and women? Babies enter into the socialization process even before they are born, when their parents decorate their nurseries, select toys, give them gendered names, and start to attribute gender characteristics to them as soon as they know the sex of the baby. Considering that the human genome is more than 99% alike in men and women, the biological differences are probably much less compelling than the effects of gender socialization (Jordan-Young, 2010).

MYTH #24: Transgender identity is rare.

FACT: Current classification systems rarely count transgender people, because questions on survey instruments and medical intakes ask only for male or female identification. Most transgender people consider themselves to be male or female based on their gender identity, and check the box that matches their identity. One study in the early 1990s (Bakker, van Kesteren, Gooren, & Bezemer, 1993) suggested that 1 in 10,000 people in the general population were male to female transsexuals (MTF or trans women) and 1 in 30,000 were female to male transsexuals (FTM or trans men). However, a more recent survey of the number of sex reassignment surgeries done in the United States revealed that 1 in 3,100 individuals undergo this procedure in their lifetimes (Horton & Goza, 2008), and the numbers of FTM and MTF transgender identities are roughly equivalent (Landen, Wålinder, Hambert, & Lundström, 1998). Gates (2011) using several population-based survey data, suggested that about 0.3% to 0.5% of the U.S. population has taken some steps toward transition and identifies as transgender. That would mean about 700,000 people in the United States identify as transgender. If these figures are correct, most healthcare professionals will work with transgender clients fairly regularly, whether they know it or not. The actual number of people who undergo sex reassignment surgery or transition is a small fraction of the transgender community, so the numbers may be much higher.

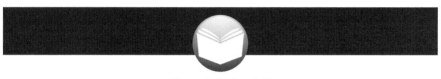

Read This 4.3

Read this short story by the BBC about pressures on lesbian and gay people in Iran to have gender reassignment surgery to "cure" their homosexuality. **https://goo.gl/MVCPDP**

MYTH #25: Transgender people are mentally ill.

FACT: Higher rates of depression and other mental disorders among transgender populations are the result of stigma: societal attitudes and negative treatment of transgender individuals (Ettner, 1996; Mallon, 2009). Newfield, Hart, Dibble, and Kohler (2006) reported significantly reduced mental health-related quality of life among 446 female to male transsexual and transgender individuals, and suggested that additional research was needed to determine the cause of this distress. Some older studies have found no increase in serious psychopathology among transsexual populations (e.g., Cole, O'Boyle, Emory, & Meyer, 1997), but the enormous amount of stigma and discrimination can certainly affect emotional adjustment—studies report very high rates of harassment and discrimination in transgender individuals. In one study, 60% of transgender individuals had experienced harassment or violence in their lifetimes and 27% had been the victim of violence. In the past year, they reported experiencing verbal abuse from strangers on the street (34%), being followed or stalked (9%), being assaulted (7%), having objects like rocks or bottles thrown at them (7%), and rape (3%) (Lombardi, Wilchins, Priesing, & Malouf, 2001). These events are certainly likely to affect one's mood and psychological well-being.

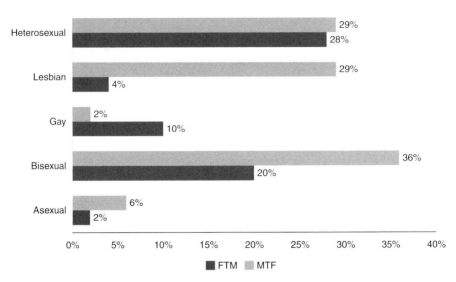

Figure 4.1 – Sexual Identification of People who Reported a Transgender Identity (Based on **Beemyn & Rankin, 2011**).

MYTH #26: Transgender people are actually lesbian and gay people who cannot accept their sexuality, so try to change their bodies to be heterosexual.

FACT: This stereotype comes from the idea that sex/gender causes sexuality and denies the possibility that gender and sexual identities can be experienced separately. In reality, transgender individuals report a wide diversity of both gender and sexual identities. Everyone has a gender and everyone has a sexual identity, and for most people, they are relatively separate. Beemyn and Rankin (2011) interviewed and/or surveyed nearly 3,500 people who fall somewhere on a trans* continuum. Figure 4.1 shows some of the data about sexual orientations, focusing just on those who identified as FTM or MTF (many were categorized as male birth sex to another gender or female birth sex to another gender, including the genderqueer and gender nonconforming groups).

MYTH #27: Transgender identity stems from a biological disorder of sex hormones, chromosome anomalies, or brain dysfunction.

FACT: There is no consensus on the origins of a transgender identity (or any sexual or gender identity for that matter). No studies have conclusively demonstrated differences in any biological structures or functions between transgender individuals and typically gendered individuals (Gooren, 2006). Most people who have been studied by researchers in the past were from university gender clinics, and identified as transsexual. They have been indistinguishable from people in the general population on dimensions of their physical bodies, hormone levels, and psychological adjustment. The only consistent difference is their perception of psychological gender. We know very little about people who identify as transgender, but have no wish to biologically alter their bodies.

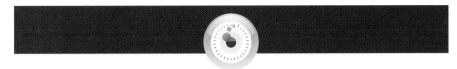

Watch This 4.2

The online miniseries "Transparent" **https://goo.gl/j6JBuX** portrays the experience of Maura, a transgender woman, and many challenges she faces in coming to terms with her identity. The series reflects the experience of many transgender individuals, who begin to experience gender dysphoria, or dissatisfaction with their physical bodies, early in childhood. As is the case for Maura, puberty was a particularly traumatic event as their bodies grow more and more out of alignment with their psychological gender. We have the medical capability to arrest pubertal development (preventing menstruation in girls, and erections and nocturnal emissions in boys), and such treatment is reversible. Watch at least one episode of this series, and consider the circumstances you think that this type of treatment could be considered.

Conclusions

Stereotypes are damaging because they remove any individuality from the person who adopts the stigmatized identity, and they are used to oppress individuals within the category and keep them powerless. Stereotypes imply that one identity completely defines the person, thus erasing their unique histories, varied temperaments and personalities, and the extraordinary diversities within any group that uses a common label. As we saw in the last chapter, stereotypes support stigma at the institutional level, and interfere with building positive relationships at the individual level. If healthcare professionals rely on myths and stereotypes rather than asking each patient about their lives, they are likely to make erroneous assumptions that can lead to inappropriate care of and disrespect toward the individual patient.

References

American Psychiatric Association (1973). *Position Statement on Homosexuality and Civil Rights*, Approved December.

American Psychiatric Association. (1998). Position statement on psychiatric treatment and sexual orientation. *The American Journal of Psychiatry*, *156*, 1131.

American Psychiatric Association. (2000). Therapies focused on attempts to change sexual orientation (reparative or conversion therapies). Position paper approved May.

Bakker, A., van Kesteren, P. J., Gooren, L. J., & Bezemer, P. D. (1993). The prevalence of transsexualism in The Netherlands. *Acta Psychiatrica Scandinavica*, *87*, 237–238.

Balsam, K. F., Beauchaine, T. P., Mickey, R. M., & Rothblum, E. D. (2005). Mental health of lesbian, gay, bisexual, and heterosexual siblings: Effects of gender, sexual orientation, and family. *Journal of Abnormal Psychology*, *114*, 471–476. Retrieved from http://doi.org/10.1037/0021–843X.114.3.471

Balsam, K. F., & Mohr, J. J. (2007). Adaptation to sexual orientation stigma: A comparison of bisexual and lesbian/gay adults. *Journal of Consulting Psychology*, *54*, 306–319.

Battle, J., & Crum, M. (2007). Black LGB health and wellbeing. In I. H. Meyer & M. E. Northridge (Eds.), *The health of sexual minorities: Public health perspectives on lesbian, gay, bisexual, and transgender populations* (pp. 320–352). New York: Springer Publishing.

Beemyn, B. G., & Rankin, S. (2011). *The lives of transgender people*. New York: Columbia University Press.

Byne, W. (2007). Biology and sexual minority status. In I. H. Meyer & M. E. Northridge (Eds.), *The health of sexual minorities: Public health perspectives on lesbian, gay, bisexual, and transgender populations* (pp. 65–90). New York: Springer. Retrieved from http://doi.org/10.1007/978–0–387–31334–4_4

Cohen, L. J., & Galynker, I. I. (2002). Clinical features of pedophilia and implications for treatment. *Journal of Psychiatric Practice, 8*, 276–289.

Cole, C. M., O'Boyle, M., Emory, L. E., & Meyer, W. J., 3rd. (1997). Comorbidity of gender dysphoria and other major psychiatric diagnoses. *Archives of Sexual Behavior, 26*, 13–26.

Coleman, E., & Rosser, B. R. S. (1996). Gay and bisexual male sexuality. In R. Cabaj & T. Stein (Eds.), *Textbook of homosexuality and mental health* (pp. 707–722). Washington, DC: APA Press.

Conger, J. J. (1975). Proceedings of the American Psychological Association, incorporated, for the year 1974: Minutes of the annual meeting of the Council of Representatives. *American Psychologist, 30,* 620–651. Retrieved from http://www.apa.org/about/policy/discrimination.aspx

D'Augelli, A. R. (2006). Developmental and contextual factors and mental health among LGB youths. In A. Omoto & H. Kurtzman (Eds.), *Sexual orientation and mental health* (pp. 37–53). Washington, DC: APA Press.

DeLeon, P. H. (1998). Proceedings of the American Psychological Association, incorporated, for the legislative year 1997: Minutes of the Annual Meeting of the Council of Representatives, August 14 and 17, Chicago, Illinois; and June, August and December 1997 meetings of the Board of Directors. *American Psychologist, 53,* 882–939.

Diamond, L. (2003). What does sexual orientation orient? A biobehavioral model distinguishing romantic love and sexual desire. *Psychological Review, 110*, 173–192.

Diamond, L. (2005). A new view of lesbian subtypes: Stable vs fluid identity trajectories over an eight-year period. *Psychology of Women Quarterly, 29*, 119–128.

Dykes, B. (2000). Problems with defining cross-cultural 'kinds of homosexuality" and a solution. *Journal of Homosexuality, 38*, 1–18.

Eagly, A. H., Diekman, A. B., Johannesen-Schmidt, M. C., & Koenig, A. M. (2004). Gender gaps in sociopolitical attitudes: A social psychological analysis. *Journal of Personality and Social Psychology, 87*, 796–816. Retrieved from http://doi.org/10.1037/0022–3514.87.6.796

Elia, J. P., & Eliason, M. J. (2010). Discourses of exclusion: Sexuality education's silencing of sexual others. *Journal of LGBT Youth, 7*(1), 29–48. Retrieved from http://doi.org/10.1080/19361650903507791

Eliason, M. J. (1998). Correlates of prejudice in nursing students. *The Journal of Nursing Education, 37*, 27–29.

Ettner, R. (1996). *Confessions of a gender defender: A psychologist's reflections on life among the transgendered*. Evanston, IL: Chicago Spectrum Press.

Fausto-Sterling, A. (1993). The five sexes. *The Sciences, 33*(2), 20–24.

Fausto-Sterling, A. (2000). *Sexing the body: Gender politics and the construction of sexuality*. New York: Basic Books.

Fieland, K., Walters, K., & Simoni, J. (2007). Determinants of health among two-spirit American Indians and Alaska Natives. In I. H. Meyer & M. Northridge (Eds.), *The health of sexual minorities: Public health perspectives on lesbian, gay, bisexual, and transgender populations* (pp. 268–300). New York: Springer Publishing.

Friedman, M. S., Koeske, G. F., Silvestre, A. J., Korr, W. S., & Sites, E. W. (2006). The impact of gender-role nonconforming behavior, bullying, and social support on suicidality among gay male youth. *The Journal of Adolescent Health: Official Publication of the*

Society for Adolescent Medicine, *38*(5), 621–623. Retrieved from http://doi.org/10.1016/j.jadohealth.2005.04.014

Gage-Davidson, M. (2000). Religion and spirituality. In R. Perez, K. DeBord, & K. Bieschke (Eds.), *Handbook of counseling and psychotherapy with LGB clients* (pp. 409–433). American Psychological Association.

Gates, G. J. (2011). How many people are lesbian, gay, bisexual and transgender? *eScholarship-UCLA: The Williams Institute.* Retrieved from https://escholarship.org/uc/item/09h684×2.pdf

Gates, G. J., & Newport, N. (2012). Gallup special report: The US adult LGBT population. Retrieved July 15, 2015, from http://williamsinstitute.law.ucla.edu/research/census-lgbt-demographics-studies/gallup-special-report-18oct-2012/

Gilman, S. E., Cochran, S. D., Mays, V. M., Hughes, M., Ostrow, D., & Kessler, R. C. (2001). Risk of psychiatric disorders among individuals reporting same-sex sexual partners in the National Comorbidity Survey. *American Journal of Public Health*, *91*(6), 933–939.

Goldberg, A. E., Gartrell, N., & Gates, G. J. (2014). Research report on LGB-parent families. Retrieved June 26, 2015, from http://williamsinstitute.law.ucla.edu/research/parenting/lgb-parent-families-jul-2014

Gooren, L. (2006). The biology of human psychosexual differentiation. *Hormones and Behavior*, *50*(4), 589–601. Retrieved from http://doi.org/10.1016/j.yhbeh.2006.06.011

Helminiak, D. A. (2012). *Sex and the sacred: Gay identity and spiritual growth*. New York: Routledge.

Herdt, G. H. (1996). *Third sex, third gender: Beyond sexual dimorphism in culture and history*. New York: Zone Books.

Herek, G. M. (2009). Hate crimes and stigma-related experiences among sexual minority adults in the United States: Prevalence estimates from a national probability sample. *Journal of Interpersonal Violence*, *24*(1), 54–74. Retrieved from http://doi.org/10.1177/0886260508316477

Horton, M. A., & Goza, E. (2008). The cost of transgender health benefits. In *Presented at Out and Equal Workplace Summit Conference.* Retrieved from http://www.spectrumwny.org/info/costbenefit.pdf

Hughes, T. L., Johnson, T., & Wilsnack, S. C. (2001). Sexual assault and alcohol abuse: A comparison of lesbians and heterosexual women. *Journal of Substance Abuse*, *13*(4), 515–532.

Jenny, C., Roesler, T. A., & Poyer, K. L. (1994). Are children at risk for sexual abuse by homosexuals? *Pediatrics*, *94*(1), 41–44.

Jordan-Young, R. M. (2010). *Brain storm: The flaws in the science of sex differences*. Cambridge, MA: Harvard University Press.

Kinsey, A. C., Pomeroy, W. B., & Martin, C. E. (1948). *Sexual behavior in the human male*. Philadelphia, PA: Saunders.

Klein, F., Sepekoff, B., & Wolf, T. J. (1985). Sexual orientation: A multi-variable dynamic process. *Journal of Homosexuality*, *11*(1–2), 35–49. Retrieved from http://doi.org/10.1300/J082v11n01_04

Kurdek, L. A. (2004). Are gay and lesbian cohabiting couples really different from heterosexual married couples? *Journal of Marriage and Family Counseling*, *66*(4), 880–900. Retrieved from http://doi.org/10.1111/j.0022–2445.2004.00060.x

Kurdek, L. A., & Schmitt, J. P. (1986). Relationship quality of partners in heterosexual married, heterosexual cohabiting, and gay and lesbian relationships. *Journal of Personality and Social Psychology*, *51*(4), 711–720.

Landen, M., Wålinder, J., Hambert, G., & Lundström, B. (1998). Factors predictive of regret in sex reassignment. *Acta Psychiatrica Scandinavica*, *97*(4), 284–289.

Laumann, E. O. (1994). *The social organization of sexuality: Sexual practices in the United States*. University of Chicago Press.

Lease, S. H., Horne, S. G., & Noffsinger-Frazier, N. (2005). Affirming faith experiences and psychological health for Caucasian lesbian, gay, and bisexual individuals. *Journal of Counseling Psychology, 52*(3), 378. Retrieved from http://doi.org/10.1037/0022–0167.52.3.378

Lombardi, E. L., Wilchins, R. A., Priesing, D., & Malouf, D. (2001). Gender violence: Transgender experiences with violence and discrimination. *Journal of Homosexuality, 42*(1), 89–101.

Mallon, G. P. (2009). *Social services with transgendered youth.* New York: Haworth.

Masters, W. H., & Johnson, V. E. (1979). *Homosexuality in perspective.* New York: Bantam Books.

Matthews, A. K., Hughes, T. L., & Tartaro, J. (2006). Sexual behavior and sexual dysfunction in a community sample of lesbian and heterosexual women. In A. M. Omoto & H. S. Kurtzman (Eds.), *Sexual orientation and mental health* (pp. 185–205). Washington, DC: American Psychological Association. Retrieved from http://doi.org/10.1037/11261–009

Meston, C. M., & Buss, D. M. (2007). Why humans have sex. *Archives of Sexual Behavior, 36*(4), 477–507. Retrieved from http://doi.org/10.1007/s10508–007–9175–2

Meyer, I. H. (1995). Minority stress and mental health in gay men. *Journal of Health and Social Behavior, 36*(1), 38–56.

Miller, S. J., & Stack, K. (2014). African-American lesbian and queer women respond to Christian-based homophobia. *Journal of GLBT Family Studies, 10*(3), 243–268. Retrieved from http://doi.org/10.1080/1550428X.2013.825219

Mock, S. E., & Eibach, R. P. (2012). Stability and change in sexual orientation identity over a 10-year period in adulthood. *Archives of Sexual Behavior, 41*(3), 641–648. Retrieved from http://doi.org/10.1007/s10508–011–9761–1

Mohr, J. J., & Rochlen, A. B. (1999). Measuring attitudes regarding bisexuality in lesbian, gay male, and heterosexual populations. *Journal of Counseling Psychology, 46*(3), 353. Retrieved from http://doi.org/10.1037/0022–0167.46.3.353

Newfield, E., Hart, S., Dibble, S. L., & Kohler, L. (2006). Female-to-male transgender quality of life. *Quality of Life Research: An International Journal of Quality of Life Aspects of Treatment, Care and Rehabilitation, 15*(9), 1447–1457. Retrieved from http://doi.org/10.1007/s11136–006–0002–3

Peplau, L. A., & Fingerhut, A. W. (2007). The close relationships of lesbians and gay men. *Annual Review of Psychology, 58*, 405–424. Retrieved from http://doi.org/10.1146/annurev.psych.58.110405.085701

Pew Research Center. (2013). A survey of LGBT Americans: attitudes, experiences and values in changing times. Retrieved July 20, 2015, from http://www.pewsocialtrends.org/2013/06/13/a-survey-of-lgbt-americans/

Ramirez-Valles, J. (2007). "I don't fit anywhere": How race and sexuality shape latino gay and bisexual men's health. In I. H. Meyer & M. E. Northridge (Eds.), *The health of sexual minorities: Public health perspectives on lesbian, gay, bisexual, and transgender populations* (pp. 301–319). New York: Springer.

Rodriguez, E. M., Lytle, M. C., & Vaughan, M. D. (2013). Exploring the intersectionality of bisexual, religious/spiritual, and political identities from a feminist perspective. *Journal of Bisexuality, 13*(3), 285–309. Retrieved from http://doi.org/10.1080/15299716.2013.813001

Rodriguez, E. M., & Ouellette, S. C. (2000). Gay and lesbian Christians: Homosexual and religious identity integration in the members and participants of a gay-positive church. *Journal for the Scientific Study of Religion, 39*(3), 333–347. Retrieved from http://doi.org/10.1111/0021–8294.00028

Rust, P. C. (1996). Sexual identity and bisexual identities: The struggle for self-description in a changing sexual landscape. In B. Beemyn & M. Eliason (Eds.), *Queer studies: A lesbian, gay, bisexual, and transgender anthology* (pp. 64–86). New York: New York University Press.

Rust, P. C. (2000). *Bisexuality in the United States: A social science reader.* New York: Columbia University Press.

Saewyc, E. M., Bauer, G. R., Skay, C. L., Bearinger, L. H., Resnick, M. D., Reis, E., & Murphy, A. (2004). Measuring sexual orientation in adolescent health surveys: Evaluation of eight school-based surveys. *The Journal of Adolescent Health: Official Publication of the Society for Adolescent Medicine, 35*(4), 345.e1–15.

Schneeberger, A. R., Dietl, M. F., Muenzenmaier, K. H., Huber, C. G., & Lang, U. E. (2014). Stressful childhood experiences and health outcomes in sexual minority populations: A systematic review. *Social Psychiatry and Psychiatric Epidemiology, 49*(9), 1427–1445. Retrieved from http://doi.org/10.1007/s00127-014-0854-8

Schroeder, M., & Shidlo, A. (2002). Ethical issues in sexual orientation conversion therapies: An empirical study of consumers. *Journal of Gay & Lesbian Psychotherapy, 5*(3–4), 131–166. Retrieved from http://doi.org/10.1300/J236v05n03_09

Szymanski, D., & Chung, B. (2003). Internalized homophobia in lesbians. In T. L. Hughes, C. Smith, & A. Dan (Eds.), *Mental health issues for sexual minority women: Redefining women's mental health* (pp. 115–126). New York: Haworth Press.

Tasker, F. (2005). Lesbian mothers, gay fathers, and their children: A review. *Journal of Developmental and Behavioral Pediatrics: JDBP, 26*(3), 224–240.

Whitley, B. E., Jr, & Kite, M. E. (1995). Sex differences in attitudes toward homosexuality: A comment on Oliver and Hyde (1993). *Psychological Bulletin, 117*(1), 146–154; discussion 155–158.

Zucker, K. (2013). The politics and science of "reparative therapy." In J. Drescher & K. J. Zucker (Eds.), *Ex-gay research: Analyzing the Spitzer study and its relation to science, religion, politics, and culture* (pp. 3–12). New York: Haworth Press.

Chapter 5

LGBTQ Families

"When we take our children to a hospital, we never know if we are going to have a problem with how we are treated as a family. One of us as a parent may be discounted, and only one parent permitted to sign consents, be listed as the parent on forms, or be allowed into the ICU or ER to visit the child. Forms that we and our children have to fill out never reflect the diversity of our families. There are checkboxes for male and female but there are some transgender parents who don't fit either box, or fit both. Rabbi Levi Alter, President of Female-To-Male International." (Wilson & Yoshikawa, 2007, p. 8)

The terms "family" and/or "family of choice" are frequently used among LGBTQs to refer to an affinity circle that has significant meaning for its members. Some LGBTQ individuals have been rejected by their families of origin so they create their own family networks composed of the people who share, support, and care for them, including partners, close friends, and often ex-lovers and/or ex-spouses (Weston, 1991). This chapter will review basic concepts related to LGBTQ families, including coming out to family members, significant other relationships, parenting, grandparenting, and family-related healthcare issues.

Defining "Family"

Despite the deep and meaningful ties that exist in LGBTQ chosen families, as the opening quote indicates, many LGBTQ families fear exclusion and discrimination from healthcare providers and institutions. These fears extend beyond self to include fear of exclusion of partners from decision-making and fear of being excluded from partner's and children's care. Hospitals and clinics often use narrow definitions of family that are sanctioned by

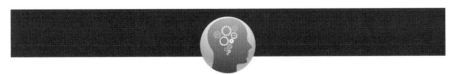

Think About It 5.1

How would you feel if this happened to you? An older lesbian underwent surgery, but died on the operating table. The doctor ignored the life partner in the waiting room while he told the biological family—not the partner—that the woman had died. To compound this tragic oversight, the biological family went home without telling the woman about the death of her partner (Saulnier, 2002, p. 360).

laws in most states, which define family as adult legal relationships between one man and one woman and the birth or adoption offspring of those unions or blood relatives. This narrow definition may exclude LGBTQ family members from critical healthcare decisions and settings if the family does not fit legal definitions. On the other hand, The Joint Commission that accredits healthcare settings (JCAHO) defines family much broader than blood or legal ties as "person(s) who plays a significant role in an individual's life. This may include a person(s) not legally related to the individual. This person(s) is often referred to as a surrogate decision maker if authorized to make care decisions for the individual should he or she lose decision-making capacity" (JCAHO Staff, 2004, p. GL–5).

Over the centuries the structures, functions, and the definitions of family have changed. In the 21st century, some of the most diverse and creative family structures have been forged by LGBTQ people. LGBTQ families can include couples in legal marriages, civil unions (see Solomon, Rothblum, & Balsam, 2004 for a description of this precursor to full marriage equality), domestic partnerships, legally unrecognized long-term, committed relationships, open relationships, or group families (e.g., a lesbian couple and a gay couple conceive and raise children together). Table 5.1 shows the changes in legal standing of same-sex couples that are happening worldwide. In many countries, some type of same-sex relationships are afforded some legal protection as of 2015.

Children can come into the family from previous heterosexual relationships, alternative insemination procedures, adoption, and co-parenting. And contrary to stereotypes about LGBTQ people as unable to reproduce and sustain relationships, many are parents. A recent review of the literature found that between 25% and 50% of transgender people are parents (Stotzer, Herman, & Hasenbush, 2014), and 37% of LGB adults have been parents—48% of women and 20% of men (Gates, 2013a). The census data also suggests that people of color in same-sex relationships are much more likely to be parents than White people in same-sex relationships. For example, in California, more African-American (43%), Asian-Pacific Islander (45%), and Latina/o (62%) same-sex couples are raising children compared to White same-sex couples (18%), but these ethnic minority households are doing so with fewer economic resources. "Latino/a same-gender couples are over three times as likely to be raising children, on less than half the average household income of White same-gender couples" (Wilson, 2007, p. 2). The high number of parents among LGBTQ people also means that most of them will be grandparents, raising questions about the uniqueness of queer grandparenting.

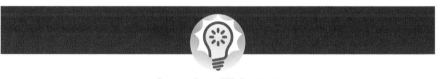

Imagine This 5.1

Peggy and Karen were legally married in California in 2008 in a civil ceremony in San Francisco City Hall not far from the room where Harvey Milk was murdered. Peggy's son and his daughters, Sophie (age 4) and Elodie (age 2) were there, along with a small group of close friends. A couple of years later, Sophie asked: "Mémé, is Karen your husband or your wife?" Peggy responded: "we call each other 'partners'." Elodie piped up with "I have a partner at school!" Imagine the world that they will grow up in, and how having a lesbian grandmother will influence their future.

Table 5.1 – Marriage Equality Worldwide (Refer to http://www.freedomtomarry .org/Landscape/Entry/C/International for the Latest Information)	
Marriage Status	**Country**
Country-wide freedom to marry	Netherlands—April 1, 2001 Belgium—June 1, 2003 Spain—July 3, 2005 Canada—July 20, 2005 South Africa—November 30, 2006 Norway—January 1, 2009 Sweden—May 1, 2009 Portugal—June 5, 2009 Iceland—June 27, 2010 Argentina—July 22, 2010 Denmark—June 15, 2012 Brazil—May 14, 2013 France—May 29, 2013 Uruguay—August 5, 2013 New Zealand—August 19, 2013 United Kingdom—England July 17, 2013 Wales—March 29, 2014 Scotland—February 4, 2014 Luxembourg—June 18, 2014 Finland—November 28, 2014 Ireland—May 23, 2015 Greenland—May, 2015 Mexico—May–June, 2015[a] United States—June 26, 2015
Taking steps toward marriage	Slovenia Australia Columbia
Broad protections for same-sex couples but not inclusive of marriage	Chile, Ecuador, Germany, Hungary, Northern Ireland, and Malta.
Limited spousal rights for same-sex couples	Andorra, Austria, Colombia, Croatia, Czech Republic, Liechtenstein, Slovenia, and Switzerland.
Marriage of same-sex couples recognized but not legal to perform in the country	Israel

[a]See these sources for the status of Mexico as of July 21, 2015:
   http://www.hrc.org/blog/entry/marriage-equality-moves-forward-in-mexico
   http://www.buzzfeed.com/lesterfeder/mexico-appears-to-have-crossed-a-major-hurdle-to-marriage-eq#.rbeA3kMWA

Language is a serious limitation when discussing LGBTQ families. There is no one widely-used term for significant others—terms such as partner, spouse, wife, husband, lover, girlfriend, boyfriend, and others are used to denote those important relationships. Ex-lovers often remain centrally involved in each other's lives. There is inadequate language to distinguish a lifelong committed partner from an intimate friendship or from a more casual relationship, and there is insufficient language for all the variety of parenting and child roles that can occur. Does a child with two fathers call them both dad? What happens when dad becomes a woman? If a child is reared in a group home, are there primary parents and secondary parents? In some cases, mom's best friend and ex-partner may play a parental role in a child's life and a biological father may have little or no role. Our language needs to be broad enough to capture the diverse relationships that two or more individuals may forge.

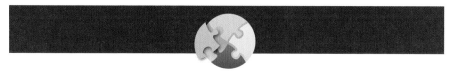

Try This 5.1

Think about how you currently ask clients about their family relationships. The most common is to ask "Are you married?" But today many people, even heterosexuals, do not marry. It is important to encourage all patients/clients to tell you about themselves and their various family situations in their own words. Ask about family relationships without necessarily referring to a "husband" or a "wife," or a "mother" or a "father." Make a list of alternative ways to ask someone about their family, and then try using several of these alternatives for at least a week. For example, you might say "Who do you count on for support?" or "Who is family to you?" Don't *ever* ask, "Who's the 'real' mother/father?"

Relationships with Families of Origin

One of the most traumatic experiences in the lives of LGBTQ people is coming out to family of origin and friends. In a recent study exploring sexual identity milestones of 396 LGB New York City residents ages 18 to 59, once a person self-identified as LG or B, disclosure to family, heterosexual friends and other LGB friends tended to happen 5 to 7 years later. Younger LGB participants reported coming out to family, friends, and other LGBs earlier than older participants, with younger participants coming out at about 17 or 18 years of age, while older participants reported coming out to others at around 24 to 25 years of age (Martos, Nezhad, & Meyer, 2014).

As noted in Chapter 6, there will be differences in the experience of coming out depending on whether a person is 13 or 33 or 73. This section reviews some of the common issues faced by individuals across the lifespan who come out to parents, children, or to partners/spouses. It is important to keep in mind that the experiences and the potential consequences may differ depending on the age/developmental stage of the person coming out, as well as the dynamics of the family relationships, racial/ethnic background, religious orientation, and many other factors, but there are some common experiences shared by many LGBTQ people such as fear of rejection and guilt for defying family expectations.

Coming Out to Parents

One of the biggest fears related to disclosure is parental rejection (Ben-Ari, 1995), so first disclosures are rarely to parents, but rather, to close friends and siblings (Savin-Williams, 1998). For most individuals, there is a gap of at least a year between coming out to self and coming out to another person (Savin-Williams & Cohen, 2007).

D'Augelli, Herschberger, and Pilkington (1998) found that most LGB youth were first aware of being different at around age 10, but did not disclose to another person until around 16. This means that the youth has had several years to think about their sexuality or gender and has come to terms with it, but their parents are often caught off guard and had not considered the possibility of having an LGBTQ child. This often forces parents into the closet themselves as they work through their own reactions. In general, mothers tend to be more accepting than fathers, but disclosure often precipitates a family crisis. Parental reactions can include guilt, loss, and shame. For youth who disclose while still living with parents, there is a potential for loss of economic support and rejection. Coming out as an adult has fewer negative consequences in some ways, but the fear of family rejection can still be very strong regardless of the age of the individual.

Some studies have suggested that coming out earlier (before 18) carries more risks. Friedman, Marshal, Stall, Cheong, & Wright (2008) found that the early disclosers among gay and bisexual men were more likely to experience victimization, forced sex, suicide attempts, and later in life, depression and HIV/AIDS than were those who came out in young adulthood. Younger individuals are developmentally more immature, have less life experience, and may have fewer support systems than young adults.

Interviews with 29 Turkish transgender individuals about their experiences coming out to their families revealed that more than half of the families were aware that the trans family member was different for more than 5 years prior to the disclosure, with most of the families aware around the time of puberty. Most of the families tried to conceal the difference (65%) and about the same number reported that they had no information about transgender issues to help them. At the time of the disclosure, most families reported severe shock (64%), tried to change the person by talking to them or force (66%), and only 28% were supportive from the beginning. However, at the time of the interviews, 40% of the families were totally accepting (Polat, Yuksel, Discigil, & Meteris, 2005).

Lev (2004) proposed four stages of reactions of family member to the disclosure of a transgender family member:

1. Discovery/disclosure: family members may react initially with betrayal, shock, fear, shame, revulsion, and anxiety.
2. Turmoil: after the initial disclosure, family members begin to wonder why, and spouses/partners may question their own sexuality.
3. Negotiation: this phase involves wishes or efforts to get the "old person" back.
4. Finding balance: finally, family members come to terms with the transition.

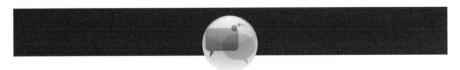

Talk About It 5.1

Share this story with a group of friends or colleagues, and discuss ways to help families work through this kind of situation:

A real story: Donna Orchard of Mobile, AL

(continued)

Eight years ago, while driving home from a movie, my 19-year-old college son began to visibly shake, white knuckles grabbing the steering wheel. The light-hearted mood suddenly changed when he said, "I have something to tell you."

"Okay." His step-dad and I nodded our heads.

"I'm gay."

I turned to look at my beautiful son who had brought me to school only once in 12 years, now on the dean's list, working his way through college as a tenor section leader in an Episcopal church in Birmingham, AL. At first there was a typical response. I squalled about AIDS and not having grandbabies. I cried those crocodile tears that he had cried in the mall when he looked up at me discovering there was no Santa. Thirty minutes later, before we got home, we hugged, and until this day I can't imagine Benjamin not being gay.

My fears, however, did not end there. Even with a supportive husband, I worried, "In the worse case scenario, my son will be considered a pedophile, at best he will be seen as a comic character on *Saturday Night Live*."

In fact, most of the attitudes about gays were not just disrespectful but downright unacceptable to me. I was scared.

"And he'll have to leave Alabama. What if he walked into the wrong bar? Well, that could happen anywhere. He'll have to live far away from me, in New York or San Francisco, forever. At least he'll be safe. What if someone does hurt him?" I was scared.

This mother found her local chapter of PFLAG and got the support she and her family needed. PFLAG (Parents, Family, Friends, & Allies United with LGBTQ People to Move Equality Forward) is a national organization with local chapters in every state in the United States. Its mission is to help family and friends learn to be supportive allies for their LGBTQ family members and peers. Visit the PFLAG web site (http://community.pflag.org/getsupport), and explore in your discussion some of the suggestions and resources offered on their Web site.

Coming Out to Children

Since individuals can come out at any point in the lifespan, some already have children before they come out, and others have families after coming out, but must decide how and when to inform their children of their sexual or gender identification. When possible, disclosure when the children are young (early childhood) is the most successful and least traumatic (Lynch & Murray, 2000; White & Ettner, 2007). If the children are adolescents, when peer pressures are greater and the child is also undergoing identity formation, the disclosure can create greater family drama (Bigner, 1996). Lynch and Murray (2000) reported that parents' decisions about disclosure to children are based on two types of concerns: potential for loss of custody and the potential effects of the disclosure on the child's life. One study found that lesbians who had children prior to coming out to themselves were somewhat less likely to be out to others because of a perceived need to protect their families (Morris, Balsam, & Rothblum, 2002). Another study found that previously "out" lesbian mothers became more discrete as their children grew into childhood and adolescents, as an attempt to protect their children (Gartrell, Deck, Rodas, Peyser, & Banks, 2005). In general, children's reactions depend on a host of factors: the comfort level of the parent when they disclose, the age and developmental stage of the child, the stability and closeness of the parent–child relationship, and others. A child's first reaction is generally, "how will this affect me?" They often worry about the reactions of their peers.

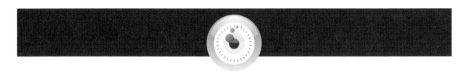

Watch This 5.1

The Amazon series, *Transparent*, shows the challenges a newly out trans woman face when trying to come out to her adult children. There was no "natural" opening in their typical exchanges to facilitate such a conversation and children can lapse back into a narcissistic mode with their parents, even as adults. It can be hard for children to see their parents as independent beings. Watch the trailer, and if possible, sign up to see the whole series! https://goo.gl/yu1u3F

Coming Out to Spouses/Partners

Many LGBTQ people marry people of the other sex prior to coming out. The stress of telling a spouse may be equal to or greater than coming out to family of origin. Most LGBTQ people marry people they genuinely love, so coming out to them feels like a major betrayal of that love.

Erhardt (2006) is a counselor who has worked with over 300 transgender and cross-dressing clients and interviewed women whose husbands had come out as transsexual or cross-dressers. One woman who found out that her husband wanted to permanently change gender had this experience:

> *"My initial reaction was one of complete shock and devastation … A lot of my discomfort was a result of the fact that I simply didn't understand. There were lots of tears and plenty of talking over the months that followed … eventually the crying stopped. I knew I loved him/her no matter what, and that I would stick by my partner."* (p. 106)

LGBTQ people may have been in heterosexual marriages prior to coming out to themselves, as an attempt to "normalize" their sexuality, and/or because they fell in love with the person. Transgender individuals, as well, often seek heterosexual relationships, or sometimes same-sex relationships, prior to initiating a transition. Many continue to feel love for their spouses/partners after they come out. Beemyn and Rankin (2011) interviewed or surveyed nearly 3,500 gender nonconforming people, and found that those who were married/partnered prior to transitioning had almost universal negative reactions from spouses because the disclosure challenged everything the spouse thought they knew about the transitioning partner and raised questions about their sexual orientation. Having a partner transition can affect the sense of identity of the partner and create a crisis of sorts. Some resolve the crisis and stay with their transitioning partners and others are not able to overcome their initial negative reactions—two-thirds of trans women who had been legally married at the time of transition ended up in divorce. Another complicated situation for many transgender people is coming out to potential partners after transition: When is the best time to do that? Should they be honest before starting dating? Come out after getting to know the person?

Intimate Relationships

Dating

When asked about her social life after a difficult breakup with her girlfriend, a lesbian told her friends "I am once again in lesbian dating hell!" Same-sex or same-gender dating has many challenges that are outside the rules and expectations imposed by heterorelational norms, and it is easy to falter, and to find oneself in an embarrassing social situation. In other words, dating evolves in heterosexual contexts based on patterns of behavior that are typical of expected male and female roles. These are depicted in the media and define patterns of flirtation and verbal/nonverbal expression of sexual attraction that provide cues to act and respond in a back-and-forth interplay that moves a romantic relationship forward. The heteronormative expectations have changed in western societies over the past several decades in that heterosexual women are now more free to initiate a dating relationship with a man, but generally there is an implicit understanding of what is going on when one person in a heterosexual pair begins to give signals of a desire to explore a relationship that might become romantic. Those signals are less clear when partners are of the same sex, where even today, women are socialized to play coy and hard to get, and men to be the initiators of dates and sex.

These patterns are not typically as reliable or common in LGBTQ interactions because of the very thin lines that can exist between friendships, casual flirtatious interactions, and serious romantic intentions. For people who are bisexual or trans* the challenges can be even greater because of the fluidity of their experience, coupled with the challenges of interacting with other people whose expectations and preconceived ideas about relationships are not typically inclusive of nongender conforming experience. Many heterosexual trans women experience the damaging stereotypes of youth and beauty that plague cisgender women, and have difficulties finding male partners. In general, LGBTQ people meet potential dates in the same types of places as heterosexual people; at work, at school, in bars, at social/recreational activities, through friends, and online. But the fact that there are fewer "rules" for dating and relationships in LGBTQ communities can lead to both frustration and challenge, but hold greater opportunities as well.

Significant Other Relationships

Are LGBTQ significant other relationships different from heterosexual relationships? So much of the traditional heterosexual relationship is based on gender stereotypes about men being breadwinners and women being the nurturers, that there are bound to be some differences, but the existing literature suggests that these differences are relatively small. Some LGBTQ individuals are engaged in family formation through polyamory, defined as the "philosophy and practice of loving more than one person at a time with honesty and integrity" (McCullough & Hall, 2003), but the majority of LGBTQ people are in monogamous couple relationships.

In regards to gay male relationships, stereotypes about gay men being promiscuous and unable to have stable relationships still abound. However, the majority of gay men forge stable, long-term relationships, although they may be more diverse than heterosexual relationships. Some gay men have "marriages" whether legal or not, that are similar to heterosexual marriage—they are monogamous and long-term commitments.

Other gay men have a primary partner, but have an open or nonmonogamous relationship, men being somewhat more likely than women to be socialized to separate love and sex. Some research has found both types of relationships to be equally satisfying and secure (LaSala, 2004). Factors that seem to predict relationship success among gay men include

- self-acceptance and being secure in one's own sexuality (Van Wormer, Wells, & Boes, 2000);
- psychological complementarity (when gender role expectations are absent, gay men are freer to select partners on individual needs and wishes (Laird, 1993); and
- extended family support.

Many male same-sex couples must negotiate sexual behavior when one or both are HIV positive. Having a secure attachment in one's relationship was found to be associated with less sexual risk behavior and greater relationship satisfaction (Starks & Parsons, 2014).

Lesbians are equally freed from gender role expectations in some regards, but also are socialized to value intimacy and connectedness more so than men. This means that lesbians may forge deep intimate relationships with other women rather quickly (Parks & Humphreys, 2006). There is a joke about lesbians taking a U-Haul on the second date, implying that the move from dating to serious relationship is very fast. Once lesbian relationships are formed, they do not differ greatly from heterosexual relationships in terms of satisfaction or challenges (Kurdek, 2001), but they do differ in terms of societal acceptance and division of labor. Lesbian relationships tend to be much more egalitarian than heterosexual relationships (Matthews, Tartaro, & Hughes, 2003). Lesbian couples are twice as likely as gay male couples to seek out civil unions where they are available, but it may have to do with parental status, because lesbian couples are also twice as likely as gay male couples to have children (Solomon et al., 2004). Some early literature about lesbian psychology suggested that many lesbian couples are pathologically close, or "fused" and debated whether this was a positive or negative characteristic. Frost and Eliason (2014) found no evidence of fusion among female same-sex couples— about the same number of female same-sex couples felt very close (or too close) as among male same-sex couples and other sex couples.

There is very little empirical research on relationships among bisexual individuals. Some of this research finds bisexual people to be more likely to engage in nonmonogamous relationships (Weinberg, Williams, & Pryor, 1994). McLean (2004) surveyed 60 Australian bisexual men and women and found that about one-fourth of the sample were in monogamous relationships, and were satisfied with those arrangements. Those in nonmonogamous relationships discussed the challenges of negotiating the ground rules for these relationships—generally, levels of trust, honesty, and a high degree of communication must be present for these relationships to thrive.

Finally, relationships are complicated for transgender individuals as well, because they represent all varieties of sexual identity from lesbian, gay, bisexual, heterosexual, and asexual. In one study, 32% of transgender respondents identified as bisexual, 20% as heterosexual, 16% as lesbian, gay, or queer, and 16% as "other" (Beemyn & Rankin, 2011). When gender and sexuality combinations are considered together, new hybrid relationships are possible.

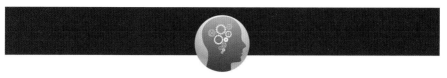

Think About It 5.2

Kate Bornstein is a performance artist, born male, and transitioned to become a woman as an adult. As a man, Kate had been married to a woman. After transitioning, Kate was in a relationship with a woman who considered herself a lesbian, but later transitioned to a male role. Currently, Kate's partner is another MTF transgender woman. So what kind of relationships has Kate had? Heterosexual, then lesbian, then heterosexual, then lesbian? These terms have little meaning when gender difference is added to the mix, and this example highlights the inadequacy of our language. Can you think of alternative language and ways of thinking about identities and relationships?

Rosser, Oakes, Bockting, and Miner (2007) in an internet survey of transgender individuals found that 28% of MTF and 6% of FTM reported that they were currently legally married. The literature does not yet contain data about other types of relationships among transgender individuals. One study addressed men who have sex with transgender women as a possible new sexual identification category (Operario, Burton, Underhill, & Sevelius, 2008)—do these men have different risk factors than men who have sex with men (MSM) or heterosexual men? We lack of information about all the unique varieties of sexual desires and sexual relationships so the basic premise of this book is especially important for healthcare providers—ASK. Healthcare providers need to remain **aware** that there is a wide diversity of relationships in LGBTQ communities, so be **sensitive** and open, without judgment, to the relationships of each person they encounter, and use the current **knowledge** that is available to inform clinical practice.

Parenting

Historically, LGBTQ people became parents through heterosexual relationships or at least heterosexual sex. In the past 20 years, increasing numbers of same-sex individuals and couples are now creating families through adoption, foster parenting, surrogate parenting, biological parenting using reproductive technologies, and step parenting. LGBTQ people are four times more likely to adopt a child than are heterosexual people, and six times more likely to have foster children (Gates, 2013a). The highest proportion of same-sex couples raising children in the United States are in states not generally known to be welcoming and inclusive of LGBTQ people: Mississippi (26% of same-sex couples raising children), Wyoming (25%), Alaska (23%), Idaho (22%), and Montana (22%) (Gates, 2013b).

Along with the rapid progress toward marriage equality in the United States, laws governing adoption for same-sex couples have also begun to change. The best resource for staying current with these changes is to consult an online source such as the Human Rights Campaign summary of changes in laws and policies, summarized in their "maps" that are updated frequently and that show what is happening in each state (http://tinyurl.com/y8fb9ofd).

The two major rights that are gradually opening up are the legal option of second-parent adoption, which grants a same sex partner of the biological or adoptive parent, equal parental rights and responsibilities; and laws that govern same-sex joint adoption. Now that same-sex marriage is legal nationwide in the United States, these laws will no longer be as concerning, but there will always be family relationships where marriage is not an option or not desired. For example, some LGBTQ people live in communal or poly relationships with three or more other adults, and often these households are raising children.

Without legal rights, parents may be denied custody, visitation, or decision-making privileges for their own child. Parenting discrimination can begin even before birth. Lesbian couples seeking coverage for fertility consultations and treatments that are necessary but expensive, are often delayed and discouraged by insurance rates that are tailored to heterosexual couples. In addition, lesbians may be denied fertility treatment altogether due to discrimination by the clinician. Gay men, bisexual, and transgender individuals may be denied outright in their applications to become foster parents or to adopt. Many states have passed religious freedom bills that allow healthcare providers and businesses to actively discriminate against people who are against their religious or moral beliefs.

Read This 5.1

Guadalupe Benitez, age 33, sought fertility treatments in San Diego in 1999 because she and her partner, Joanne Clark, wanted to have a family. She was denied artificial insemination because the doctor said it was against her religious beliefs to perform the procedure for a lesbian. Benitez sued the doctor and the clinic. Ms. Benitez went outside of her insurance plan to find a physician who would provide treatment and she subsequently gave birth to a son. Her case, hoping to set precedent for other LGBTQ people seeking to have children, was reviewed by the California Supreme Court, who ruled in favor of Benitez. Read the details of this case and the final ruling handed down in August, 2008, that made it clear that California's state law prohibiting discrimination must be followed (https://goo.gl/a1ymcC).

This case illustrates the importance of continuing to pursue nondiscrimination for LGTBQ individuals and families in all areas.

Most early studies about LGBTQ individuals and parenting were directed toward the physical and psychosocial outcomes for the children. More recent work has included the experiences of the parents themselves (Epstein, 2002; Ross, Steele, & Sapiro, 2005; Tasker, 2005). The Committee on Lesbian, Gay, and Bisexual Concerns, the Committee on Children, Youth and Families, and the Committee on Women in Psychology of the American Psychological Association conducted a comprehensive review of the published research about lesbian and gay parenting since the 1960s. The report concluded that "there is no evidence to suggest that lesbian women or gay men are unfit to be parents or that psychosocial development among children of lesbian women or gay men is compromised relative to that among the offspring of heterosexual parents" (American Psychological Association, 2005, p. 15).

LGBTQ parents are as diverse as heterosexual parents. They face many of the same challenges and have the same desires for themselves and their children. What is different, as we have seen in previous chapters, is that prejudice affects their lives and restricts many of their choices. For example, even becoming parents may be complicated (Baetens, Camus, & Devroey, 2003). Although all parents consider where and how to raise their children, LGBTQ parents must also consider the effects that stigma may have on play dates, preschool, and all of the years of schooling to follow. These parents may face additional worries about their children being bullied because of the sexual orientation of the parents (Clarke, Kitzinger, & Potter, 2004). Prejudice may result in negative outcomes whether from judges, legislators, professionals, or the public (Cooper & Cates, 2006). And, when there are multiple diversities as with ethnicity and economic circumstances, the situation can become even more complicated.

Even among individuals who believe that LGBTQ adults should be allowed the same civil rights as others, there are a subset who believe that LGBTQ people should not be allowed to be parents based on religious doctrine or other beliefs, such as it would be unfair to the children because they might be teased or harassed or that children need a male and a female parental role model. When those attitudes are present in the family of origin, the new LGBTQ parents may feel less support from their families, although in many cases, the family ties improve after the arrival of the child (Goldberg, Gartrell, & Gates, 2014).

In the court arguments that led to the U.S. Supreme Court decision making marriage legal for all same-sex couples, both sides have used arguments involving the welfare of children raised by LGBT parents. Most of the arguments that claimed that children are harmed by LGBT parents were based on religious beliefs, stereotypes, and myths. The arguments favoring marriage equality drew on strong research evidence that overwhelmingly indicates scientific consensus that being raised by LGBT parents does not harm children (Columbia Law School, 2015).

Child Outcomes

"My parents divorced when I was four, and my mom came out as a lesbian. When I was young I went through a lot of teasing. I changed schools, then changed again. At my school now, only a few people know and they're very supportive. My mom has taught me to love all types of people. Because of my mom, I'm not like everyone else I'm different and I love it. —Claire V. (15 yrs), Berkeley. (Wilson, 2007)

In addition to research about LGBTQ parents, there is some information from the children's perspective about what it is like to have lesbian or gay parents (Howey & Samuels, 2000; Perrin, 1998; Rafkin, 1990). Also, in the comprehensive review published by the American Psychological Association (2005) described above, there is a section about children of lesbian and gay parents. The authors focused on research about the children's sexual identity, social relationships, and other aspects of personal psychological development. Within sexual identity they included gender identity, gender role behavior, and sexual orientation. The development of gender identity among children of lesbian parents followed expected patterns with most children identifying as male or female, although there were no reported studies of gender identity formation for the children of gay fathers. There were no differences between children of lesbian and heterosexual parents on gender role behavior; again no studies about gay fathers were reported. In most studies the majority of children of both lesbian mothers and gay fathers described themselves as heterosexual. The authors reported that these children have "positive relationships with peers and that their relationships with adults of both sexes are also satisfactory" (American Psychological Association, 2005, p. 12). They concluded that there was no evidence to date to indicate that children of lesbian and gay parents are disadvantaged relative to children of heterosexual parents (p. 15). It is important to note that although studies about lesbian mothers and gay fathers have been conducted, they are relatively few and research about bisexual or transgendered parents has rarely been reported. One recent review (Stotzer, Herman, & Hasenbush, 2014) found 51 studies that concerned transgender parenting at least partly. They reported that children's gender identity and sexual orientation development do not seem to be affected, and most have good relationships with their transgender parents.

Most of the research has focused on lesbian mothers, probably because lesbians are more likely to be parents than gay men (Solomon et al., 2004). The National Lesbian Family Study (NLFS) started in 1986 with lesbians who enrolled during their insemination experiences or pregnancies, and they have been followed since (Gartrell et al., 2005). This is the largest prospective study of lesbian families in the literature, but must be viewed with some caution, because the participants are 93% White and highly educated, and because they all had children via donor insemination (that is, planned families). One report from this study summarizes the interviews done when the children were age 10. In general, the children were healthy and well-adjusted. They had comparable rates of developmental disorders (15%) such as learning and attention problems, as the general population of children (17%), but lower rates of sexual abuse experiences (5% of the girls, none of the boys), and none reported physical abuse. They were also comparable to children in the general population on the Child Behavior Checklist (CBCL), with one exception. Girls in lesbian families had fewer externalizing behavior problems than girls in the general population. The majority (85%) of the children were doing well academically, but 43% had experienced homophobic instances, mostly at school. Those who reported homophobia had slightly higher rates of behavior problems than those who did not experience homophobia. Many of the children, however, had been prepared for these incidents by their mothers and coped well with teasing or homophobic comments.

> *"One kid said one time that he didn't like gays and lesbians and I said, 'You mean like my mom?' and he said, 'I didn't know your mom was.' So I told him that if he had a friend and he was Black, would he stop being his friend and he said, 'No.' I told him it was the same thing."* (Gartrell et al., 2005, p. 522)

When the children were adolescents (age 17), they were surveyed again (Gartrell, Bos, Peyser, Deck, & Rodas, 2012) and were still doing well. They reported a mean grade point average of 3.56 and 90% expected to go to college. The vast majority (90%) were comfortable bringing friends home and 81% said most or all of their friends knew their mother was a lesbian. At this point, 13% identified somewhere on the LGB spectrum.

In another study (Bliss & Harris, 1999) teachers of children raised by lesbian and gay parents reported that the children had more problems with social interactions, but were more mature, tolerant, and self-confident than their peers from heterosexual parents. As one respondent said about school:

> *"Teachers don't allow kids to make negative comments about skin color or gender, but they don't stop them from saying negative things about gays."* (Gartrell et al., 2005, p. 522)

Divorce

The legal right to domestic partner status in states early to recognize same-sex unions, and now to marriage in all 50 states of the United States and in many other countries, brings with it the legal right to divorce. This may not seem like much of a benefit in some ways, but it provides legal protections that help to bring about equitable settlements related to property, children, and other economic issues. Since this legal status is very new, it is not yet clear if there are any unique factors for same-sex couples, compared to that of heterosexual couples. A 2014 report from the Williams Institute shows that at the time of the report, same-sex couples had an annual divorce rate of 1.1% compared to 2% for other-sex couples. Future research will provide a much better understanding of this important relationship dynamic (Badgett & Mallory, 2014).

LGBTQ Grandparenting

If 35% of LGBTQ people have children, the chances are high that they will live to become grandparents. LGBTQ people serve the same role in their grandchildren's lives of offering emotional, caregiving, and material support. In some research, not being out to grandchildren was a source of stress for lesbian and bisexual grandmothers (Orel & Fruhauf, 2006). Qualitative interviews with 11 gay grandfathers (Fruhauf, Orel, & Jenkins, 2009) showed that adult children were critical in the process of grandparents coming out to their grandchildren, and with that support of adult children, coming out to grandchildren was considerably easier than coming out to their children had been. Those who were partnered found it easier to come out, and some said that coming out was a

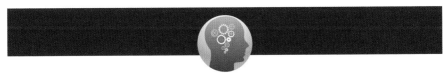

Think About It 5.3

One study (Gartrell et al., 2000) found that 17% of the grandparents of children with lesbian mothers had refused to recognize them as full-fledged grandchildren. In another study a gay grandfather is quoted as saying "The thing that hits me is that for grandchildren there's the great opportunity to grow up with it and have it become part of the fabric … but to stay hidden and not have that be part of the fabric of grandchildren's life denies them then the opportunity to get rid of one piece of intolerance and prejudice that is part of the culture" (Fruhauf et al., 2009, p. 110). Think about the implications of these different situations, and how these extended family dynamics influence the children involved.

way of educating their grandchildren about tolerance. In many cases, the adult children had informed the children of their grandparent's sexual orientation. In other cases, a grandparent does not come out to grandchildren to honor the wishes of the adult child (Orel & Fruhauf, 2006).

Health-Related Family Issues

There are three categories of legal concerns related to healthcare for same-sex parents with children: consent for medical procedures/treatment, involvement in sharing of information and decision-making, and visitation rights. These issues are discussed in Chapter 13. On top of the legal concerns are the issues we discuss elsewhere in this book concerning the potential for poor quality treatment or even refusals of treatment based on one's perceived sexuality or gender—or in this case, the parents' sexuality or gender. Here is one example of the type of challenges that LGBTQ families face in the healthcare system:

> "My partner and I were vacationing and my daughter became ill and had to be taken to the emergency room at a local hospital. Even though she was sitting in my lap, calling me mommy, and I had her insurance card, the professional staff all looked to my partner (who is not her biological mother) when they talked about my daughter. I look androgynous, and I believe it made them uncomfortable and unable to "see" me as her mother. It's not the first time it happened, and it probably won't be the last, but it still makes me angry." (DeJoseph, personal communication, 2007)

Conclusion

LGBTQ people come from families of origin that vary in how they respond to the person's disclosure of sexuality and gender, and they create their own families. Sometimes these new families are indistinguishable from the kinds of families created by heterosexual couples, and sometimes they differ. However, all families deserve support, respect, and validation in healthcare settings. If our society is truly committed to "traditional family values" then it must encourage laws and policies that support all families.

References

American Psychological Association. (2005). Lesbian and gay parenting. Retrieved June 27, 2015, from http://www.apa.org/pi/lgbt/resources/parenting-full.pdf

Badgett, M. V. L., & Mallory, C. (2014). Patterns of relationship recognition for same-sex couples: Divorce and terminations. Retrieved July 20, 2015, from http://williamsinstitute.law.ucla.edu/wp-content/uploads/Badgett-Mallory-Divorce-Terminations-Dec-2014.pdf

Baetens, P., Camus, M., & Devroey, P. (2003). Counseling lesbian couples: Requests for donor insemination on social grounds. *Reproductive Biomedicine Online, 6*, 75–83.

Beemyn, B. G., & Rankin, S. (2011). *The lives of transgender people.* New York: Columbia University Press.

Ben-Ari, A. (1995). The discovery that an offspring is gay: parents', gay men's, and lesbians' perspectives. *Journal of Homosexuality, 30*, 89–112.

Bigner, J. J. (1996). *Working with gay fathers: Developmental, postdivorce parenting, and therapeutic issues*. Jossey-Bass.

Bliss, G. K., & Harris, M. B. (1999). Teachers' views of students with gay or lesbian parents. *Journal of Gay, Lesiban, and Bisexual Identity, 4*, 149–171.

Clarke, V., Kitzinger, C., & Potter, J. (2004). "Kids are just cruel anyway": Lesbian and gay parents' talk about homophobic bullying. *British Journal of Social Psychology, 43*, 531–550.

Columbia Law School. (2015). What does the scholarly research say about the wellbeing of children with gay or lesbian parents? Retrieved June 27, 2015, from http://whatweknow. law.columbia.edu/topics/lgbt-equality/what-does-the-scholarly-research-say-about-the-wellbeing-of-children-with-gay-or-lesbian-parents/

Cooper, L., & Cates, P. (2006). *ACLU Lesbian and Gay Rights Project: Too high a price: The case against restricting gay parenting* (2nd ed.). New York: American Civil Liberties Union Foundation. Retrieved from https://www.aclu.org/lgbt-rights_hiv-aids/too-high-price-case-against-restricting-gay-parenting

D'Augelli, A. R., Hershberger, S. L., & Pilkington, N. W. (1998). Lesbian, gay, and bisexual youth and their families: Disclosure of sexual orientation and its consequences. *The American Journal of Orthopsychiatry, 68*, 361–371.

Epstein, R. (2002). Butches with babies: Reconfiguring gender and motherhood. *Journal of Lesbian Studies, 6*, 41–57.

Erhardt, V. (2006). *Head over heels: Wives who stay with cross-dressers and transsexuals*. New York: Routledge.

Friedman, M. S., Marshal, M. P., Stall, R., Cheong, J., & Wright, E. R. (2008). Gay-related development, early abuse and adult health outcomes among gay males. *AIDS and Behavior, 12*(6), 891–902. Retrieved from http://doi.org/10.1007/s10461–007–9319–3

Frost, D. M., & Eliason, M. J. (2014). Challenging the assumption of fusion in female same-sex relationships. *Psychology of Women Quarterly, 38*(1), 65–74. Retrieved from http://doi.org/10.1177/0361684313475877

Fruhauf, C. A., Orel, N. A., & Jenkins, D. A. (2009). The coming-out process of gay grandfathers: Perceptions of their adult children's influence. *Journal of GLBT Family Studies, 5*(1–2), 99–118. Retrieved from http://doi.org/10.1080/15504280802595402

Gartrell, N., Banks, A., Reed, N., Hamilton, J., Rodas, C., & Deck, A. (2000). The national lesbian family study: 3. Interviews with mothers of five-year-olds. *The American Journal of Orthopsychiatry, 70*(4), 542–548. Retrieved from http://www.ncbi.nlm.nih.gov/pubmed/11086532

Gartrell, N., Bos, H. M. W., Peyser, H., Deck, A., & Rodas, C. (2012). Adolescents with lesbian mothers describe their own lives. *Journal of Homosexuality, 59*(9), 1211–1229. Retrieved from http://doi.org/10.1080/00918369.2012.720499

Gartrell, N., Deck, A., Rodas, C., Peyser, H., & Banks, A. (2005). The national lesbian family study: 4. Interviews with the 10-year-old children. *The American Journal of Orthopsychiatry, 75*(4), 518–524. Retrieved from http://doi.org/10.1037/0002–9432.75.4.518

Gates, G. J. (2013a). LGBT parenting in the United States. eScholarship-UCLA: The Williams Institute. Retrieved from http://escholarship.org/uc/item/9xs6g8xx.pdf

Gates, G. J. (2013b). Same sex and different sex couples in the American Community Survey: 2005–2011. eScholarship-UCLA: The Williams Institute. Retrieved from http://escholarship.org/uc/item/8dk71277.pdf

Goldberg, A. E., Gartrell, N., & Gates, G. J. (2014). Research report on LGB-parent families. Retrieved June 26, 2015, from http://williamsinstitute.law.ucla.edu/research/parenting/lgb-parent-families-jul-2014/

Howey, N., & Samuels, E. (Eds.). (2000). *Out of the ordinary: Essays on growing up with gay, lesbian, and transgender parents*. New York: St Martins Press.

Kurdek, L. A. (2001). Differences between heterosexual-nonparent couples and gay, lesbian, and heterosexual-parent couples. *Journal of Family Issues*, *22*(6), 727–754. Retrieved from http://doi.org/10.1177/019251301022006004

Laird, J. (1993). Lesbian and gay families. In F. Walsh (Ed.), *Normal family processes: Growing diversity and complexity* (pp. 238–283). New York: Guilford Press.

LaSala, M. C. (2004). Extradyadic sex and gay male couples: Comparing monogamous and nonmonogamous relationships. *Families in Society: The Journal of Contemporary Social Services*, *85*(3), 405–412.

Lev, A. I. (2004). *Transgender emergence: Therapeutic guidelines for working with gender-variant people and their families*. New York: Haworth.

Lynch, J. M., & Murray, K. (2000). For the love of the children: The coming out process for lesbian and gay parents and stepparents. *Journal of Homosexuality*, *39*(1), 1–24. Retrieved from http://doi.org/10.1300/J082v39n01_01

Martos, A. J., Nezhad, S., & Meyer, I. H. (2014). Variations in sexual identity milestones among lesbians, gay men, and bisexuals. *Sexuality Research & Social Policy: Journal of NSRC: SR & SP*, *12*, 24–33. Retrieved from http://doi.org/10.1007/s13178-014-0167-4

Matthews, A. K., Tartaro, J., & Hughes, T. L. (2003). A comparative study of lesbian and heterosexual women in committed relationships. *Journal of Lesbian Studies*, *7*(1), 101–114. Retrieved from http://doi.org/10.1300/J155v07n01_07

McCullough, D., & Hall, D. S. (2003). Polyamory—What it is and what it isn't. *The Electronic Journal of Human Sexuality*, *6*. Retrieved from http://www.ejhs.org/volume6/polyamory.htm

McLean, K. (2004). Negotiating (Non) monogamy: Bisexuality and intimate relationships. In R. Fox (Ed.), *Current research on bisexuality* (pp. 83–98). New York: Haworth. Retrieved from http://doi.org/10.4324/9780203057117

Morris, J. F., Balsam, K. F., & Rothblum, E. D. (2002). Lesbian and bisexual mothers and nonmothers: Demographics and the coming-out process. *Journal of Family Psychology: JFP: Journal of the Division of Family Psychology of the American Psychological Association*, *16*(2), 144–156.

Operario, D., Burton, J., Underhill, K., & Sevelius, J. (2008). Men who have sex with transgender women: Challenges to category-based HIV prevention. *AIDS and Behavior*, *12*(1), 18–26. Retrieved from http://doi.org/10.1007/s10461-007-9303-y

Orel, N. A., & Fruhauf, C. A. (2006). Lesbian and bisexual grandmothers' perceptions of the grandparent-grandchild relationship. *Journal of GLBT Family Studies*, *2*(1), 43–70. Retrieved from http://doi.org/10.1300/J461v02n01_03

Parks, C. A., & Humphreys, N. A. (2006). Lesbian relationships and families. In D. F. Morrow & L. Messinger (Eds.), *Sexual orientation and gender expression in social work practice* (pp. 216–242). Columbia University Press.

Perrin, E. C. (1998). Children whose parents are lesbian or gay. *Contemporary Pediatrics*, *15*, 113–132.

Polat, A., Yuksel, S., Discigil, A. G., & Meteris, H. (2005). Family attitudes toward transgendered people in Turkey: Experience from a secular Islamic country. *International Journal of Psychiatry in Medicine*, *35*(4), 383–393.

Rafkin, L. (1990). *Different mothers: Sons and daughters of lesbians talk about their lives*. Pittsburgh, PA: Cleis Press.

Ross, L. E., Steele, L., & Sapiro, B. (2005). Perceptions of predisposing and protective factors for perinatal depression in same-sex parents. *Journal of Midwifery & Women's Health*, *50*(6), e65–e70. Retrieved from http://doi.org/10.1016/j.jmwh.2005.08.002

Rosser, B. R. S., Oakes, J. M., Bockting, W. O., & Miner, M. (2007). Capturing the social demographics of hidden sexual minorities: An Internet study of the transgender population in the United States. *Sexuality Research & Social Policy: Journal of NSRC: SR & SP*, *4*(2), 50–64.

Saulnier, C. F. (2002). Deciding who to see: Lesbians discuss their preferences in health and mental health care providers. *The Social Worker*, *47*(4), 355–365.

Savin-Williams, R. C. (1998). The disclosure to families of same-sex attractions by lesbian, gay, and bisexual youths. *Journal of Research on Adolescence: The Official Journal of the Society for Research on Adolescence, 8*(1), 49–68. Retrieved from http://doi.org/10.1207/s15327795jra0801_3

Savin-Williams, R. C., & Cohen, K. M. (2007). Development of same-sex attracted youth. In I. H. Meyer & M. E. Northridge (Eds.), *The health of sexual minorities: Public health perspectives on lesbian, gay, bisexual, and transgender populations* (pp. 27–47). New York: Springer. Retrieved from http://doi.org/10.1007/978–0–387–31334–4_2

Solomon, S. E., Rothblum, E. D., & Balsam, K. F. (2004). Pioneers in partnership: Lesbian and gay male couples in civil unions compared with those not in civil unions and married heterosexual siblings. *Journal of Family Psychology: JFP: Journal of the Division of Family Psychology of the American Psychological Association, 18*(2), 275–286. Retrieved from http://doi.org/10.1037/0893–3200.18.2.275

JCAHO Staff. (2004). *2005–2006 comprehensive accreditation manual for integrated delivery systems (CAMIDS)*. Joint Commission Resources. Retrieved from http://books.google.com/books/about/2005_2006_Comprehensive_Accreditation_Ma.html?hl &id P0SCVcq_bMwC

Starks, T. J., & Parsons, J. T. (2014). Adult attachment among partnered gay men: Patterns and associations with sexual relationship quality. *Archives of Sexual Behavior, 43*(1), 107–117. Retrieved from http://doi.org/10.1007/s10508–013–0224–8

Stotzer, R. L., Herman, J. L., & Hasenbush, A. (2014). Transgender parenting: A review of existing research. Retrieved June 26, 2015, from http://williamsinstitute.law.ucla.edu/research/parenting/transgender-parenting-oct-2014/

Tasker, F. (2005). Lesbian mothers, gay fathers, and their children: A review. *Journal of Developmental and Behavioral Pediatrics: JDBP, 26*(3), 224–240.

Van Wormer, K. S., Wells, J., & Boes, M. (2000). Social work with lesbians, gays, and bisexuals: A strengths perspective. Boston, MA: Allyn & Bacon.

Weinberg, M. S., Williams, C. J., & Pryor, D. W. (1994). *Dual attraction: Understanding bisexuality*. Oxford: Oxford University Press.

Weston, K. (1991). *Families we choose: Lesbians, gays, kinship*. New York: Columbia University Press.

White, T., & Ettner, R. (2007). Adaptation and adjustment in children of transsexual parents. *European Child & Adolescent Psychiatry, 16*(4), 215–221. Retrieved from http://doi.org/10.1007/s00787–006–0591-y

Wilson, B. D. (2007). Our families: Attributes of Bay Area lesbian, gay, bisexual, and transgender parents and their children. Retrieved July 27, 2015, from http://www.sccoe.org/depts/csh/CSH%20SB48%20Doc%20Library/BT%20Parents%20and%20Their%20Children.pdf

Wilson, P. A., & Yoshikawa, H. (2007). Improving access to health care among African-American, Asian and Pacific Islander, and Latino lesbian, gay, and bisexual populations. In I. H. Meyer & M. E. Northridge (Eds.), *The health of sexual minorities: Public health perspectives on lesbian, gay, bisexual, and transgender populations* (pp. 607–637). New York: Springer. Retrieved from http://doi.org/10.1007/978–0–387–31334–4_25

Chapter 6

Developmental Transitions

"I went through the labels … tomboy in childhood, dyke in my life after divorce from a man, butch in middle age, then trans as I become aware of it." (Respondent in Beemyn & Rankin, 2011, p. 109)

Most of the health-related research on LGBTQ individuals has focused on risk factors, such as victimization, HIV risk, suicide, substance abuse and mental health, and very little research has focused on "normal" developmental transitions, resilience, and whether or not there are unique differences in common experiences such as dating, negotiating relationships, or aging. Many human characteristics unfold in a predictable, linear manner, such as language development, motor skills, and cognitive development. Others, like social identities, are cyclical or nonlinear, more bound by social context, and influenced by overall developmental stage in the lifespan. Children, adolescents, young adults, midlife adults, and older adults have different priorities and varied experiences with life transitions, some established by our biology but most by our culture (Dunlap, 2014). In this chapter, we discuss what is currently reflected in the literature related to LGBTQ developmental transitions, and suggest important avenues that need to be explored further.

Table 6.1 summarizes some of the ways that having a minority sexual or gender identification might impact those common developmental transitions. These developmental issues are discussed in more detail below, but keep in mind that people come out at a wide variety of ages, from childhood to elder years. The age of coming out intersects with a person's general maturation level. Someone who is 30 when they come out has very different emotional, interpersonal, and material resources available to them than someone who is 12. A person who has been out for less than 1 year has more challenges related to their sexual and gender identities than a person who has been out for 10 years, regardless of their chronological age.

There is more research on LGBTQ youth (adolescents and young adults) than any other age group, but much of it does not address other forms of diversity, such as racial/ethnic identity. Social identities always intersect in unique ways for individual development, so we are still limited in our ability to say definitively how sexual orientation or gender identity impacts human development. We are all the product of multiple, unique differences ranging from genetic factors and biological bodies to family histories, life experiences, cultural influences, and relationships. We also have unique combinations of social identities that affect how others treat us.

	Table 6.1 – Developmental Milestones and LGBTQ Identities/Stigma	
Stage	**Milestones/ Characteristics**	**Possible Effects of LGBTQ Identity**
Childhood	Concrete thinkers Families are strong influence Development of peer relationships Learning about power dynamics through bullying School (Industry)	May be deeply impacted by stereotypes, which may be considered "the truth." Fear family rejection. Avoid close peer relationships for fear of others finding out. May be bullied/teased (especially gender nonconforming youth). Preoccupation with sex/gender may affect ability to concentrate in school. May lack language to describe their difference.
Adolescence	Moving into abstract thought Conformity/fitting in Identity exploration Experimenting with sexuality and/or gender Homophobia as part of masculine socialization Still dependent on families Experimenting with ATOD use	Starting to recognize oppression, social justice issues. Some desperately want to fit in (act heterosexual/gender normative); others rebel. May experiment with sexuality and gender expression without accurate information on risks. Greatest risks of victimization from family and male peers.
Young adulthood	Independence from family of origin Developing intimate relationships Starting families Exploring and settling into careers	Freer to live an open life. Serious dating, relationships impacted by lack of validation of same-sex relationships. Difficulty finding others with high self-acceptance for good relationships. Deciding if/how/when to have children. Career choices might be impacted—finding careers that are more accepting of LGBTQ people (often lower paying).
Middle adulthood	Stability Generativity/mentoring Midlife crisis/transitions Spirituality	Maintaining relationships and family of choice in the face of societal pressures. For those without children, finding other ways to leave a legacy for the next generation. Worrying about the future. Deepening spirituality may require seeking alternative practices/communities and/or reconciling sexuality and religion.
Older adulthood	Integrity Wish to remain independent Desire for good health Facing mortality Wisdom	Current LGBTQ elders are less likely to be out than younger generations because they grew up in a more hostile climate. More likely to be single than heterosexual elders—fear of becoming dependent on strangers for care. Minority stress has increased the risk of physical and mental health disorders that accumulate over the years into serious chronic illnesses. Youth-oriented gay male culture may not be inclusive of elders and miss out on their wisdom; lesbian/bisexual women's culture less so, but lack of opportunities to share the wisdom.

LGBTQ Childhood

The developmental tasks of childhood include achieving autonomy, developing peer relationships, and achieving success in social and cognitive tasks at school and elsewhere. In the past, there was a common belief that sexual orientation did not emerge until adolescence with the onset of puberty, but this is just not true for either LGBTQ or heterosexual youth. Until recently, children did not have access to information that would allow them to label their feelings. As children are exposed more to communication technologies, particularly the internet, and as media portrayals of LGBTQ people proliferate, they are able to adopt labels for their perceived differences earlier than ever before. The age of first coming out has declined over the past 20 years, primarily because of this greater exposure to LGBTQ people in our culture, not because more children are LGBTQ than in previous generations.

How does coming out prior to puberty affect the achievement of developmental milestones of an individual? We know very little about this, but can speculate that the individual might meet great resistance from family, teachers, and peers because of a widespread belief that sexual identities develop at puberty or later. Many children are told that someone so young could not possibly know if they are LGBTQ. Yet, if you ask LGBTQ people when they first were aware of their sexual or gender difference, many will tell you that they knew before puberty. One longitudinal study found that three-fourths of LGB individuals reported feeling different as children, at an average age of 8 (D'Augelli & Grossman, 2001). Another study found an average age of coming out to self at about 10. Figure 6.1 shows coming out milestones for 224 respondents who were young adults when they completed a survey (Ryan, Huebner, Diaz, & Sanchez, 2009). These data show that although an awareness of same-sex attraction began in childhood, the individual typically did not begin to label it or reveal it to others until adolescence, contributing to the myth that sexual orientation emerges in adolescence.

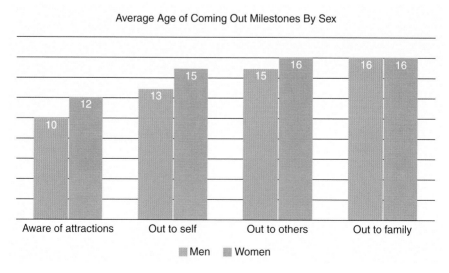

Average Age of Coming Out Milestones By Sex

■ Men   ■ Women

Figure 6.1 – Sexual Identity Milestones by Gender in LGB Youth (Based on **Ryan et al., 2009**).

People who identify as transgender later in life often report similar ages of being aware of their difference (Pazos, 1999). Younger children who are aware of their differences from others may feel that they have no one to talk to, and may fear parental and peer rejection or resistance. We can only speculate about their experiences, because human subjects review panels and funding agencies are very sensitive about research that asks young children about issues related to sexuality, so we have very little empirical data on this age group. We have to rely on retrospective memories of youth or adults. Beemyn and Rankin (2011) found that people who reported a transgender or gender nonconforming identity as adults were likely to have felt different from childhood, with 83% saying they were aware of their difference before the age of 18. Some never felt identified with the sex assigned to them at birth.

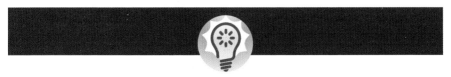

Imagine This 6.1

Imagine yourself as a child who feels different. You have a male body, but are not interested in typical boy activities like sports, war games, or playing with trucks and cars. Instead, you like music, dancing, and playing house with your sister. At school, you are harassed by bullies who call you "sissy," and "fag." At home, your father disapproves of you playing with your sister, and sometimes punishes you by sending you to your room. As you move into your adolescent years, your mother tries to arrange dates for you through her church network. She and your father bring you to a minister who talks to you about your "manly responsibilities." School is becoming an increasingly hostile place for you as the bullies now do more than taunt you. You have experienced physical attacks twice this year. You form a close friendship with a girl who encourages you to join the Gay Straight Alliance (GSA) with her. Instead of giving up, you resolve that you will survive school and throw yourself into your studies hoping to get a scholarship for college to get you out of your neighborhood. At 17, you fall in love for the first time. It feels glorious, but the only people you can tell are the members of the GSA because your parents and other family members, the minister, and most of your peers at school would be appalled. You long for the escape to college where you can start living an authentic, open life.

LGBTQ Adolescence

Developmental tasks of adolescence often include identity exploration, dating and first sexual experiences, individuating from parents, and dealing with the strong influence of peers on behavior and attitudes. Some think that a degree of risk-taking is a normal part of adolescent development, such as experimenting with sex, drugs, and alcohol. Much of the research about LGBTQ youth is focused on how their sexual orientation or gender identity is related to unhealthy choices such as tobacco use, unsafe sexual behaviors, mental health disorders, or suicide (Birkett, Newcomb, & Mustanski, 2015; Remafedi, 2007; Spirito & Esposito-Smythers, 2006). LBGTQ adolescents also face the potential for violence from others because of their sexual orientation, gender identity, or gender expression. One frequently cited example is the Matthew Shepard case. Matthew Shepard, a 21-year-old college student, was murdered in an anti-gay hate crime in Laramie Wyoming in October of 1998. His death raised awareness of LGBTQ issues on an international scale. Transgender youth are also vulnerable to violence and disruption of their physical and mental health (Mallon & DeCrescenzo, 2006). In one study of transgender youth from age 15 to 21, participants noted that there were four major problems in health-related areas, including lack of safe environments, poor access to physical health services, inadequate resources to address their mental health concerns, and a lack of continuity of caregiving by their families and communities (Grossman & D'Augelli, 2006). Whereas violence is at one end of the anti-LGBTQ continuum, bullying and harassment are nearly everyday events for most youth. Experiencing bullying and homophobic/biphobic/transphobic remarks at school have been linked to higher rates of suicidal ideation (Rivers, 2004) and poorer school achievement (Kosciw, Greytak, Palmer, & Boesen, 2014).

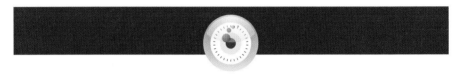

Watch This 6.1

Watch the powerful documentary, "Valentine Road," that traces the murder of Lawrence King, a mixed-race transgender youth shot to death at school by a fellow student, Brandon. The documentary shows the intersections of race, class, sexuality, and gender and also shows the chilling comments of teachers and jurors who sided with Brandon because of Larry's "flamboyant" nature. You can watch the trailer on YouTube here: **https://goo. gl/rndYQ1**. The full-length documentary is available for streaming through HBO (**http:// www.hbo.com/documentaries/valentine-road**); the DVD is available for purchase through Amazon.com

There is some information about the protective factors and resilience of LGBTQ adolescents (Eisenberg & Resnick, 2006; Poteat, Scheer, Marx, Calzo, & Yoshikawa, 2015; Sanders & Kroll, 2000), particularly related to having social support from parents and school. Perhaps the most encouraging factor is that the broad range of issues of LGBTQ youth are now being studied, including the structural issues that are created by stigma to create hostile environments at home and school. For example, family acceptance versus rejection has been studied in terms of health outcomes of LGBT youth. Instead of focusing on the youth who comes out, the emphasis is on how families react. When families show rejecting behaviors, the odds of suicide ideation (Odds ratio of 5.6 compared to accepting parents), suicide attempts (8.4), depression (6.0), illicit drug use (3.3), and unprotected sex (3.4) are much higher than for families with accepting behaviors (Ryan et al., 2009). In terms of school, several studies report that the presence of gay-straight alliances (GSAs) and policies that protect LGBT youth result in better health and well-being outcomes for sexual minority youth (Hatzenbuehler, Keyes, Hamilton, & Hasin, 2014; Poteat, Sinclair, DiGiovanni, Koenig, & Russell, 2013).

In the latest school climate study conducted by the Gay, Lesbian, Straight Education Network (GLSEN), nearly 8,000 youth of ages 13 to 21 were surveyed, finding that 56% felt unsafe at school because of their sexual orientation, and 38% because of their gender expression. This fear led to missing school, avoiding gender-segregated spaces (like bathrooms and locker rooms), and avoiding school functions and extracurricular activities because of safety concerns (Kosciw, Greytak, Palmer, & Boesen, 2014). In terms of harassment, 74% had been verbally harassed, 36% physically harassed, 17% physically assaulted, and 49% cyberbullied, but of those who reported an incident, 62% said nothing was done about it. Most schools still have LGBTQ-discriminatory policies and practices (56%) and 42% of transgender students had been prevented from using their preferred name. Students who were harassed often had a lower grade point average than those with less harassment and were less likely to report wanting to go to college. Those who experienced discrimination were more likely to be depressed and have lower self-esteem. Only half of the students reported having a GSA in their school, but those with a GSA felt safer, heard fewer negative comments, felt more connected to their schools, and were more likely to report that school personnel intervened when hearing homophobic remarks. Very few schools had any content on LGBTQ issues in the school curriculum (only 19% of students were taught any positive representations of LGBT people or issues and 15% had been taught negative content). School policies are slowly changing, and more schools now have anti-bullying policies (82%), but only 10% said that the policy covered both sexual orientation and gender identity/expression. GLSEN has been conducted these surveys for over 10 years, and comparing across the years, the 2013 results showed a slow, but steady improvement in nearly all categories, although there is much more work to be done to make middle and high schools safer for LGBTQ students.

One sign that we are beyond a mere focus on risk factors is that there is a growing body of research on dating experiences of LGBTQ youth. According to stereotypes, LGBTQ youth are isolated and afraid to come out, and if they do, face victimization in their schools, families, and communities. Do LGBTQ youth, then, miss out on dating, a developmental milestone that allows youth to rehearse intimate relationships and explore their gender, sexuality, and communication skills? Diamond (2002) found that most young lesbian and bisexual women (like their heterosexual peers) have intense, passionate same-sex friendships in adolescence, and most of these are nonsexual. When they do become sexual relationships, they provide a catalyst for exploring sexual identity labels. Diamond noted that many women reported having an intense same-sex relationship in youth that is never repeated, and therefore, does not affect the sexual identity label of the person in adulthood (Diamond, 2002). These intense emotional relationships may play the same role as dating in rehearsing communication, emotional intimacy, and physical affection for those who later adopt a lesbian or bisexual identity. Elze (2002) studied 112 lesbian and bisexual female youth aged 13 to 18 from New England, and found that contrary to stereotypes, most of them do date. Lesbian and bisexual women sometimes met their partners at sexual minority youth meetings (22%), but more typically found those partners at the same venues as heterosexual youth—at school (24%), through friends (13%), and at events or recreational settings (27%). Some of the risks that Elze identified were the intensity of breakups: about one-fourth of those who had experienced a breakup in the past 6 months reported that they felt suicidal in response to the breakup. In addition, about 44% of bisexual women's relationships and 25% of lesbian relationships had involved physical or verbal abuse, suggesting that LGBTQ youth as much as heterosexual youth, need education about healthy relationships to guard against intimate partner violence. Finally, one study examined the characteristics of adolescent same-sex couples, finding that they faced challenges in addressing sexual risk and protective factors, communication, finding role models and social support, and dealing with family and relationship violence (Greene, Fisher, Kuper, Andrews, & Mustanski, 2015).

Ritch Savin-Williams (2005) noted that youth are "increasingly redefining, reinterpreting, and renegotiating their sexuality such that possessing a gay, lesbian, or bisexual identity is practically meaningless" (p. 1). In fact, youth are constantly creating a whole new language to refer to gender and sexuality: gayish, metrosexual, boidyke, polygendered, onmisexual, queerboi, genderqueer, and a host of other creative labels. Some do continue to use labels such as LGBT or Q, so those who work with youth must stay open to a wide and shifting continuum of labels, refusals to use labels, and new combinations of sexual attractions and gender expressions.

LGBTQ Young Adulthood

The developmental transitions of young adulthood focus on the establishment of careers and worklife, and the development of intimate relationships and families. Research literature about LGBTQ adults has addressed some of the same issues as the research conducted among heterosexual adults. One issue is related to parenting (see Chapter 5), and another to specific disease states such as breast cancer or HIV (see Chapter 10). However, some of the research is associated specifically with being LGBTQ: for example, dealing with heterosexism (Burn, Kadlec, & Rexer, 2005) and the processes of coming out (D'Augelli, 2006a, 2006b; Floyd & Bakeman, 2006). There is also a growing body of research about multiple and intersecting identities among LGBTQ individuals, such as culture and ethnicity with sexual orientation (Balsam, Huang, Fieland, Simoni, & Walters, 2004; Cochran, Mays, Alegria, Ortega, & Takeuchi, 2007; Guarnero, 2007; Parks, Hughes, & Matthews, 2004). Chapter 7 provides more detail on the intersections of oppression among LGBTQ people.

Other investigators have noted the effect that an individual's level of being "out" has on health (Huebner & Davis, 2005; Koh & Ross, 2006; Ragins, Singh, & Cornwell, 2007). About two-thirds of LGB adults report that they had come out to parents by the age of 24, and two-thirds of those reported a positive response and adequate emotional and social support. For women, those who did not disclose to parents had greater illicit drug use, were more likely to be in fair or poor health, and more were depressed than those who did come out to parents. Those who came out to unsupportive parents also had higher rates of depression and drug use than those who came out to accepting parents. For men, there were no adverse effects associated with nondisclosure, but those who came out to unsupportive parents had higher levels of current binge drinking and depression (Rothman, Sullivan, Keyes, & Boehmer, 2012). It appears that parents continue to exert considerable influence on individuals even in adulthood.

Some research about LGBTQ adults focuses on the experiences of violence, whether from anti-gay hate bias (Russell & Richards, 2003), the long-term effects of bullying during adolescence (Rivers, 2004), or violence within intimate partner relationships (Bornstein, Fawcett, Sullivan, Senturia, & Shiu-Thornton, 2006; Ristock, 2003).

There are some encouraging trends in recent research about LGBTQ adults. The first is recognition about the relationship and family similarities between LGBTQ and heterosexual individuals (Kurdek, 2004; Means-Christensen, Snyder, & Negy, 2003). Another trend is a decrease in the number of studies that consider sexual orientation or gender identity as the reason for all physical, mental, emotional, and social difficulties experienced by LGBTQ people (the "blame the victim" approach). Instead, there is a deepening understanding that minority stress may offer a conceptual framework for understanding mental health issues and other health-related experiences among LGBTQ adults (Durso & Meyer, 2013; Meyer, 2003). Population sampling techniques are also being employed to place the experiences of LGBTQ individuals in the same nonclinical groups as heterosexuals (Bradford & McKay, 2004; Case et al., 2004; Cochran & Mays, 2007). Another trend is a consideration of the amazing resilience of many LGBTQ individuals (Bowleg, Craig, & Burkholder, 2004; Kwon, 2013; Oswald, 2002).

Developmental transitions for young adulthood include career development and relationships and family. We addressed relationship and family issues in Chapter 5, so will focus on career here. It appears that being LGBTQ influences both academic and career choices. In one study, 45% of college students thought that their sexual orientation/gender identity had a positive effect on their career choices, but 12% thought it had a negative impact, and 18% felt it narrowed their career options. Gay men and transgender students were more likely to report negative influences, and lesbians to suggest that their sexuality opened up new possibilities (Schneider & Dimito, 2010).

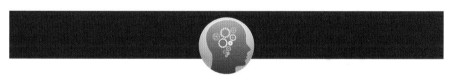

Think About It 6.1

Trevor Halley, lesbian and former navy nurse, founded the top-rated Castro Walking Tours in San Francisco in 1989. On her tours, she provided visitors with a fascinating account of how the Castro district became a "gay" neighborhood—a fact that she attributed in part to both the Gold Rush, and the opening of the Panama Canal, both of which brought large numbers of traveling men (cowboys, explorers, and navy men) to the area. Although the gender-segregated occupations of these groups landing on the west coast gave rise female sex workers and entertainers who catered to the men, Trevor maintained that for many, the choice of leaving home to travel with a group of same-sex comrades attracted many who preferred to occupy their time with others of the same sex. She told of a group of "Lavender Cowboys," and shared her own experience of choosing the navy as her career, not only because as a nurse she worked mostly with other women, but because of the attraction of putting on a uniform, being independent, and perhaps even driving a big truck. She made some of these comments in jest playing with lesbian stereotypes, but also as a way of emphasizing how, for many LGBTQ people, career choice is influenced by sexual and gender identity. Trevor retired in 2005, but Kathy Amendola continues to offer these fascinating tours. For more information, see **http://www.cruisinthecastro.com/about_us.html**

Think about the factors that influenced your own choice of career, and the extent to which your sexual and gender identities entered into this choice.

How do LGBTQ adults decide whether or not to be out at work? Being out at work can increase the potential for harassment and verbal and physical threats (Bradford, Ryan, & Rothblum, 1994; Herek, 1995), and for job loss (Badgett & Williams, 1992). Some researchers have noted that hiding one's sexuality is draining and results in lost work productivity and decreased job satisfaction (Boatwright, Gilbert, Forrest, & Ketzenberger, 1996). Rostosky and Riggle (2002), in a study of lesbian and gay adults, found that being out was related to an individual's level of self acceptance (interpreted as having low levels of internalized homophobia), having a nondiscrimination policy at work, and having a partner who also worked in a setting with a nondiscrimination policy. Figure 6.2 shows the experiences that some LGBT people have on the job, as reported by the Human Rights Campaign (2014). How difficult is it to focus on one's job and career development in the face of anti-LGBT jokes and uncomfortable coworkers? LGBTQ employees generally report higher work-related stress than heterosexual people because of the potential stigma from bosses and coworkers, and lack of institutional support such as health insurance and sick leave policies.

Transgender individuals may have more difficulty with obtaining and keeping "legitimate" employment than nearly any group of people. Xavier, Honnold, and Bradford (2007) reported that many transgender Virginians reported being denied a job (21% of MTF and 18% of FTM) or being fired from a job (15% of MTF and 9% of FTM) because of their gender expression. Many male-to-female transgender people, especially those with less education and who come from racial/ethnic minority groups, end up in sex work to survive (Nemoto, Operario, Keatley, Han, & Soma, 2004; Reback, Simon, Bemis, & Gatson, 2001). A survey of over 6,400 transgender and gender nonconforming individuals in 2011 showed staggering rates of employment discrimination: double the rate of unemployment compared to the general population; 90% of those who were employed had experienced harassment, mistreatment, or discrimination on the job; 47% had been fired, not

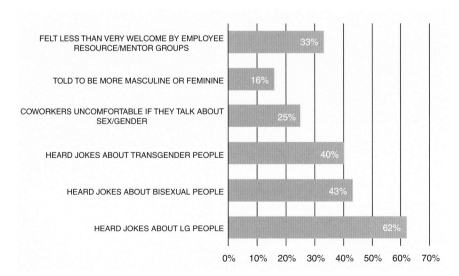

Figure 6.2 – Employment Issues for LGBT People (Based on Human Rights Campaign, 2014).

hired, or denied a promotion because of their gender identity; and 16% had been forced into sex work or selling drugs to survive (Grant et al., 2010).

LGBTQ Midlife

Discussions of midlife transitions in the general population often focus on menopause and "empty nest" syndrome for women, and career and goal aspirations and "midlife crisis" for men. It is sometimes described as a time of reflection on earlier life, of deepening spirituality, and of "generativity." How does having a minority sexual or gender identification impact the midlife phase of life?

Starting with women, menopause may have different meanings for lesbian, bisexual, and transgender women. There may be less concern about the physical appearance changes of aging among those in same-sex relationships, as in general, lesbian, and bisexual women's communities do not place as much emphasis on youth as other groups. Bisexual and transgender women who are in relationships with men or dating men may experience pressures more like heterosexual women experience. LBT women without children do not experience empty nest syndrome, whereas those with children may experience the launching of the children in similar ways to heterosexual women. One difference might be related to the co-parent, who is often not acknowledged as having a parental role, and thus may not receive any validation or recognition of the difficulties she experiences when the children leave home. Another potential difference is the experience of menopause for those with same-sex partners. Jennifer Kelly (2005) interviewed 20 lesbians about menopause experiences. One respondent summed up views of many in the study that another woman is likely to be able to relate to menopause transitions better than men:

> *"I think that the lesbian community would provide the atmosphere for sharing about menopause that heterosexual women may not have. Having a woman partner and lesbian friends makes it so normal to talk about it, and not only talk about it, but understand from a woman's point of view. I can't imagine a heterosexual woman in menopause would get the same support and understanding from a male partner."* (p. 168)

Another respondent noted that menopause might actually be a positive experience for many lesbians:

> *"For lesbians who are childless, being past childbearing is no consequence. Losing your attractiveness to males isn't within our reality, and menopause—a sign of getting older—does not bring the same fears as hets [heterosexuals] would feel. As a feminist lesbian the experience is a positive one."* (p. 171)

Some respondents noted that the deepened reflection and scrutinizing of one's life prompted by menopause may result in coming out. A woman who came out while in menopause talked of her experience of letting go of the expectations of others and learning to focus on her own needs and desires (Kelly, 2005, p. 181). Coming out at 50 may be a very different experience from coming out at 16 or 25 or even 40.

Gay, bisexual, and trans men are less likely than heterosexual men or women of any sexuality to have children, so career and aging concerns may be greater than family concerns. "Gay male culture" tends to be more youth and beauty-oriented than lesbian/bisexual women's culture, so GBT men may have more difficulty adapting to the changes of aging than lesbian/bisexual women. One study found that midlife gay men reported more concern with a perceived change in their bodily appearance as they aged, than did heterosexual men (Lodge & Umberson, 2013). As Kooden and Flowers (2000) noted, "Gay men are deeply invested in their bodies, and many feel that their body is their best asset—not only for sex, but for feelings of attractiveness, power, and success" (p. 28). This focus on the body can result in significant loss of self-esteem during midlife, but can be balanced by focusing on cultivating emotional intimacy and de-emphasizing the purely physical aspects of sexuality. Recent studies are showing that having a domestic partner or legal marriage for gay/bisexual men is a protective factor against stress and depression (Wight, Leblanc, & Badgett, 2013).

Career concerns and evaluating whether one has achieved their goals in life are common themes for midlife heterosexual men, and are likely experienced by GBT men as well. If workplaces have been hostile or not accepting, career satisfaction may be lower (Drydakis, 2012; Velez, Moradi, & Brewster, 2013), and if oppression has affected one's ability to achieve life goals, there may be a greater experience of a midlife "crisis." One interesting study examined the intersections of sexual identity and race in employment. Pedulla (2014) showed that gay male stereotypes related to perceptions of weakness and being effeminate counteracted Black male stereotypes of aggression and criminality, resulting in gay Black men being rated more highly as job applicants than straight Black men or White gay men. How people are perceived in the workplace is a complicated issue.

Very little is known about midlife experiences of bisexuals, as they are subsumed under the category of lesbian or gay if in same-sex relationships and heterosexual if in other-sex relationships. Weinberg, Williams, and Pryor (2001) followed a group of bisexual individuals over 20 years, and at midlife they found that about half reported being sexually active with only one gender of partner: 1/3 were exclusively heterosexual and 1/5 exclusively with same-sex partners, but the majority were firm in their bisexual identities—that is, the type of relationship did not affect their individual sense of sexual identification as bisexual. For some, the stresses of biphobia that come from both heterosexual and lesbian and gay communities might continue to affect their health and well-being into midlife (Grossman, D'Augelli, & Hershberger, 2000).

For transgender individuals, midlife may be the time of transition or discovery/ adoption of a transgender identity, or it may be a later stage in the process. Xavier, Honnold, & Bradford (2007) reported that 33% of MTF and 16% of FTMs began their transition after the age of 40. Ironically, women assigned female at birth can easily get hormones in midlife if they wish to treat menopause symptoms, but a transgender woman must get a letter from a mental health provider confirming that she is "sane" before she can receive the same hormones at the same doses as a perimenopausal person assigned female at birth. Cook-Daniels (2006) outlined five potential concerns of transgender individuals as they move from midlife to older adulthood:

1. Chronic health problems: The onset of heart disease, diabetes, and other chronic illnesses may affect gender-related treatments such as hormonal therapies and surgeries.
2. Entrenched social roles: the older we get, the greater the chance that we find it difficult to make changes in our social roles (such as relationships with

partners, spouses, and family members) and our behaviors (speech patterns, physical mannerisms), therefore, an older transgender person may not learn to "pass" as the other sex as well as a younger person.

3. Dating: the combined stigmas of transphobia and ageism may severely limit dating opportunities, and the trans person often must learn dating patterns of the other sex.

4. Legal concerns: changing one's sex on legal documents can be costly and time-consuming. As a person ages, it is imperative to make sure that documents such as social security records, VA records, hospital and clinic reports, and pensions are accurate and up-to-date so that health care is not delayed.

5. Employment (see the previous section).

For all individuals at midlife, one major milestone is the development of generativity, the feeling that one has left a legacy that will live on after them. For some LGBTQ people, generativity can be achieved through parenting, whereas others address this need through mentoring, teaching, cultural production (novels, plays, art work, nonfiction work, research), and/or community activism. Midlife is often a time of giving back to one's community. Some LGBTQ people at midlife may want to work with youth, to share their wisdom about coming out and living a life of integrity in a hostile world, but may hesitate because of the stereotypes about LGBTQ people, especially gay men, as sexual predators or trying to "recruit" young people. Sadly, many LGBTQ people who could be powerful mentors and role models are unable to satisfy generativity needs because of the stereotypes.

Finally, another common change in midlife is a greater seeking of spirituality. As an individual processes issues of mortality, there is a need to make sense of the world and have hope for the future. Among many LGBTQ people, the AIDS epidemic heightened awareness of mortality even in younger people. A section in the next chapter addresses spirituality and religion.

LGBTQ Elders

> *"As strong as I am today ... when I'm at the gate of the nursing home, the closet door is going to slam shut behind me." (Fred Riley, age 75, gay male quoted in the New York Times)* (Gross, 2007)

Developmental transitions of older adulthood are related to dealing with losses and accepting one's own mortality. In the last two decades in the United States the number of people over the age of 65 has been increasing twice as fast as the rest of the population. It also means that there are now more LGBTQ individuals over the age of 65 than there have ever been. How do stereotypes about aging and about LGBTQ people intersect to affect the lives of LGBTQ elders? Adjustment to aging is heavily influenced by the sociocultural context in which the person came out, and for many LGBTQ elders, this was the period prior to the gay liberation movement. The experiences of much greater societal stigma and need for secrecy may deeply affect LGBTQ elders today, but as the current baby boomer generation ages into maturity, they will be more open and out about their identities than the current generation (Wierzalis, Barret, Pope, & Rankins, 2006). The percentage of same-sex couples in the over age 65 population in the United States increased from 4.9% in 2005 to over 6% in 2011 (Gates, 2013).

Some researchers are concerned about what the accumulated lifetime of stigma and stress might to do the health of LGBTQ elders. Stigma throughout one's lifetime may limit employment opportunities, leaving LGBTQ people with fewer resources for old age. Poverty is one of the major predictors of poor health at any age, and several studies find more LGBTQ people living in poverty than heterosexual people at any age (summarized in Center for American Progress & Movement Advancement Project, 2015). One study examined population-based data from Washington state (Fredriksen-Goldsen, Kim, Barkan, Muraco, & Hoy-Ellis, 2013). LGB elders over 50 had higher rates of disability, mental health disorders, smoking and drinking, than did age-matched heterosexuals. These health problems are all confounded with poverty.

LGBTQ elders have many of the same issues related to aging that other elders have (Brotman, Ryan, & Cormier, 2003; Claes & Moore, 2000; Fox, 2007; McMahon, 2003). They have concerns about their present and their future. They are worried about their physical and mental health, their safety, their families of origin and/or choice, loneliness, and perhaps most of all, their economic security. Unlike heterosexual elders, stigma and prejudice may affect many of their decisions. They may have additional concerns about where they will live, since many retirement communities will not allow a same-sex couple to live together in the same unit. LGBTQ elders may also face ostracism from others living in those centers (Johnson, Jackson, Arnette, & Koffman, 2005) and/or the staff in these centers who have little or no training about LGBTQ elders. Advance care planning and end of life care may be more complicated for them than for heterosexuals (Stein & Bonuck, 2001). Elders face what every LGBTQ individual faces daily about coming out and its consequences. It may be even more difficult for elders since their choices may be decreased, or coming out may place them in a highly vulnerable or even dangerous situation. However, it would be incorrect to ignore the vibrant contributions many LGBTQ elders make daily to their families and communities. Many LGBTQ elders have lived through times that young people today cannot imagine. Those life experiences need to be shared so we do not lose this history. LGBTQ historical associations, archives, and story projects are vital in capturing these experiences.

> *"Whenever I looked for employment, though I was willing and eager, people did not usually want to employ 'someone like me.' Because the jobs that I could get were usually at gay bars, working as a bartender 'off the books' I have nothing in my social security account, which means that when I turn 65 I will have no financial security. As a result of the discrimination that I have experienced, I have often had to depend on public assistance like welfare to survive." (Tina Donovan, 61 year old transgender woman)* (Donovan, 2001, p. 20)

Because so many LGBTQ people have had to fight gender stereotypes all of their lives, they often highly value independence—many have learned to cook, clean, change the oil in the car, and fix the toilet as they are more free of gender stereotypes that drive the division of labor in many heterosexual couples. Therefore, any loss of independence may be felt even more keenly by LGBTQ elders than heterosexual people who adhered more to gender stereotypes. Disability may be considered even more negatively by LGBTQ seniors as a result (O'Toole, 2000). This overvaluing of independence may serve as a barrier in inclusion of people with disabilities into LGBTQ communities, and may interfere with seeking help for those who need it, but feel it is a threat to their independence to ask for assistance.

Chapter 10 deals with some of the chronic health problems that are reported at higher rates among LGBTQ people; most of these are age-related as well. Most of the population-based studies have not had sufficiently large samples to examine the rates of illness by age group, but as in the general population, the rate of chronic illness increases with age. One study (Grossman, D'Augelli, & O'Connell, 2001) specifically examined the health and well-being of LGB elders (people ranging from 60 to 91 with a mean age of 68.5). The authors reported that although half of the sample reported that they were in a current relationship, many of the couples did not live together. Two-thirds lived alone. Factors associated with greater physical health problems included living alone, having less income, having more experiences of victimization in their lifetimes, and having a more limited social network. Factors associated with greater mental health problems included living alone, less income, and lifetime victimization experiences. Mental health disorders were also associated with greater suicide ideation, lower self-esteem, loneliness, alcohol and drug problems, and more negative views of their own sexuality. It is important to note, however, that living alone is not always associated with loneliness. Many LGBTQ elders may have significant others and rich social support networks, but choose to live alone (Appelbaum, 2007), so assessments should address perceptions of loneliness, not just living status.

Retirement is one of the transitions that many older adults will face, if they are lucky enough to be financially stable. A recent Prudential poll asked adults ages 25 to 68, "Are you prepared for retirement?" Of the heterosexual respondents, 29% were ready, but of LGBT, only 14%. Financially, heterosexuals had on average $88,000 saved for retirement, compared to $66,000 saved by LGBT respondents (Prudential, 2012). Similarly, a poll conducted on behalf of SAGE found that 51% of LGBT adults age 45 and older are concerned about having enough money to live on, compared to 36% of heterosexual people, but less likely to use a financial planner to make decisions (28% of LGBT and 37% of heterosexual) (Espinoza, 2014). HIV/AIDS decimated the savings of many gay/bisexual men diagnosed in the 1970s and 80s. Many spent what

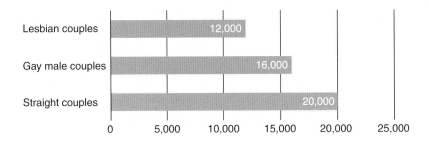

Figure 6.3 – Social Security Income of Same-Sex and Other Sex Couples Over 65 (Based on Data From the Williams Institute [**Gates, 2013**]).

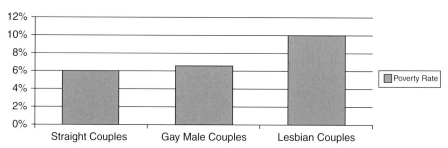

Figure 6.4 – Poverty Rates of Older Couples in the United States (Based on data from the Williams Institute [**Gates, 2013**]).

they had, thinking they would not live long, only to find themselves today with costly medications and an impaired ability to work. Metlife surveyed LGB respondents and found that over half did not have a will, living will, or long-term care policies. Lesbian and bisexual women were less financially prepared for end of life than gay/bisexual men (Metlife, 2010). This is understandable, since the combination of sexism and heterosexism have more severely limited financial opportunities for lesbian/bisexual women compared to gay/bisexual men. Figures 6.3 and 6.4 show data on social security income and poverty rates for adults over the age of 65 in male same-sex couples, female same-sex couples, and heterosexual couples.

Conclusion

In summary, although there is a growing body of literature on the developmental transitions of LGBTQ people, there are many gaps in our knowledge. Most of the research has focused on the negative: on the risk factors or the adverse outcomes experienced by many LGBTQ people because of stigma, but certainly not all LGBTQ people have any adverse outcomes and the majority live long and happy lives. We know a lot less about resilience and why and how so many LGBTQ people do thrive at all ages and stages of life in spite of the challenges. It is useful for healthcare professionals to consider sexual identity milestones such as coming out and disclosure along with other age/developmental transitions that everyone experiences, as these do influence health and well-being.

References

Appelbaum, J. (2007). Late adulthood and aging: Clinical approaches. In Makadon, H. J., Mayer, K. H., Potter, J., & Goldhammer, H (Eds.), *The Fenway guide to lesbian, gay, bisexual, and transgender health* (pp. 135–158). Philadelphia, PA: American College of Physicians Press.

Badgett, M. V. L., & Williams, R. M. (1992). The economics of sexual orientation: Establishing a research agenda. *Feminist Studies: FS, 18*(3), 649–657. Retrieved from http://doi.org/10.2307/3178091

Balsam, K. F., Huang, B., Fieland, K. C., Simoni, J. M., & Walters, K. L. (2004). Culture, trauma, and wellness: A comparison of heterosexual and lesbian, gay, bisexual, and two-spirit native Americans. *Cultural Diversity & Ethnic Minority Psychology, 10*, 287–301. Retrieved from http://doi.org/10.1037/1099–9809.10.3.287

Beemyn, B. G., & Rankin, S. (2011). *The lives of transgender people*. New York: Columbia University Press.

Birkett, M., Newcomb, M. E., & Mustanski, B. (2015). Does it get better? A longitudinal analysis of psychological distress and victimization in lesbian, gay, bisexual, transgender, and questioning youth. *The Journal of Adolescent Health: Official Publication of the Society for Adolescent Medicine, 56*(3), 280–285. Retrieved from http://doi.org/10.1016/j.jadohealth.2014.10.275

Boatwright, K. J., Gilbert, M. S., Forrest, L., & Ketzenberger, K. L. (1996). Impact of identity development upon career trajectory: Listening to the voices of lesbians. *Journal of Vocational Behavior, 48*, 210–228.

Bornstein, D. R., Fawcett, J., Sullivan, M., Senturia, K. D., & Shiu-Thornton, S. (2006). Understanding the experiences of lesbian, bisexual and trans survivors of domestic violence: A qualitative study. *Journal of Homosexuality, 51*, 159–181. Retrieved from http://doi.org/10.1300/J082v51n01_08

Bowleg, L., Craig, M. L., & Burkholder, G. (2004). Rising and surviving: A conceptual model of active coping among Black lesbians. *Cultural Diversity & Ethnic Minority Psychology, 10*, 229–240.

Bradford, J. B., & McKay, T. (2004). Foundations for sexual minority health. Retrieved July 25, 2015, from http://sph.unc.edu/files/2013/07/bradford_slides_2004.pdf

Bradford, J. B., Ryan, C., & Rothblum, E. D. (1994). National lesbian health care survey: Implications for mental health care. *Journal of Consulting and Clinical Psychology, 62*, 228–242.

Brotman, S., Ryan, B., & Cormier, R. (2003). The health and social service needs of gay and lesbian elders and their families in Canada. *The Gerontologist, 43*, 192–202.

Burn, S. M., Kadlec, K., & Rexer, R. (2005). Effects of subtle heterosexism on gay, lesbians, bisexuals. *Journal of Homosexuality, 49*, 23–38.

Case, P., Austin, S. B., Hunter, D. J., Manson, J. E., Malspeis, S., Willett, W. C., & Spiegelman, D. (2004). Sexual orientation, health risk factors, and physical functioning in the Nurses' Health Study II. *Journal of Women's Health, 13*, 1033–1047. Retrieved from http://doi.org/10.1089/jwh.2004.13.1033

Center for American Progress, & Movement Advancement Project. (2015). Paying an unfair price: The financial penalty for LGBT women in America. Retrieved June 24, 2015, from http://lgbtmap.org/file/paying-an-unfair-price-lgbt-women.pdf

Claes, J. A., & Moore, W. (2000). Issues confronting lesbian and gay elders: the challenge for health and human services providers. *Journal of Health and Human Services Administration, 23*, 181–202.

Cochran, S. D., Mays, V. M., Alegria, M., Ortega, A. N., & Takeuchi, D. (2007). Mental health and substance use disorders among Latino and Asian American lesbian, gay, and bisexual adults. *Journal of Consulting and Clinical Psychology, 75*, 785–794.

Cochran, S. D., & Mays, V. M. (2007). Physical health complaints among lesbians, gay men, and bisexual and homosexually experienced heterosexual individuals: Results from the California Quality of Life Survey. *American Journal of Public Health, 97*, 2048–2055. Retrieved from http://doi.org/10.2105/AJPH.2006.087254

Cook-Daniels, L. (2006). Trans aging. In D. Kimmel, T. Rose, & S. David (Eds.), *Lesbian, gay, bisexual, and transgender aging: Research and clinical perspectives* (pp. 20–35). New York: Columbia University Press.

D'Augelli, A. R. (2006a). Coming out, visibility, and creating change: empowering lesbian, gay, and bisexual people in a rural university community. *American Journal of Community Psychology, 37*, 203–210. Retrieved from http://doi.org/10.1007/s10464-006-9043-6

D'Augelli, A. R. (2006b). Developmental and contextual factors and mental health among LGB youths. In A. Omoto & H. Kurtzman (Eds.), *Sexual orientation and mental health* (pp. 37–53). Washington, DC: APA Press.

D'Augelli, A. R., & Grossman, A. H. (2001). Sexual orientation victimization of lesbian, gay, and bisexual youth. In *2001 Proceedings: American Psychological Association*, San Francisco, CA.

Diamond, L. (2002). "Having a girlfriend without knowing it": The relationships of adolescent lesbian and bisexual women. *Journal of Lesbian Studies, 6*, 5–16.

Donovan, T. (2001). Being transgender and older: A first person account. In D. C. Kimmel & D. L. Martin (Eds.), *Midlife and aging in gay America* (pp. 19–22). New York: Haworth.

Drydakis, N. (2012). Men's sexual orientation and job satisfaction. *International Journal of Manpower, 33*(8), 901–917. Retrieved from http://doi.org/10.1108/01437721211280371

Dunlap, A. (2014). Coming-out narratives across generations. *Journal of Gay & Lesbian Social Services, 26*(3), 318–335. Retrieved from http://doi.org/10.1080/10538720.2014.9 24460

Durso, L. E., & Meyer, I. H. (2013). Patterns and predictors of disclosure of sexual orientation to healthcare providers among lesbians, gay men, and bisexuals. *Sexuality Research & Social Policy: Journal of NSRC: SR & SP, 10*(1), 35–42. Retrieved from http://doi.org/10.1007/s13178–012–0105–2

Eisenberg, M. E., & Resnick, M. D. (2006). Suicidality among gay, lesbian and bisexual youth: The role of protective factors. *Child Welfare, 85*, 299–316.

Elze, D. (2002). Against all odds: The dating experiences of adolescent lesbian and bisexual women. *Journal of Lesbian Studies, 6*, 17–29.

Espinoza, R. (2014). *Out and visible: The experiences and attitudes of lesbian, gay, bisexual, and transgender older adults, ages 45–75*. New York: Sage.

Floyd, F. J., & Bakeman, R. (2006). Coming-out across the life course: Implications of age and historical context. *Archives of Sexual Behavior, 35*(3), 287–296. Retrieved from http://doi.org/10.1007/s10508–006–9022-x

Fox, R. C. (2007). Gay grows up: An interpretive study on aging metaphors and queer identity. *Journal of Homosexuality, 52*(3–4), 33–61.

Fredriksen-Goldsen, K. I., Kim, H. J., Barkan, S. E., Muraco, A., & Hoy-Ellis, C. P. (2013). Health disparities among lesbian, gay, and bisexual older adults: Results from a population-based study. *American Journal of Public Health, 103*, 1802–1809. Retrieved from http://doi.org/10.2105/AJPH.2012.301110

Gates, G. J. (2013). Same sex and different sex couples in the American Community Survey: 2005–2011. *eScholarship-UCLA: The Williams Institute*. Retrieved from http://escholarship.org/uc/item/8dk71277.pdf

Grant, J. M., Mottet, L. A., Tanis, J., Herman, J. L., Harrison, J., Keisling, M., & Others. (2010). National transgender discrimination survey report on health and health care. Retrieved July 25, 2015, from http://www.kwncbxw.thetaskforce.org/downloads/resources_and_tools/ntds_report_on_health.pdf

Greene, G. J., Fisher, K. A., Kuper, L., Andrews, R., & Mustanski, B. (2015). "Is this normal? Is this not normal? There's no set example": Sexual health intervention preferences of LGBT youth in romantic relationships. *Sexuality Research & Social Policy: Journal of NSRC: SR & SP, 12*(1), 1–14. Retrieved from http://doi.org/10.1007/s13178–014–0169–2

Gross, J. (2007). *Aging and gay, and facing prejudice in twilight*. The New York Times. Retrieved from http://02b655a.netsolhost.com/gen_silent_press_room_files/Aging%20and%20Gay,%20and%20Facing%20Prejudice%20in%20Twilight%20-%20New%20York%20Times.pdf

Grossman, A. H., & D'Augelli, A. R. (2006). Transgender youth: invisible and vulnerable. *Journal of Homosexuality, 51*(1), 111–128. Retrieved from http://doi.org/10.1300/J082v51n01_06

Grossman, A. H., D'Augelli, A. R., & Hershberger, S. L. (2000). Social support networks of lesbian, gay, and bisexual adults 60 years of age and older. *The Journals of Gerontology. Series B, Psychological Sciences and Social Sciences, 55*(3), P171–P179. Retrieved from http://doi.org/10.1093/geronb/55.3.P171

Grossman, A. H., D'Augelli, A. R., & O'Connell, T. S. (2001). Being lesbian, gay, bisexual, and 60 or older in North America. In D. C. Kimmel & D. L. Martin (Eds.), *Midlife and aging in gay America* (pp. 23–40). New York: Haworth Press.

Guarnero, P. A. (2007). Family and community influences on the social and sexual lives of Latino gay men. *Journal of Transcultural Nursing: Official Journal of the Transcultural Nursing Society/Transcultural Nursing Society, 18*(1), 12–18. Retrieved from http://doi.org/10.1177/1043659606294195

Hatzenbuehler, M. L., Keyes, K. M., Hamilton, A., & Hasin, D. S. (2014). State-level tobacco environments and sexual orientation disparities in tobacco use and dependence in the USA. Tobacco Control, 23(e2), e127–e132. Retrieved from http://doi.org/10.1136/tobaccocontrol-2013-051279.

Herek, G. M. (1995). Psychological heterosexism in the United States. In A. R. D'Augelli & C. J. Patterson (Eds.), *Lesbian, gay, and bisexual identities over the lifespan: Psychological perspectives* (pp. 321–346). Oxford: Oxford University Press.

Huebner, D. M., & Davis, M. C. (2005). Gay and bisexual men who disclose their sexual orientations in the workplace have higher workday levels of salivary cortisol and negative affect. *Annals of Behavioral Medicine: A Publication of the Society of Behavioral Medicine, 30*(3), 260–267. Retrieved from http://doi.org/10.1207/s15324796abm3003_10

Johnson, M. J., Jackson, N. C., Arnette, J. K., & Koffman, S. D. (2005). Gay and lesbian perceptions of discrimination in retirement care facilities. *Journal of Homosexuality, 49*(2), 83–102. Retrieved from http://doi.org/10.1300/J082v49n02_05

Kelly, J. M. (2005). *Zest for life: Lesbians' experiences of menopause.* Melbourne, Australia: Spinifex Press.

Koh, A. S., & Ross, L. K. (2006). Mental health issues: A comparison of lesbian, bisexual and heterosexual women. *Journal of Homosexuality, 51*(1), 33–57. Retrieved from http://doi.org/10.1300/J082v51n01_03

Kooden, H., & Flowers, C. (2000). *Golden men: The power of gay midlife.* New York: Avon.

Kosciw, J. W., Greytak, E. A., Palmer, N. A., & Boesen, M. J. (2014). The 2013 National School Climate Survey: The experiences of LGBT youth in our nation's schools *(A Report from the Gay, Lesbian & Straight Education Network).* Retrieved July 26, 2015, from http://www.glsen.org/sites/default/files/2013%20National%20School%20Climate%20Survey%20Full%20Report_0.pdf

Kurdek, L. A. (2004). Are gay and lesbian cohabiting couples really different from heterosexual married couples? *Journal of Marriage and Family Counseling, 66*(4), 880–900. Retrieved from http://doi.org/10.1111/j.0022–2445.2004.00060.x

Kwon, P. (2013). Resilience in lesbian, gay, and bisexual individuals. *Personality and Social Psychology Review: An Official Journal of the Society for Personality and Social Psychology, Inc, 17*, 371–383. Retrieved from http://doi.org/10. 1177/1088868313490248

Lodge, A. C., & Umberson, D. (2013). Age and embodied masculinities: Midlife gay and heterosexual men talk about their bodies. *Journal of Aging Studies, 27*(3), 225–232. Retrieved from http://doi.org/10.1016/j.jaging.2013.03.004

Mallon, G. P., & DeCrescenzo, T. (2006). Transgender children and youth: A child welfare practice perspective. *Child Welfare, 85*(2), 215–241.

McMahon, E. (2003). The older homosexual: Current concepts of lesbian, gay, bisexual, and transgender older Americans. *Clinics in Geriatric Medicine, 19*(3), 587–593.

Means-Christensen, A. J., Snyder, D. K., & Negy, C. (2003). Assessing nontraditional couples: Validity of the marital satisfaction inventory–revised with gay, lesbian, and cohabiting heterosexual couples. *Journal of Marital and Family Therapy, 29*(1), 69–83.

Metlife. (2010). Still out, still aging: The metlife study of lesbian, gay, bisexual and transgender baby boomers. Retrieved July 25, 2015, from https://www.metlife.com/assets/cao/mmi/publications/studies/2010/mmi-still-out-still-aging.pdf

Meyer, I. H. (2003). Prejudice, social stress, and mental health in lesbian, gay, and bisexual populations: Conceptual issues and research evidence. *Psychological Bulletin, 129*(5), 674–697. Retrieved from http://doi.org/10.1037/0033–2909.129.5.674

Nemoto, T., Operario, D., Keatley, J., Han, L., & Soma, T. (2004). HIV risk behaviors among male-to-female transgender persons of color in San Francisco. *American Journal of Public Health, 94*(7), 1193–1199.

O'Toole, C. J. (2000). The view from below: Developing a knowledge base about an unknown population. *Sexuality and Disability, 18*(3), 207–224. Retrieved from http://doi.org/10.1023/A:1026421916410

Oswald, R. F. (2002). Resilience within the family networks of lesbians and gay men: Intentionality and redefinition. *Journal of Marriage and Family Counseling, 64*(2), 374–383. Retrieved from http://doi.org/10.1111/j.1741–3737. 2002.00374.x

Parks, C. A., Hughes, T. L., & Matthews, A. K. (2004). Race/ethnicity and sexual orientation: Intersecting identities. *Cultural Diversity & Ethnic Minority Psychology, 10*(3), 241–254. Retrieved from http://doi.org/10.1037/1099–9809.10.3.241

Pazos, S. (1999). Practice with female-to-male transgendered youth. In G. Mallon (Ed.), *Social services with transgendered youth* (pp. 65–82). New York: Taylor & Francis.

Pedulla, D. S. (2014). The positive consequences of negative stereotypes: Race, sexual orientation, and the job application process. *Social Psychology Quarterly, 77*(1), 75–94. Retrieved from http://doi.org/10.1177/0190272513506229

Poteat, V. P., Scheer, J. R., Marx, R. A., Calzo, J. P., & Yoshikawa, H. (2015). Gay-straight alliances vary on dimensions of youth socializing and advocacy: Factors accounting for individual and setting-level differences. *American Journal of Community Psychology, 55*(3–4), 422–432. Retrieved from http://doi.org/10.1007/s10464–015–9722–2

Poteat, V. P., Sinclair, K. O., DiGiovanni, C. D., Koenig, B. W., & Russell, S. T. (2013). Gay-straight alliances are associated with student health: A multischool comparison of LGBTQ and heterosexual youth. *Journal of Research on Adolescence: The Official Journal of the Society for Research on Adolescence, 23*(2), 319–330. Retrieved from http://doi.org/10.1111/j.1532–7795.2012.00832.x

Prudential. (2012). The LGBT financial experience 2012–2013 prudential research study. Retrieved June 28, 2015, from http://www.prudential.com/media/managed/Prudential_LGBT_Financial_Experience.pdf

Ragins, B. R., Singh, R., & Cornwell, J. M. (2007). Making the invisible visible: Fear and disclosure of sexual orientation at work. *The Journal of Applied Psychology, 92*(4), 1103–1118. Retrieved from http://doi.org/10.1037/0021–9010.92.4.1103

Reback, C. J., Simon, P. A., Bemis, C. C., & Gatson, B. (2001). The Los Angeles transgender health study: Community report. Retrieved July 26, 2015, from http://friendscommunitycenter.org/documents/LA_Transgender_Health_Study.pdf

Remafedi, G. (2007). Lesbian, gay, bisexual, and transgender youths: Who smokes, and why? *Nicotine & Tobacco Research: Official Journal of the Society for Research on Nicotine and Tobacco, 9*(*Suppl 1*), S65–71. Retrieved from http://doi.org/10.1080/14622200601083491

Ristock, J. L. (2003). Exploring dynamics of abusive lesbian relationships: Preliminary analysis of a multisite, qualitative study. *American Journal of Community Psychology, 31*(3–4), 329–341.

Rivers, I. (2004). Recollections of bullying at school and their long-term implications for lesbians, gay men, and bisexuals. *Crisis, 25*(4), 169–175. Retrieved from http://doi.org/10.1027/0227–5910.25.4.169

Rostosky, S. S., & Riggle, E. D. B. (2002). " Out" at work: The relation of actor and partner workplace policy and internalized homophobia to disclosure status. *Journal of Counseling Psychology, 49*(4), 411.

Rothman, E. F., Sullivan, M., Keyes, S., & Boehmer, U. (2012). Parents' supportive reactions to sexual orientation disclosure associated with better health: Results from a population-based survey of LGB adults in Massachusetts. *Journal of Homosexuality*, *59*(2), 186–200. Retrieved from http://doi.org/10.1080/00918369.2012.648878

Russell, G. M., & Richards, J. A. (2003). Stressor and resilience factors for lesbians, gay men, and bisexuals confronting antigay politics. *American Journal of Community Psychology*, *31*, 313–328.

Ryan, C., Huebner, D., Diaz, R. M., & Sanchez, J. (2009). Family rejection as a predictor of negative health outcomes in white and Latino lesbian, gay, and bisexual young adults. *Pediatrics*, *123*(1), 346–352. Retrieved from http://doi.org/10.1542/peds.2007–3524

Sanders, G. L., & Kroll, I. T. (2000). Generating stories of resilience: helping gay and lesbian youth and their families. *Journal of Marital and Family Therapy*, *26*(4), 433–442.

Savin-Williams, R. C. (2005). *The New gay teenager*. Cambridge, MA: Harvard University Press. Retrieved from http://doi.org/10.4159/9780674043138

Schneider, M. S., & Dimito, A. (2010). Factors influencing the career and academic choices of lesbian, gay, bisexual, and transgender people. *Journal of Homosexuality*, *57*(10), 1355–1369. Retrieved from http://doi.org/10.1080/00918369.2010.517080

Spirito, A., & Esposito-Smythers, C. (2006). Attempted and completed suicide in adolescence. *Annual Review of Clinical Psychology*, *2*, 237–266. Retrieved from http://doi.org/10.1146/annurev.clinpsy.2.022305.095323

Stein, G. L., & Bonuck, K. A. (2001). Attitudes on end-of-life care and advance care planning in the lesbian and gay community. *Journal of Palliative Medicine*, *4*(2), 173–190.

Velez, B. L., Moradi, B., & Brewster, M. E. (2013). Testing the tenets of minority stress theory in workplace contexts. *Journal of Counseling Psychology*, *60*(4), 532–542. Retrieved from http://doi.org/10.1037/a0033346

Weinberg, M. S., Williams, C. J., & Pryor, D. W. (2001). Bisexuals at midlife commitment, salience, and identity. *Journal of Contemporary Ethnography*, *30*(2), 180–208.

Wierzalis, E. A., Barret, B., Pope, M., & Rankins, M. (2006). Gay men and aging: Sex and intimacy. In D. Kimmel, T. Rose, & S. David (Eds.), *Lesbian, gay, bisexual, and transgender aging: Research and clinical perspective* (pp. 91–109). New York: Columbia University Press.

Wight, R. G., Leblanc, A. J., & Lee Badgett, M. V. (2013). Same-sex legal marriage and psychological well-being: Findings from the California Health Interview Survey. *American Journal of Public Health*, *103*(2), 339–346. Retrieved from http://doi.org/10.2105/AJPH.2012.301113

Xavier, J., Honnold, J. A., & Bradford, J. B. (2007). *The health, health-related needs, and life-course experiences of transgender Virginians*. Richmond, VA: VA Department of Health.

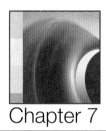

Chapter 7

Cultures Within Cultures: Diversity and LGBTQ Communities

"Since every identity has meaning only because it is named against other identities, there can never be an identity that is all-inclusive. By saying who we are and what we are fighting for, we are necessarily saying what we are not and what we are not fighting for." (Kumashiro, 2001, p. 6)

As Kumashiro so astutely noted, our focus on LGBTQ identities in this book can have the effect of rendering other social identities invisible, or to seem less important. No individual can be characterized by only one of their multitude of identities, but is, in reality, an amalgam of many sometimes conflicting, and constantly shifting identities. Which identities a person chooses to evoke in any given situation depends on the context. LGBTQ people represent every form of diversity known within human experience. Thus far, however, LGBTQ health research is still in an infancy stage, and little attention has been paid to subgroup variations or the influence of intersecting identities within LGBTQ populations. It is likely that some demographic and personal characteristics are equally or more important in influencing health outcomes than sexual and gender identities. Consider the potential differences among these individuals, all of whom might be lumped together in a study of the effects of sexual stigma on health:

- Tony is a 15-year-old Asian-American (second-generation Japanese) youth who thinks he might be gay, but fears more harassment at school (he is already harassed for being Asian in a predominately White high school). Tony has a family that does not discuss topics related to sexuality openly and he relies completely on his parents for healthcare services.
- Lee, a 66-year-old American Indian who does not use terms like male/female or LGBTQ, has been considered "two-spirit" since childhood and serves a healer role in the community. Lee, by western standards, has a male body, but by traditional standards, is a "third gender." Lee, who is severely disabled with emphysema and mobility problems, lives on a reservation with a 45% unemployment rate.
- Lauretta is 50, African American, and was raised as a devout Catholic. She entered a convent at age 18, but left a few years later when she fell in love with a fellow nun. She works as a receptionist in a small business in a Black neighborhood and does not talk about her personal life to coworkers. She just got health insurance for the first time because of the Affordable Care Act. Her partner of 18 years, Joyce, is a bus driver with insurance, but it does not cover domestic partners.

- George is a 26-year-old Latino, bisexual man who contracted HIV in his youth, before he was employed. He is relatively healthy now and works full time, but could not get insurance for the past 6 years because of the "pre-existing condition." He lives in a rural area with few services for people with HIV.
- Rami is a 22-year-old Arab man who fell in love with his roommate in college, Jim. They were together for 4 years, but now Rami's visa is up and he cannot stay in the United States. Jim would not be welcomed by Rami's family or community; in fact, they would risk severe violence in Rami's homeland.
- Rachel is a 34-year-old Jewish lesbian with cerebral palsy. She uses a wheelchair to get around, and is frustrated by the lack of accessible events in the lesbian community. She also attends a support group for women with disabilities, but is the only lesbian in the group and must constantly challenge their heterosexism. She fights the stereotype of the asexual disabled woman constantly within the larger society and the lesbian community.
- Samantha is a 10-year-old Latina from a large Catholic family. From as long as she can remember, Samantha has thought of herself as a boy and has rebelled against her family's efforts to make her into a "girly-girl." She wants her family to call her Sam and treat her like a boy. Her family thinks she is far too young to know these things, and is ashamed of her difference.

Each of these individuals has multiple identities or characteristics that affect their ability to access health care and that affect how others perceive and treat them. They may or may not use terms like LGBT or Q to describe themselves. The forms of oppression are intersecting in contemporary society, and stress related to multiple diverse identifications is not merely additive, but instead, the identities intersect to create unique situations. Historically, LGBTQ identity politics have sometimes inadvertently, and sometimes deliberately, excluded discussion of other oppressed minorities in an attempt to unify under one label (usually the sexuality label). Kumashiro (2001) pointed out that

"any attempt to focus on 'queer' is simultaneously a process of separating queer genders and sexualities from other identities, thereby leaving unmarked those (nonqueer) identities that are traditionally privileged (such as White American and male identities) … Similarly, some civil rights movements based on race or ethnicity have excluded gender and sexual minority identifications, sometimes in a deliberate move to 'normalize.' LGBTQ identities are labeled as 'a white thing' and to adopt an LGBTQ identity as a person of color is to be a 'race traitor.'" (p. 4)

A truly inclusive approach to health disparities takes into account many different identities that impact one's health status, a challenging but necessary task for those who work in healthcare settings. One useful model for doing this is intersectionality. This theory arose out of Black feminist writing as a way of viewing both race and sex/gender as powerful influences on a woman's life (Hill-Collins, 2005).

Racism and heterosexism have long been linked, as Somerville (2000) noted:

"it was not merely historical coincidence that the classification of bodies as either 'homosexual' or 'heterosexual' emerged at the same time that the United States was aggressively constructing and policing the boundary between 'black' and 'white' bodies." (p. 3)

Eugenics and sexology colluded to produce messages about deviance that affected cultural stigma about race and sexuality simultaneously. In health studies, intersectionality has been used to study the effects of the multiple intersecting influences and identities on health (e.g., Thomeer, 2013; Veenstra, 2013).

In this chapter, we will address just a few of the common forms of diversity within any LGBTQ community. We addressed sex, gender, and age in other chapters, so in this one, will briefly discuss race/ethnicity, religion/spirituality, ability/disability status, and gender expression. Keep in mind that the divisions are artificial, and that in reality, all people experience all of their identities more or less simultaneously and often cannot sort out the influence of any one identity in isolation of the others.

Race/Ethnicity

"White male doctors make it their job to see to it that Black women do not have any more babies ... Whenever I went in [to a doctor's office] they would never let up when I said, no, I don't need birth control. So sometimes I would come out as a lesbian, just to get them to move on to other things. The doctors would fumble around and say something like, 'Oh ... I'm sorry.' It was so awkward ... I always felt harassed because I am black and because I am a lesbian." (Stevens, 1998, p. 84)

It is difficult to make any definitive statements about how LGBTQ identities are expressed among the different racial/ethnic cultures of the world and within the United States. Some cultures do not even have terms or concepts that are equivalent to our western notions of sexual identity and gender identity. In academic circles in the west, we differentiate sex/gender from sexual identity/orientation, but many other cultures do not. A good example of this is the noncorrespondence of western sex/gender/sexuality terms to the North American indigenous people's concept of "two-spirit." There are vast tribal differences in concepts of sex/gender, but in the 1990s, the term two-spirit was adopted by many as a unifying label for indigenous people who experienced their sex/gender/ sexuality as a spiritual identity, and as a means of rejecting western concepts that were irrelevant to their own heritages and experiences. The identity of "two-spirit" represents a blending of gender and sexuality (Gilley, 2010; Walters, Simoni, & Horwath, 2001).

At least within the United States, we can be fairly certain that LGBTQ people exist in all racial/ethnic groups at about the same rate as in the heterosexual population. U.S. Census data has collected information about same-sex households in recent years. Figure 7.1 shows how same-sex households were distributed by race/ethnicity compared to other-sex households in the 2000 U.S. census (Romero, Baumle, Badgett, & Gates, 2007). Every racial/ethnic group had same-sex couples to about the same percentage as the general population data, for example 10% of the U.S. population was Latino/a and 11% of same-sex couples were Latino/a. Figure 7.2 shows how racism affects healthcare access by comparing those who have health insurance by race/ethnicity and within same-sex or different-sex couples (Kastanis & Wilson, 2014).

Racial/ethnic minority communities are extraordinarily diverse, varying by immigration status, language, degree of acculturation, income levels, education, religion, and a host of other dimensions. Any discussion of the impact of race/ethnicity, like discussions of sexuality and gender, are generalizations that may or may not apply to

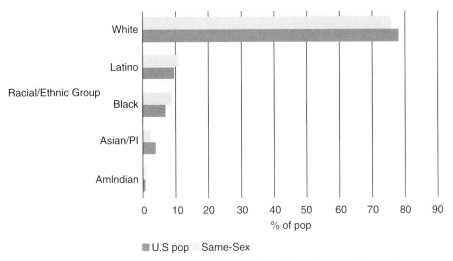

Figure 7.1 – Racial/ethnic Distribution of Households: Other-Sex and Same-Sex Couples in 2000 Census (Based on **Romero, Baumle, Badgett, & Gates, 2007**).

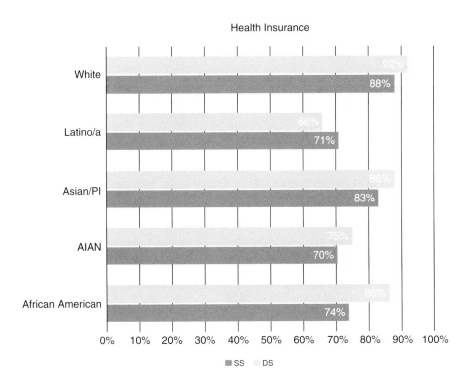

Figure 7.2 – Health Insurance in Same-Sex (SS) and Different-Sex (DS) Couples by Race/Ethnicity in U.S. 2008 (Based on **Kastanis & Wilson, 2014**).

any given individual. The differences in households of same-sex people of color may (or may not) be related to:

- Being less "out," because potential costs of being out are much higher. Support from family and community, religious leaders, and ethnic social justice organizations may be critical to support oneself against racism and classism (Aranda et al., 2015; Grov, Bimbi, Nanín, & Parsons, 2006).
- There may be rejection of terms considered to be "White" concepts, such as L,G,B,T, and Q, and therefore, they may not use these labels or use different ones, such as "same-gender loving," "family," "two-spirit," and others.
- Political affiliations may be with groups that focus on race/ethnicity rather than sexuality/gender, since there are few that truly integrate both identities (Rosario, Schrimshaw, & Hunter, 2004). One study found "conflicts in allegiance" to be more likely among LGB people of color, who have to reconcile allegiance to communities of color with allegiance to LGBTQ communities (Sarno, Mohr, Jackson, & Fassinger, 2015).
- Racism affects income status, thus LGBTQ individuals and their families of color are more likely to live in poverty, be unemployed, and have less access to quality health care—and experience more discrimination when they do access health services than do White LGBTQs (Kastanis & Wilson, 2014).
- People of color are more likely to have been raised in and continue to belong to conservative religions, such as the Catholic faith (many Latinos, Filipinos), evangelical Christian protestant denominations (African Americans), and Islam (African Americans and Arab Americans). Religious affiliation may be a more potent marker of homophobia in these communities than race/ethnicity per se.
- People of color are more likely to be raising children, which increases family stress and the financial burden on the family. In the 2008–10 American Community Survey, 16% of White, 17% of Asian and Pacific Islanders, 26% of American Indian/Alaska Natives, 30% of Latino/a, and 41% of Black same-sex households contained children (Kastanis & Wilson, 2014).
- Some cultures have taboos against talking openly about topics related to sexuality to avoid public conflicts and/or to maintain harmony (save face). Other cultures have attitudes that private sexual behaviors are one's own business as long as in public they fulfill their familial "duties" that are common in more collectively oriented cultures, such as many Asian groups (Mao, McCormick, & van de Ven, 2002).

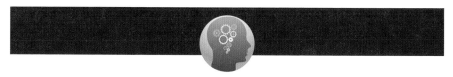

Think About It 7.1

The media furor a few years ago about African-American men on the "down low" is an example of "racialized sexism" (Miller, Andre, Ebin, & Bessonova, 2007). It targets Black men who have sex with men without telling their female partners. The issue is that some people from all cultural backgrounds engage in this behavior. Why have Black men been

(continued)

targeted in this media attention? Battle and Crum (2007) proposed that poverty is the major factor in the higher rates of HIV among African Americans, not men on the "down low." Binson, Michaels, Stall, and Coates (1995) found that Black men were only slightly more likely to be behaviorally bisexual than White men, however, these numbers are still very small and cannot account for the higher rates of HIV (see also Mays, Cochran, & Zamudio, 2004). The down-low media frenzy uses Black men, who are an already marginalized population, as scapegoats to deflect attention from the real issues of racism, sexism, and heterosexism.

Anti-gay campaigns have often deliberately pitted communities of color against LGBTQ communities, making them seem mutually exclusive (e.g., implying that there are no LGBTQ people of color) and in competition for scarce resources. The recent anti-gay campaigns and public policies have disproportionately affected Black and Latino same-sex families, because they are twice as likely to have children, to have more limited income, to work in the public sector, to be affected by immigration policies, and to serve, and be discharged, from the military (Cahill, 2008).

Religion/Spirituality/Moral Beliefs

"I was scared because the preacher would say stuff like, 'We ain't hatching no faggots up in here.' And the whole church, including my mother, would scream, 'Amen!' I knew what a faggot was because my brothers called me that." (Respondent in a study of African American gay men) (Miller, 2007, p. 57)

LGBTQ people are born into families that represent the entire continuum of religious and spiritual belief systems, but as adults, LGBTQ people are more likely to report being "nonreligious." Table 7.1 shows religious affiliations of people in the United States.

The influences of religion and spirituality are difficult to study because of the multitiered sets of influences. We will begin with a discussion of religion. For example, let's say that Ray, an African-American bisexual man, was raised in a southern Baptist church. The message from minister and elders of the church may or may not reflect the doctrine of the larger Baptist organization, and Ray's family may or may not model or

Table 7.1 – Religious Affiliations of LGBTQ Compared to the General Public (Based on Data From the Pew Research Center, 2013)		
Affiliation	**LGBTQ**	**General Public**
Christian	42%	73%
Protestant	27%	49%
Catholic	14%	22%
Jewish	2%	2%
Atheist/Agnostic	17%	6%
None	31%	14%

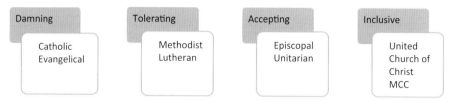

Damning	Tolerating	Accepting	Inclusive
Catholic Evangelical	Methodist Lutheran	Episcopal Unitarian	United Church of Christ MCC

Figure 7.3 – Examples of a Continuum of Formal Christian Religion Positions on LGBTQ Identities/Behaviors.

espouse the beliefs of the larger church doctrines or even their local church. The church leaders who teach Sunday school or bible study classes may present yet another interpretation. Perhaps the choir leader is known to be gay, but is widely liked and accepted in the church. Maybe that gay choir leader is Ray's uncle. If Ray gets a stronger message of "love thy neighbor" than "homosexuals will go to hell," he may have an easier time of reconciling his faith with his sexuality than if the "hell" message is emphasized.

Figure 7.3 shows the continuum of Christian churches' stands on sexual orientation. Fewer of them have direct policies about gender identity. Ex-gay ministries (programs designed to "cure" homosexuality) are found primarily in the "damning" category. LGBTQ people are raised in, and sometimes remain steadfast to the beliefs of religions across the entire continuum from damning to welcoming.

In the general population, religion has been found to have positive health benefits and affect quality of life (Koenig, McCullough, & Larson, 2001), but less is known about the impact of religious involvement for LGBTQ people. Many LGBTQ people are affiliated with religious denominations or groups and often seek out LGBTQ-specific or welcoming congregations or advocacy groups. Maher (2006) documented over 450 LGBTQ religious groups located between the west coast and the Mississippi River from 1989 to 1993. He defined "gay group" as a group focused on LGBT issues in religion or a group/congregation consisting of 50% or more LGBTQ people. Historically, in 1962 the first LGBT ministry within a mainstream church was at the Glide Memorial Church in San Francisco, headed by the Reverend Cecil Williams, a tireless heterosexual ally/advocate for LGBTQ people. In 1968, the Metropolitan Community Church (MCC), an LGBTQ affirmative nondenominational Christian church, was created in Los Angeles by gay male Reverend Troy Perry. MCC churches are now found in nearly every state in the United States, and 24 other countries. In 1969, Dignity, a group of LGBTQ and supportive ally Catholics was formed, and went national in 1973. The United Church of Christ ordained the first openly gay pastor in 1972. The same year, the first LGBTQ Jewish synagogue opened in Los Angeles. The purpose of these congregations and groups was to help people integrate their faith and their sexuality/ gender. Gorman (1997) suggested that the increase in LGBTQ religious groups in the 1980s and 90s may be related to two factors. The first is the aging of the baby-boomer, post-Stonewall generation, which may share in common with their heterosexual counterparts an increased search for spirituality and meaning in their lives as they age. The second factor is the AIDS epidemic which highlighted issues of mortality and search for meaning in people across the lifespan.

Bishop Gene Robinson was the first openly gay person to be ordained to the position of bishop in the Episcopal Church, but his ordination was not without great controversy. Robinson was married and had two children before coming out. He has the full support of his family. In 2003, he was elected to the position of bishop in New Hampshire, a move which has forced considerable discussion of the position of the church on homosexuality.

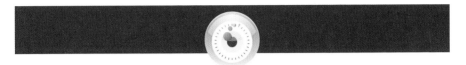

Watch This 7.1

Watch this 15-minute video in which Bishop Robinson shares the story of his life from early childhood, through his journey coming to terms with his sexuality and his religious faith. https://www.youtube.com/watch?v=HqvcPa-BbLc

Race/ethnicity and religion intersect in the lives of many LGBTQ people. For example, the "black church" has been described as a homophobic environment for LGBTQ people by some, but as an "open closet" by others who describe the common scene of "gay men singing in the choir while homosexuality is denounced from the pulpit" (Miller, 2007, p. 53). Leaders among some of the more conservative religious/cultural institutions of the African American community are strongly homophobic, as this quote from the leader of the Nation of Islam, Louis Farakhan indicates:

> *"Now brother, in the Holy world you can't switch [mimicking an effeminate man]. No, no no ... in the Holy world you better hide that stuff 'cause see if God made you for a woman, you can't go with a man ... You know what the penalty of that is in the Holy land? Death ... Sisters get to going with another sister—both women [are decapitated]."* (Simmons, 1991, p. 222)

Among Latinos, involvement in the Catholic Church is high, and may be associated with more negativity about LGBTQ people or at least same-sex behaviors. The paradox of "love the sinner, hate the sin" is important to highlight. Among LGBTQ people, same-sex expression and gender expression are parts of the person's core identity, so to be construed as "sin" means a rejection of the person as well as the behavior. In addition, many people may not truly make this distinction of love the sinner and hate the sin. In a study of substance abuse counselors (Eliason, 2000), scores on a homophobia scale did not differ between the groups that endorsed statements "Love the sinner but hate the sin" and "LGBT people are sinful and immoral." Both groups were equally negative and significantly more homophobic than people who endorsed, "I accept LGBT people and behavior as normal."

In some cases, religious affiliation may have harmful effects on the LGBTQ person. In a study of college students, those who were not heterosexual had higher rates of substance use, depression, and suicide thoughts if they were affiliated with a religion than those LGBTQ people who were not religious. For students who identified as "spiritual but not religious" there was no difference by sexual orientation in average number of drinks per week (heterosexual = 4.0; LGBTQ = 3.8), but for students who identified as "religious," LGBTQ students had significantly higher rates of drinking (7.2) than heterosexual students (3.2). This makes religion a risk factor for some LGBTQ youth, rather than the protective factor that it is for heterosexual youth (Eliason, Burke, Van Olphen, & Howell, 2011).

Other world religions also vary on their doctrines related to sexual orientation. Most religions have a conservative/traditional and a more liberal branch, with the conservative wing being more negative about gender and sexual minorities than the liberal branch. Some LGBTQ people have turned to Buddhism, because it is more of a life philosophy than a formal religion, but there are certainly segments of the Buddhist community that are anti-LGBTQ as well. Some of the most anti-LGBTQ countries in the world base their objections on religion (many Arab nations, for example).

Because of the difficulties that many LGBTQ people have experienced in the religions of their childhood, some of them have rejected religion entirely and sought out alternative ways to express their spirituality. Some join existing groups such as Wiccan and Neopagan movements that are open and affirming to all genders and sexualities. Others form their own groups, develop highly individual spiritual practices, and/or adopt Buddhism as philosophy rather than a religion. Having a strong spiritual belief system and practices may be protective against the stresses of oppression, whether that spirituality is accessed through a formal religion or other means.

Ability/Disability Status

> *"People ask me which I am: Woman, disabled, Asian. I tell them I am all three, it's like a triangle. It just depends on what is on top right now."* (Cupolo, Corbett, & Lewis, 1982, p. 3)

There is very little research on disability and LGBTQ people, for both disability and sexuality are taboo topics. In fact, the Institute of Medicine (2011) report on LGBT health, that reviewed all the literature on health-related issues, has only one sentence about disability: "Disability among LGBT elders is a topic rarely considered in research." It is rarely considered as a topic at any age, although the inclusion of sexual orientation questions on the big health surveillance instruments is beginning to change that.

Like any other persons, LGBTQ people might be born with disabilities or acquire them at any point in life. Some of the recent data suggest that among LGBTQ adults, minority stress might combine with chronic health problems to create greater risk for disability and debilitation (Cochran & Mays, 2007; Fredriksen-Goldsen, Kim, Barkan, Muraco, & Hoy-Ellis, 2013; Fredriksen-Goldsen, Kim, & Barkan, 2012; Garland-Forshee, Fiala, Ngo, & Moseley, 2014; Wallace, Cochran, Durazo, & Ford, 2011), suggesting that LGBTQ people may be even more likely than people in the general population to become disabled. People with HIV/AIDS may also be more likely to suffer disabilities than those without HIV/AIDS. One study of lesbian/bisexual women with and without disabilities found many similarities in term of educational level, whether partnered, and mental health quality of life, but significant differences on income level and sense of connection to LGBT and women's communities (Eliason, Martinson, & Carabez, 2015).

O'Toole (2000) noted several issues that disabled lesbians might have to deal with. These issues are probably relevant for other sexual and gender minority individuals as well:

- There is a presumption of heterosexuality or asexuality by caregivers, healthcare professionals, and potential dates, making the LGBTQ person invisible.
- The invisibility is in both LGBTQ communities and disability communities.
- Many able-bodied LGBTQ people place high value on self-reliance and independence, making people with disabilities feel inadequate or excluded.
- There is an absence of relevant sexuality education/information for people with disabilities.
- There is very high potential for sexual abuse and/or exploitation of people with disabilities who may be more vulnerable because of physical, intellectual, or mental health disabilities.
- There is an absence of LGBTQ role models with disabilities.
- There are many complicated legal issues (e.g., guardianship, ability to freely choose partners if institutionalized, etc.).

On the other hand, the goals of the LGBTQ and the disability communities overlap to a great extent. As a disabled lesbian poet put it "There is a disability culture and at the core of this culture is empowerment, pride, and a flat-out, no apologies celebration of difference" (Cheryl Marie Wade, quoted in (O'Toole, 2000, p. 215)). LGBTQ communities often try to make their events accessible and to be more inclusive of the diversity found within the community, but for many organizations and groups, disability issues are overlooked because of the invisibility of disability communities with the larger LGBTQ population. Able-bodied LGBTQ people may benefit greatly from the inclusion of people with disabilities in communities and social networks as role models for learning to adapt to changing health and physical mobility challenges that are inevitable as we age.

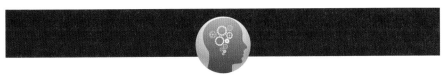

Think About It 7.2

Bring to mind an experience you have had with a patient who was different from you in at least two ways: a different sexual or gender identity *and* a different racial/ethnic background, a different religion, or different physical ability. How did you feel about the encounter? Did you feel comfortable that you knew the right terminology to use? How did the person respond to you?

Gender Expression Within Sexual Identities

We discussed gender expression in an earlier chapter in regards to transgender identity, but there is also much greater diversity of gender expression among people who are not transgender, but label their sexuality as lesbian, gay, or bisexual. Being on the margins of society can be liberating in some ways, and being freed, to some extent, from the social pressures to conform to heterosexual forms of femininity and masculinity, LGBQ people may express themselves in a variety of ways.

Among lesbian and bisexual women, there is an entire subculture built around the practices of "butch–femme" identities. Historically, these practices arose in the 19th century (Faderman, 1991) and were codified in urban working class cultures of the 1940s and 50s as an erotic style, with butch women more masculine in appearance and behavior and defined by their desire for femme women (Kennedy & Davis, 1993). With the rise of feminism in the late 1960s and 70s, White butch–femme couples were denounced as "mimicking" heterosexual relationships, and there was pressure on lesbian and bisexual women to appear more androgynous (Faderman, 1991). However, butch–femme relationships only superficially looked like heterosexual relationships— they were polarized by gender, masculine and feminine, but a masculine woman is not a man and division of labor did not follow typical heterosexual patterns (Kennedy & Davis, 1993).

Another shift in thinking occurred in the 1990s with the rise of queer theory and postmodern feminism movements that encouraged individual expression of gender and sexuality (Inness & Lloyd, 1996). Now butch–femme relationships are considered a form of self-identification, are mostly accepted, and not related to class status, although many women do not identify with these labels. In addition, there are butch–butch relationships and femme–femme relationships. It seems that sexual attractions are quite unique and varied from one person to another—what one person finds erotic, another might find a turn-off. Some lesbians/bisexual women are attracted to others with a particular kind of gender presentation and some are not. There is a stereotype that all same-sex female relationships need to have one partner play the "man" and the other the "woman," however, butch-femme is not equivalent to male-female, and the majority of lesbians do not seek out butch–femme relationships.

In one examination of personal ads (Smith & Stillman, 2002), 75% of the ads had no mention of butch–femme identities or preferences. Of the self-identified femmes ($n = 55$ out of 388), most requested femme partners (56%). Among self-identified butch lesbians ($n = 45$), 74% requested femme partners. All women fall somewhere on a continuum between extremely masculine and extremely feminine, and whereas most lesbian/bisexual women can categorize themselves, the majority do not seek partners who are on the "opposite" end of the spectrum. Being more "masculine" or gender-nonconforming can lead to an earlier adoption of a lesbian identity. Levitt & Horne (2002) reported that femme women recognized their sexuality at a later age (22) than did butch women (15).

Only a handful of studies have examined health outcomes or risk factors related to women's gender expression. One study found that butch-identified lesbians tend to prefer and value a larger body size (Ludwig & Brownell, 1999). Another study found a stronger desire for muscularity among butch lesbians (Yean et al., 2013). Greater masculinity in women may be associated with a rejection of feminine beauty standards, so butch lesbians may feel less pressure to conform to feminine body norms, and be satisfied or even desire a greater weight. Femme-identified women may share concerns about weight and body appearance with heterosexual women, since they have similar values about projecting a feminine appearance.

Lesbians with butch identities were more likely to report childhood traumas than femme-identified women, who experienced more victimization in adulthood (Lehavot, Molina, & Simoni, 2012). Butch-identified women tend to come out at earlier ages and experience more discrimination, minority stress, and substance use (Lehavot & Simoni, 2011; Rosario, Schrimshaw, & Hunter, 2008). On the other hand, femme-identified women can more readily conceal their sexual identity, so they may suffer greater levels of internalized homophobia related to guilt about passing (Hie-stand & Levitt, 2005; Lehavot & Simoni, 2011).

Gay and bisexual men do not have the same political history with feminism that women do, but they also benefited from feminist and queer movements that opened up the concepts of gender. Some men choose to adopt a hypermasculine physique, with almost pathological devotion to the gym (Blashill, 2010). However, this masculine physical appearance may or may not be paired with traditional masculine behaviors. Other men express their feminine natures more, and at the extreme end of the continuum, might be described as "queens." Yet others shift roles and deliberately play with their gender. Sanchez and Vilain (2012) found that masculinity was more highly valued among gay men, both in themselves and others, than femininity, and that feeling less "masculine" might be related to internalized homophobia. The majority of LGBTQ people, however, fit into some vaguely defined "typical" gender expression, conforming at least to some extent to gender stereotypes for their biological sex or gender identity.

Resiliency

It is rather amazing that in the face of so much societal pressure to be heterosexual and to be clearly male/masculine or female/feminine that so many LGBTQ people thrive and are psychological and physically healthy. The concept of resiliency may be pertinent here. Facing and surviving adversity may make a person stronger. They must learn coping strategies and build creative and strong social support networks. LGBTQ people have found ways to have loving and strong families in the absence of legal and societal support. They have built community structures, such as LGBTQ community centers, bookstores, restaurants, coffee shops, religious and spiritual groups, political advocacy organizations, and a host of local community events from pride festivals to weekly potlucks and dances. In addition, the internet opened up the world to more isolated LGBTQ people, who have built social support and found information to help them survive. Growing media coverage of LGBTQ issues and portrayal of those who live their lives in very similar ways to heterosexual people, has increased the acceptability of being LGBTQ in families and communities at large.

Russell and Richards (2003) studied resiliency factors in LGB people in Colorado following a yearlong campaign for an anti-gay referendum that created deep emotional responses in many citizens. The authors found that there were five major sources of resilience for dealing with the anti-gay sentiment:

1. The ability to place anti-gay comments and actions into a political context (of oppression)
2. Confronting internalized homophobia
3. Being able to express one's anger and other emotions about the stress, which often propelled people to action
4. Being witnessed—having support from family, friends, coworkers, public officials and others, especially heterosexual people who stepped up to challenge the anti-gay rhetoric
5. Support and validation from the LGBTQ community

Kwon (2013) developed a model of resiliency for LGBTQ individuals that may have relevance for healthcare professionals. He proposed that resilience has three overarching factors: (1) social support (of friends, family, coworkers, institutions like religion and schools); (2) emotional openness (the ability to accept and process emotions and see the connections between unfair situations and systemic oppression); and (3) a sense of optimism or hopefulness (seeing stress as a challenge rather than a threat). Mental health providers can help individuals to develop better coping mechanisms that help them deal with stress, but it is critical that we do not focus all of our attention on putting band-aids on LGBTQ people, making them more equipped to deal with oppressive situations. Instead, healthcare systems and providers can work to reduce the stressful situations that result from societal stigma and feelings of exclusion. Only structural change ultimately will reduce minority stress.

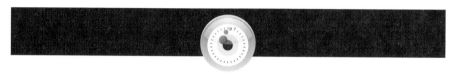

Watch This 7.2

On June 26, 2015, the U.S Supreme Court ruled that it is unconstitutional for any state to ban same-sex marriage, a decision that brought marriage equality to all in the United States. The comments of Jim Obergefell, the lead plaintiff in the case, in response to the ruling, are an inspiring example of the sources of resilience that are so important in overcoming stigma and discrimination. Watch his comments here: **https://www.youtube.com/watch?v=qMxWLJGuPJk**

Conclusions

There is enormous diversity among LGBTQ people and their families. The fact that people may experience stress and oppression on multiple levels makes the study of the origins, processes, and prevention of health disparities very difficult. All the various social identities tend to coexist in the individual, and a person often cannot sort out the sources of stress or resiliency among these different identities. Life is usually perceived as a whole, not broken down into aspects of the personality or specific identities. On the other hand, these multiple identities are what bring texture to life and make us all unique. The key to successful inclusion of all persons in healthcare settings is to be open to this diversity and complexity and see each person as unique.

References

Aranda, F., Matthews, A. K., Hughes, T. L., Muramatsu, N., Wilsnack, S. C., Johnson, T. P., & Riley, B. B. (2015). Coming out in color: Racial/ethnic differences in the relationship between level of sexual identity disclosure and depression among lesbians. *Cultural Diversity & Ethnic Minority Psychology*, *21*(2), 247–257. Retrieved from http://doi.org/10.1037/a0037644

Battle, J., & Crum, M. (2007). Black LGB health and wellbeing. In I. H. Meyer & M. E. Northridge (Eds.), *The health of sexual minorities: Public health perspectives on lesbian, gay, bisexual, and transgender populations* (pp. 320–352). New York: Springer Publishing.

Binson, D., Michaels, S., Stall, R., & Coates, T. J. (1995). Prevalence and social distribution of men who have sex with men: United States and its urban centers. *Journal of Sex Reearch, 32*, 245–254.

Blashill, A. J. (2010). Elements of male body image: Prediction of depression, eating pathology and social sensitivity among gay men. *Body Image, 7*(4), 310–316. Retrieved from http://doi.org/10.1016/j.bodyim.2010.07.006

Cahill, S. (2008). The disproportionate impact of antigay family policies on black and latino same-sex couple households. *Journal of African American Studies, 13*(3), 219–250. Retrieved from http://doi.org/10.1007/s12111–008–9060–7

Cochran, S. D., & Mays, V. M. (2007). Physical health complaints among lesbians, gay men, and bisexual and homosexually experienced heterosexual individuals: Results from the California Quality of Life Survey. *American Journal of Public Health, 97*, 2048–2055. Retrieved from http://doi.org/10.2105/AJPH.2006.087254

Cupolo, A., Corbett, K., & Lewis, V. (1982). *No more stares*. Berkeley, CA: Disability Rights Education and Defense Fund, Inc.

Eliason, M. J. (2000). Substance abuse counselor's attitudes regarding lesbian, gay, bisexual, and transgendered clients. *Journal of Substance Abuse, 12*(4), 311–328. Retrieved from http://doi.org/10.1016/S0899–3289(01)00055–4

Eliason, M. J., Burke, A., Van Olphen, J., & Howell, R. (2011). Interactions of sexual identity, sex/gender, and religious/spiritual beliefs on college student substance use. *Sexuality Research & Social Policy: Journal of NSRC: SR & SP, 8*, 117–125.

Eliason, M. J., Martinson, M., & Carabez, R. (2015). Disability among sexual minority women: Descriptive data from an invisible population. *Journal of LGBT Health Research. Journal of LGBT Health research, LGBT Health, 2*(2), 113–120. Retrieved from http://doi.org/10.1089/lgbt.2014.009

Faderman, L. (1991). *Odd girls and twilight lovers: A history of lesbian life in twentieth-century America*. New York: Columbia University Press.

Fredriksen-Goldsen, K., Kim, H., & Barkan, S. (2012). Disability among lesbian, gay, and bisexual adults: Disparities in prevalence and risk. *American Journal of Public Health, 102*, 16–21.

Fredriksen-Goldsen, K. I., Kim, H. J., Barkan, S. E., Muraco, A., & Hoy-Ellis, C. P. (2013). Health disparities among lesbian, gay, and bisexual older adults: Results from a population-based study. *American Journal of Public Health, 103*, 1802–1809. Retrieved from http://doi.org/10.2105/AJPH.2012.301110

Garland-Forshee, R. Y., Fiala, S. C., Ngo, D. L., & Moseley, K. (2014). Sexual orientation and sex differences in adult chronic conditions, health risk factors, and protective health practices, Oregon, 2005–2008. *Preventing Chronic Disease, 11*, E136. Retrieved from http://doi.org/10.5888/pcd11.140126

Gilley, B. J. (2010). Native sexual inequalities: American Indian cultural conservative homophobia and the problem of tradition. *Sexualities, 13*(1), 47–68. Retrieved from http://doi.org/10.1177/1363460709346114

Grov, C., Bimbi, D. S., Nanín, J. E., & Parsons, J. T. (2006). Race, ethnicity, gender, and generational factors associated with the coming-out process among gay, lesbian, and bisexual individuals. *Journal of Sex Research, 43*(2), 115–121. Retrieved from http://doi.org/10.1080/00224490609552306

Hiestand, K. R., & Levitt, H. M. (2005). Butch identity development: The formation of an authentic gender. *Feminism & Psychology, 15*(1), 61–85. Retrieved from http://doi.org/10.1177/0959353505049709

Hill-Collins, P. (2005). *Black sexual politics: African Americans, gender, and the new racism*. New York: Routledge.

Inness, S. A., & Lloyd, M. E. (1996). Joes in Barbieland: Recontextualizing butch in twentieth-century lesbian culture. In B. Beemyn & M. J. Eliason (Eds.), *Queer studies: A lesbian, gay, bisexual, and transgender anthology* (pp. 9–34). New York: NYU Press.

Institute of Medicine. (2011). *The health of lesbian, gay, bisexual, and transgender people: Building a foundation for better understanding.* Washington, DC: National Academies Press. Retrieved from http://www.iom.edu/Reports/2011/The-Health-of- Lesbian-Gay-Bisexual-and-Transgender-People.aspx

Kastanis, A., & Wilson, B. D. (2014). Race/ethnicity, gender and socioeconomic wellbeing of individuals in same-sex couples. eScholarship: The Williams Institute. Retrieved from http://escholarship.org/uc/item/71j7n35t

Kennedy, E. L., & Davis, M. (1993). *Boots of leather, slippers of gold: A history of a lesbian community.* New York: Routledge.

Koenig, H. G., McCullough, M., & Larson, D. B. (2001). *Handbook of religion and health: A century of research reviewed (see article).* New York: Oxford University Press.

Kumashiro, K. (2001). *Troubling intersections of race and sexuality: Queer students of color and anti-oppressive education.* Lanham, MD: Rowman & Littlefield Publishers, Inc.

Kwon, P. (2013). Resilience in lesbian, gay, and bisexual individuals. *Personality and Social Psychology Review: An Official Journal of the Society for Personality and Social Psychology, Inc, 17,* 371–383. Retrieved from http://doi.org/10. 1177/1088868313490248

Lehavot, K., Molina, Y., & Simoni, J. M. (2012). Childhood trauma, adult sexual assault, and adult gender expression among lesbian and bisexual women. *Sex Roles, 67*(5–6), 272–284. Retrieved from http://doi.org/10.1007/s11199–012–0171–1

Lehavot, K., & Simoni, J. M. (2011). The impact of minority stress on mental health and substance use among sexual minority women. *Journal of Consulting and Clinical Psychology, 79*(2), 159–170. Retrieved from http://doi.org/10.1037/a0022839

Levitt, H. M., & Horne, S. G. (2002). Explorations of lesbian-queer genders: Butch, femme, androgynous, and "other." *Journal of Lesbian Studies, 6*(2), 25–39. Retrieved from http://doi.org/10.1300/J155v06n02_05

Ludwig, M. R., & Brownell, K. D. (1999). Lesbians, bisexual women, and body image: An investigation of gender roles and social group affiliation. *The International Journal of Eating Disorders, 25*(1), 89–97. Retrieved from http://doi.org/10.1002/(SICI)1098–108X(199901)25:13.0.CO;2-T

Maher, M. J. (2006). A voice in the wilderness: Gay and lesbian religious groups in the Western United States. *Journal of Homosexuality, 51*(4), 91–117. Retrieved from http://doi.org/10.1300/J082v51n04_05

Mao, L., McCormick, J., & van de Ven, P. (2002). Ethnic and gay identification: Gay Asian men dealing with the divide. *Culture, Health & Sexuality, 4,* 419–430.

Mays, V. M., Cochran, S. D., & Zamudio, A. (2004). HIV prevention research: Are we meeting the needs of African American men who have sex with men? *The Journal of Black Psychology, 30*(1), 78–105. Retrieved from http://doi.org/10.1177/0095798403260265

Miller, M., Andre, A., Ebin, J., & Bessonova, L. (2007). *Bisexual health: An introduction and model practices for HIV/STI prevention programming.* New York: National Gay & Lesbian Task Force Policy Institute, Fenway Institute, and BiNetUSA.

Miller, R. M. (2007). Lincoln and the American Manifesto. *Library Journal, 132,* 131–132.

O'Toole, C. J. (2000). The view from below: Developing a knowledge base about an unknown population. *Sexuality and Disability, 18,* 207–224.

Pew Research Center. (2013). A survey of LGBT Americans: attitudes, experiences and values in changing times. Retrieved July 20, 2015, from http://www.pewsocialtrends.org/2013/06/13/a-survey-of-lgbt-americans/

Romero, A. P., Baumle, A. K., Badgett, M. V., & Gates, G. J. (2007). Census snapshot: United States. eScholarship: The Williams Institute. Retrieved from https://escholarship.org/uc/item/6nx232r4

Rosario, M., Schrimshaw, E. W., & Hunter, J. (2004). Ethnic/racial differences in the coming-out process of lesbian, gay, and bisexual youths: A comparison of sexual identity development over time. *Cultural Diversity & Ethnic Minority Psychology*, *10*(3), 215–228. Retrieved from http://doi.org/10.1037/1099–9809.10.3.215

Rosario, M., Schrimshaw, E. W., & Hunter, J. (2008). Butch/femme differences in substance use and abuse among young lesbian and bisexual women: examination and potential explanations. *Substance Use & Misuse*, *43*(8–9), 1002–1015. Retrieved from http://doi.org/10.1080/10826080801914402

Russell, G. M., & Richards, J. A. (2003). Stressor and resilience factors for lesbians, gay men, and bisexuals confronting antigay politics. *American Journal of Community Psychology*, *31*, 313–328.

Sanchez, F. J., & Vilain, E. (2012). "Straight-acting gays": The relationship between masculine consciousness, anti-effeminacy, and negative gay identity. *Archives of Sexual Behavior*, *41*, 111–119. Retrieved from http://doi.org/10.1007/s10508–012–9912-z

Sarno, E. L., Mohr, J. J., Jackson, S. D., & Fassinger, R. E. (2015). When identities collide: Conflicts in allegiances among LGB people of color. Cultural diversity & ethnic minority psychology. Retrieved from http://doi.org/10.1037/cdp0000026

Simmons, R. (1991). Some thoughts on the challenges facing black gay intellectuals. In E. Hemphill (Ed.), *Brother to brother* (pp. 211–228). Boston, MA: Alyson.

Smith, C. A., & Stillman, S. (2002). What do women want? The effects of gender and sexual orientation on the desirability of physical attributes in the personal ads of women. *Sex Roles*, *46*(9–10), 337–342. Retrieved from http://doi.org/10.1023/A:1020280630635

Somerville, S. B. (2000). *Queering the color line: Race and the invention of homosexuality in American culture*. Durham, NC: Duke University Press.

Stevens, P. E. (1998). The experiences of lesbians of color in health care encounters. *Journal of Lesbian Studies*, *2*, 77–94. Retrieved from http://doi.org/10.1300/J155v02n01_06

Thomeer, M. B. (2013). Sexual minority status and self-rated health: the importance of socio-economic status, age, and sex. *American Journal of Public Health*, *103*, 881–888. Retrieved from http://doi.org/10.2105/AJPH.2012.301040

Veenstra, G. (2013). Race, gender, class, sexuality (RGCS) and hypertension. *Social Science & Medicine*, *89*, 16–24. Retrieved from http://doi.org/10.1016/j.socscimed.2013.04.014

Wallace, S. P., Cochran, S. D., Durazo, E. M., & Ford, C. L. (2011). The health of aging lesbian, gay, and bisexual adults in California. Retrieved July 26, 2015, from http://www.ncbi.nlm.nih.gov/pmc/articles/PMC3698220/

Walters, K. L., Simoni, J. M., & Horwath, P. F. (2001). Sexual orientation bias experiences and service needs of gay, lesbian, bisexual, transgendered, and two-spirited American Indians. *Journal of Gay & Lesbian Social Services*, *13*, 133–149.

Yean, C., Benau, E. M., Dakanalis, A., Hormes, J. M., Perone, J., & Timko, C. A. (2013). The relationship of sex and sexual orientation to self-esteem, body shape satisfaction, and eating disorder symptomatology. *Frontiers in Psychology*, *4*, 887. Retrieved from http://doi.org/10.3389/fpsyg.2013.00887

Chapter 8

The Effects of Stigma on Health

"The study of why some people swim well and others drown when tossed into a river displaces the study of who is tossing whom into the current—and what else might be in the water." (Krieger, 2001, p. 670)

In Chapter 3, we reviewed the effects of stigma on the everyday lives of LGBTQ people, including lack of recognition of significant others and family, hate crimes, social rejection, and employment discrimination. This chapter addresses the effects of stigma on the health of LGBTQ people. It is easy to fall into an individual focus when discussing health problems and assign individual responsibility for overcoming these problems, such as telling LGBTQ people that they should seek out health care earlier, comply with healthcare prescriptions, and/or learn better coping strategies. Nancy Krieger's astute comment that begins the chapter grounds the discussion, reminding us that stigma arises from societal level influences that impact the individual. Not all LGBTQ people will have overt health problems related to stigma, but the overall hostile climate of society in general and healthcare institutions in particular, creates the conditions for health disparities to develop and fester.

Social stigma refers to severe disapproval and discrimination that is directed by one group toward others based on their perceived or actual membership in a particular group. The disapproval may be manifest in such diverse behaviors as ignoring, invalidating, avoiding, harassing, or even violent actions. Discrimination can occur in education, housing, employment, public services, religious organizations, and health care. Stigma is based on prejudice and stereotypes that unjustly judge the other as deficient, evil, abnormal, inferior, sick, subhuman, immoral, or criminal. These attitudes and stereotypes, reviewed in Chapters 3 and 4, marginalize LGBTQ people from the mainstream of society, deny them basic and fundamental rights of citizenship, create an atmosphere of fear and hatred, and endanger their well-being. Stigma affects society as a whole, because it creates an atmosphere of hatred, hostility, and intolerance, robs the community of the benefits that could be gained by full participation and contribution of those who are stigmatized, increases the health burden of the LGBTQ community, and interferes with the development of potentially supportive relationships among people of differing sexualities and genders.

Stigma can result from visible or relatively invisible human characteristics. Some authors argue that individuals with a concealable stigma can easily hide and therefore avoid the prejudice and resultant discrimination that goes along with visible differences (Goffman, 1963). Recent research suggests, however, that the effort of hiding a stigmatized identity takes an enormous toll and may adversely impact the individual's life. Whereas people with visible differences (such as obvious skin color differences or in a wheelchair) are constantly "out," people with hidden forms of difference must continually make decisions about disclosure, sometimes multiple times in the course of a day. LGBTQ people must weigh "whether, when, how, and to whom to disclose their stigma" (Pachankis, 2007, p. 328), always wondering whether the reaction will be positive or negative. Some authors refer to this internal cognitive processing as "stigma management" (Meyer, 2007) and it adds a level of stress to daily life that heterosexual people may never have imagined.

Sources of Stigma

In the United States, stigma regarding sexual and gender identities stems primarily from one of two sources. The first is from medical discourses based on ideas of disease or biological abnormality, particularly beliefs drawn from the field of psychiatry about sickness, abnormality, or mental illness. The second is the stigma that results from religious or moral beliefs, including the idea of sin or immorality. Sin and sickness discourses coexist in much of the anti-LGBTQ rhetoric throughout the past century, and continue today in the cultural clashes about LGBTQ civil rights. Medical sciences have focused on a search for the cause of minority sexual and gender orientations, but not for the cause of heterosexuality, and for a biological basis for male/female differences rather than focusing on the similarities. By not equally studying how heterosexuality arises, and by making the assumption that men and women have different skill sets, personalities, or behaviors because of biological differences, medical sciences tend to reify sexual and gender difference rather than highlight the myriad similarities among people with differing gender and sexuality (Jordan-Young, 2010). In 1973, the American Psychiatric Association removed sexual orientation from their diagnostic categories of mental illness from the Diagnostic and Statistical Manual of Mental Disorders (DSM), but there continues to be a minority of psychiatrists and psychologists who advocate "reparative" therapies (also called conversion therapy) to attempt to change the sexual orientation of LGB people (see e.g., NARTH: the National Association for Research and Therapy for Homosexuality). The presence of reparative therapy, which has considerable overlap with fundamentalist religious beliefs and religious conversion experiences, perpetuates the myth that minority sexual/gender identifications are associated with mental illness and abnormality, and this contributes to the stigma of being openly LGBTQ.

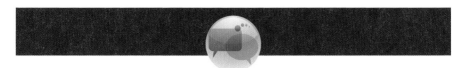

Talk About It 8.1

Most people cannot even imagine someone advising them that they need to change their sexual identity, because most people identify as heterosexual, and take for granted that this could never be challenged or changed. Read this summary of the history of so-called "therapies" to change the sexual identity of people who identify as gay, lesbian or bisexual, then discuss with friends and colleagues.

(continued)

Therapies to change one's sexual orientation stem from psychoanalytic theories in the late 1880s. Although Freud himself was not a supporter of such therapies, his daughter Anna reported that she had successfully changed men's sexual orientation through therapy. Psychoanalytic therapies were common in the United States in the early 1900s and well into the 1960s. The first edition of the Diagnostic and Statistical Manual of Mental Disorders, published in 1952, listed homosexuality as a mental disorder. The three types of therapy still used today include (1) long-term psychoanalysis, (2) forms of behavior modification, particularly aversion therapies, some of which resembled torture in their methods, and (3) ex-gay ministries that focus on gender issues, relationships with same-sex role models/ parents, and/or prayer.

One of the first challenges to the pathologizing of homosexuality came from psychologist Evelyn Hooker in a 1957 publication that corrected the problems with older research based on mostly institutionalized or incarcerated populations. Hooker found normal psychological development in homosexual men. Psychologists who were vocal about the ability to change sexual orientation included Irving Bieber, Albert Ellis, Charles Socarides, Elizabeth Moberly, and Joseph Nicolosi. In the 1990s, the Christian right became much more involved in sponsoring reparative therapies (see Family Research Council, for example), with programs such as Love Won Out and Exodus International.

In 2001, the Surgeon General of the United States, David Satcher, issued the first government-sponsored report condemning reparative therapy. The same year, a study by Robert Spitzer claimed that highly motivated individuals could change their sexual orientation— years later in 2012, Spitzer recanted his study and apologized to the LGBT community. Nearly every professional association in health fields have issued statements against reparative therapy.

California became the first state to ban reparative therapy for minors (2012), followed by New Jersey, the District of Columbia, and Oregon. In mid 2015, several other states had such legislation in the works. These laws only protect minors from being coerced into therapy, but there are still desperate adults and youth who have suffered much rejection and trauma related to their sexual orientation or gender identity that are vulnerable to claims of therapists or religious groups that they can "cure" them.

We discussed the role of religion on attitudes about LGBTQ people briefly in Chapters 4 and 7. A recent rise in fundamentalism has resulted in renewed attacks on the civil liberties of LGBTQ people, most notably focusing on the battles around marriage equality. But there has also been an increase in the number of "ex-gay" ministries (Hedges, 2008), which are ministries devoted to changing people from LGBTQ to heterosexual through prayer, isolation, and pseudo-psychological techniques. Erzen (2006) studied men in one of the oldest ex-gay ministries in the United States and proposed that "ex-gay" had become yet another social identity in place of LGBTQ, and that few of the men actually converted to or considered themselves as heterosexual even after years of prayer, social isolation, and religious intervention. Rather, they learned to suppress their sexual desires by associating only with "safe" people—mostly other "ex-gays" and to deal with frequent relapses and persistent same-sex desires. Research on conversion and reparative therapies confirms Erzen's position—few if any people engaging in these therapies are able to change their sexual attractions or desires (Shidlo, Schroeder, & Drescher, 2002).

The overwhelming lack of evidence that reparative therapy, whether based on religion or psychological theory, changes sexual orientation, and the mounting evidence of the harm inflicted by the attempt to change one's sexuality have led the majority of medical and psychological associations in the United States to denounce reparative therapy as unethical (e.g., The American Medical Association, the American Psychiatric Association, the American Psychological Association, the National Association of Social Workers). California became the first state to ban reparative therapy for nonconsenting youth, making it illegal for parents or religious leaders to force youth into therapy.

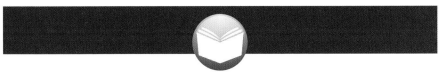

Read This 8.1

Read the full text of the California law banning reparative therapies for youth (**https://goo.gl/4LJKFP**). The Web site has tabs that provide interesting information about the bill, including the history of the bill and an analysis of the bill.

The United States is supposedly built upon a separation of church and state, meaning that public institutions that serve the needs of the population are not to inflict any particular religious viewpoint upon their clients or constituents. This separation of church and state has eroded considerably in the past 10 years, with right to religious freedom laws in several states affecting businesses and healthcare institutions. For example, the Supreme Court's ruling on the Hobby Lobby case opened the door for states to say that individual businesses and people within agencies could refuse to serve people based on their religious beliefs. This allowed magistrates to refuse to marry same-sex couples. Indiana passed such a bill in 2014, but it was softened after national outcry against it and threats to boycott the state. North Carolina in summer of 2015 passed a similar law, in spite of the considerable backlash against the Indiana law. Civil

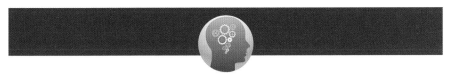

Think About It 8.1

Whereas most healthcare professionals may not conduct or refer clients to reparative therapy or refuse to serve LGBTQ patients (although a small number do), some of them impose their religious beliefs in other ways. Unfortunately, far too many clients are exposed to unwanted proselytizing when they attempt to access health care, as the following example illustrates.

When J. went to the doctor's office in her Florida town, the last thing she expected to receive was a packet of anti-gay propaganda referring to homosexuality as "sinful" and "impure" and advising lesbians and gay men to change their sexual orientation. "When I opened the sealed packet, I was shocked and outraged," says J. "I was extremely offended and I felt like I had been violated." J. made a formal complaint with the office manager, who informed her that their office routinely disseminates the anti-gay materials to patients. When she retrieved her medical records, J. was in for yet another shock. On her chart was written "Scripture references were given regarding homosexuality and lesbianism."

If you were J., what would you have done?

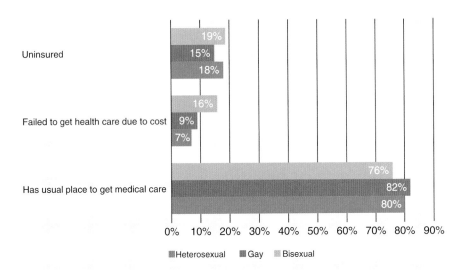

Figure 8.1 – Healthcare Access for Men in the NHIS (Based on **Ward et al., 2014**).

rights work is a constant process of progress and backlash, but as Martin Luther King said, "The arc of the moral universe is long, but it bends toward justice."

The sin and sickness discourses have impacted healthcare institutions in other ways as well, limiting access to healthcare services and affecting the quality of care received once in the system. The National Health Interview Survey (NHIS) included a sexual orientation question for the first time in their 2013 survey and reported indicators of healthcare access including insurance coverage, having a regular provider, and failing to get care because of cost (Ward, Dahlhamer, Galinsky, & Joestl, 2014). Figure 8.1 depicts data for men and Figure 8.2 for women, showing somewhat greater

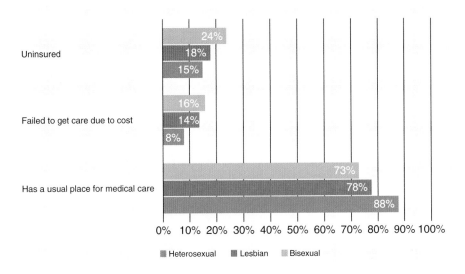

Figure 8.2 – Healthcare Access for Women in the NHIS (Based on **Ward et al., 2014**).

disparities for sexual minority women who simultaneously suffer the stigmas of sexism and heterosexism. Bisexual men and women also suffer more health access issues than do gay/lesbian or heterosexual people.

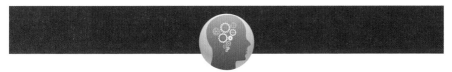

Think About It 8.2

Marion is a male-to-female postoperative transgender woman, and is a pediatrician in a large suburban practice in the Midwest. She is concerned that being "out" would jeopardize her career in her conservative community, so she has told no-one of her gender identity. She lives with her partner of 5 years, a lesbian named Shelly, who has been introduced at work as Marion's roommate. They have a very small circle of friends in the lesbian community, but restrict their public social activities with those friends for fear of being seen by patients or coworkers. Marion needs to find a primary care physician for herself, and is in turmoil about finding a discrete provider who will not reveal her gender and sexual identities to colleagues. The stress of concealing her identities has affected Marion in many ways—she is paranoid and suspicious at work and coworkers think of her as "stand-off-ish." She occasionally has panic attacks, and the secrecy is affecting her relationship with Shelly, who wants to be out and open about their relationship, but fears rejection by the lesbian community as well as by Marion's heterosexual coworkers. If Marion worked in the healthcare setting where you work or receive care, how do you think she would be treated if her gender and sexual identities were known?

Effects of Stigma on Health

"So, you know, in the lesbian community and being gay and being a person of color, being a big person, you know, it's all those stresses. They take a toll on you. And sometimes you just don't want to feel it. You just want to, like, be out and have fun. And sometimes you need alcohol or drugs or whatever, because then you don't feel so self-conscious about being who you are. And that's sad ..." (Respondent in Gruskin, Byrne, Kools, & Altschuler, 2006, p. 110)

The stress related to minority identification can affect people from any disenfranchised or oppressed group. *Minority Stress* refers to the additional stresses experienced specifically because of identification with an oppressed minority group. Minority stress is

1. unique, and adds more stress on top of the general life stressors that many people experience;
2. chronic; and
3. comes from social processes, institutions or structures rather than from individual risk factors such as biological or genetic variables (Meyer, 2007, pp. 243–244).

Mays and Cochran (2001) found that LGB people were more likely to report discrimination in jobs, housing, education, health care, and other settings than heterosexual people. Being denied health care or receiving inferior care was reported by 7% of lesbian/bisexual women, 3% of gay/bisexual men, 3% of heterosexual women, and 4% of heterosexual men (Mays & Cochran, 2001). Xavier, Honnold, and Bradford (2007) reported that 27% of transgender Virginians had no health insurance, 38% did not have a regular physician, 36% felt uncomfortable talking to healthcare professionals about transgender-specific health issues, and 24% had experienced discrimination from a healthcare professional. Much less is known about bisexual people's experiences with health care (Miller, Andre, Ebin, & Bessonova, 2007), but there is mounting evidence that the even greater stigma of bisexuality affects healthcare access (Ward et al., 2014).

Minority stress can come from internal and external sources. Some authors discuss the internalized effects of stigma, called variously in the literature internalized homophobia, internalized oppression, or internalized heterosexism. Internalization occurs when individuals believe the negative stereotypes related to their identities and as a consequence, develop shame, guilt, and self-hatred (Meyer, 2013). They may expect poor treatment from others. However, even well-adjusted LGBTQ people who have rejected the negative stereotypes must deal with minority stress from external sources, such as discrimination, harassment, and threat of violence from others who hold the negative stereotypes. Minority stress results in a heightened sense of vigilance in situations where the person anticipates that discrimination, harassment, or violence may occur. Unfortunately, healthcare settings are among the places where that increased vigilance is at play (Eliason & Schope, 2001; Hitchcock & Wilson, 1992; Stevens, 1994). The increased vigilance takes its toll. It is stressful and energy-draining to always be on one's guard. Of all places, a healthcare setting should be one where patients feel safe and protected.

The high level of internal and external stress can result in new disorders or worsen existing health problems, and may be compounded by lack of access to quality health care. Emotional status and reactions to the environment can have enormous impact on physical and mental health. It is important to recognize when stress is causing or contributing to illness because conventional treatments may not be as effective if the root source of stress is not addressed. People who have experienced chronic stress may no longer recognize the stress because it has become part of their daily existence, so helping them to become aware of stress and finding ways to reduce the stress are important components of treatment. Recognizing that they are not to blame for the negative attitudes of other people is another critical aspect of treatment.

Stress can impact nearly any organ system, but we will focus on the areas where there is a substantial evidence-base about the impact of minority stress related to sexual and gender identification (Frost, Lehavot, & Meyer, 2015; Hatzenbuehler, Slopen, & McLaughlin, 2014). In the next two chapters, we discuss these adverse effects on health in two general categories: mental and physical health problems, although we recognize that there is considerable overlap among these categories. Mental health problems include substance abuse, depression, anxiety, suicide attempts, and body image and eating disorders, and physical health disorders include chronic physical ailments such as diabetes, asthma, heart disease, cancer, and sexually transmitted infections. In this chapter, we focus on the more general effects of stigma on well-being, including intimate partner violence (IPV), effects of living in more restrictive geographic regions without LGBTQ legal protections, and the stress of interacting in healthcare settings.

The Effects of Living in Fear/Uncertainty

There has been increased study of the structural effects of stigma on LGBTQ people's health in recent years. This research has linked increased rates of sexual risk behavior to country-level stigma in an international study (Pachankis et al., 2015) and was also found for differing structural stigma in states in the United States where MSM in more stigmatized states reported less use of HIV-prevention strategies and higher sexual risks (Oldenburg et al., 2015). Among youth, living in an area with fewer protections and resources for LGBTQ people leads to higher drug use (Hatzenbuehler, Jun, Corliss, & Bryn Austin, 2015). Suicide behaviors are also higher among youth who live in neighborhoods with higher rates of hate crimes against LGBT people (Duncan & Hatzenbuehler, 2014) and for youth in schools without gay-straight alliances or protective policies (Hatzenbuehler, Birkett, Van Wagenen, & Meyer, 2014). Finally, one study linked anti-gay prejudice in heterosexual respondents to higher mortality rates. Those with anti-gay attitudes died on average 2.5 years earlier than those with low levels of anti-gay prejudice, suggesting that stigma adversely affects heterosexuals as well as LGBTQ people (Hatzenbuehler, Bellatorre, & Muennig, 2014).

Domestic Violence/Intimate Partner Violence

Much of the literature on domestic violence, or IPV in heterosexual relationships, particularly by feminist researchers, has focused on power imbalances based on gender and explores why men are overwhelmingly the perpetrators of violence and women the victims. This focus on power imbalance based on sexism rendered the possibility of same-sex IPV invisible for years. As more research examined IPV, it has been noted that the incidence of IPV in same-sex couples is about equal to or higher than in other-sex couples (Balsam, Beauchaine, Mickey, & Rothblum, 2005; Greenwood et al., 2002; Tjaden, Thoennes, & Allison, 1999, 2000; Walters, Chen, & Breiding, 2013).

Gender is not the only source of power imbalance in relationships, and it is rare to find couples that are truly equal in all ways. Imbalances in finances, social support outside the relationship, drug and alcohol abuse, the degree of "neediness," fear of being outed, and the stress of stigma (minority stress), as well as sexism and heterosexism, are factors in same-sex IPV. In addition, in heterosexual couples, depression and alcohol use are associated with higher rates of abuse, particularly bidirectional partner violence, and since both depression and alcohol use are higher among LGBTQ people, they may drive the higher rates of partner abuse seen in some studies (Lewis et al., 2015).

A systematic review of the literature on lesbians and IPV (Badenes-Ribera, Bonilla-Campos, Frias-Navarro, Pons-Salvador, & Monterde-I-Bort, 2015) pointed out that the majority of studies in the past have methodological flaws, with the majority employing convenience samples of mostly White and well-educated women. The victimization rates reported in these studies ranged from 10% to 73% and the perpetration rates from 17% to 75%, probably because of the different definitions and measures of violence used across these studies. Walters et al. (2013) reported prevalence rates from a probability sample from the CDC, as shown in Figure 8.3. This data show that bisexual women have the highest rates of lifetime victimization (with 95% of that from male partners). These data are even more shocking when one considers the definition of victimization

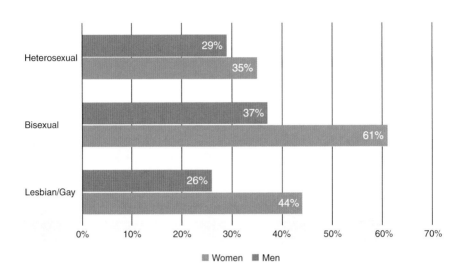

Figure 8.3 – Prevalence of Intimate Partner Victimization in a Lifetime by Sexual Orientation and Gender (Based on **Walters et al., 2013**).

here: lifetime experience of rape, physical violence, or stalking. Emotional abuse and verbal abuse are not included in this data, yet we know they are even more common occurrences.

One study found higher rates of IPV among transgender people (52%) compared to cis gender people (34%) (Langenderfer-Magruder, Whitfield, Walls, Kattari, & Ramos, 2014). HIV positive and younger men were more vulnerable to violence than HIV negative and older men. In addition, LGBTQ people are more likely to experience psychological and physical violence within their intimate relationships, presumably because the stresses of same-sex relationships are greater (Badenes-Ribera et al., 2015; Balsam et al., 2005). One way that domestic violence might differ in same-sex relationships is that the abusive partner may use the threat of outing the individual to their boss, parents, or other people, and use that threat to isolate the partner from potential social support (Pitt & Dolan-Soto, 2001). Additionally, the abusing partner might use the threat of stigma to deter the victim from seeking help ("the police never believe queers") or state that no one would believe the victims story ("no one is going to believe that a woman could be the perpetrator" or "no one would believe that men can be victims").

The underlying reasons for violence are often the same as in other-sex relationships (such as power, finances, fears of abandonment), but the resources for intervention/treatment are much more limited (Calton, Cattaneo, & Gebhard, 2015). Battered women's shelters often do not know how to deal with female same-sex relationship issues, where the line between perpetrator and victim is sometimes more blurred. Women's shelters usually do not accept men or transgender individuals at all, and one study found that 62% of LGBTQ victims of abuse who sought assistance in a domestic violence shelter were refused services (National Coalition of Anti-Violence Programs [NCAVP], 2013). Men who are battered have very few or no community resources, and may face ridicule or denial that a man could be a victim of abuse. Men who are victimized are seen as "sissies" and stereotyped as inferior men. They often experience secondary victimization from police, courts, hospital staff, social workers, and other healthcare professionals (National Coalition of Anti-Violence Programs [NCAVP], 2013).

Transgender individuals who are sex workers, much like cisgender women sex workers, face much higher risks for abuse from strangers/clients, but little is known about their risk for violence within their intimate relationships. One study reported that 10% of transgender people had experienced intimate relationship violence (Xavier et al., 2007), but many more experience verbal abuse and harassment from parents (22%), siblings (17%), and other relatives (14%) as well as police officers (37%) (Reback, Simon, Bemis, & Gatson, 2001). The National Gay & Lesbian Task Force commissioned a report on issues of transgender individuals in homeless shelters that addresses some of the same problems that transgender people would encounter in domestic violence shelters—this may serve as a useful starting point for those healthcare professionals who work in any kind of residential setting (Mottet & Ohle, 2003). An unexplored potential source of domestic violence among transgender individuals may be their significant others at the time that they "come out" as transgender. As one partner of a trans person put it,

> *"I don't always think staying together is the most positive outcome for a couple. Some SOs [significant others] are much happier when they leave, and it's right for them to do so. Often the transperson is happier too, especially vis-à-vis transition ... especially those who had wives who denigrated them for the cross-dressing for a long time. There's a huge potential for (mostly verbal) abuse of transpeople by partners that no one is really talking about much yet."* (Erhardt, 2006, p. 5)

The Role of Stress/Distress on Health

It appears that minority stress is one of the major factors that influence the health of LGBTQ people. In a study of physical health symptoms and disorders (Cochran & Mays, 2007) when the analysis controlled for psychological distress, most of the differences by sexual orientation on physical health for women nearly disappeared, suggesting that stress was the major underlying factor. For men, physical health problem differences remained even after controlling for psychological distress. Sandfort, Bakker, Schellevis, and Vanwesenbeeck (2009) found that the type of coping strategies for stress in gay men accounted for a considerable portion of their excess mental and physical health problem when compared to heterosexual men. Amadio (2006) found internalized heterosexism to be associated with greater number of adverse consequences from drinking (see also McKirnan & Peterson, 1989). Reilly and Rudd (2007) found an association between internalized oppression and body image in gay men. Warner et al. (2004) found that mental health disorders were associated with demographic factors but also conflict between religion and sexuality and being insulted in school in the past 5 years—these same factors predicted suicide risk. These studies and more suggest that minority stress or stigma is the primary culprit in LGBTQ health disparities of all sorts, from mental health to chronic physical problems.

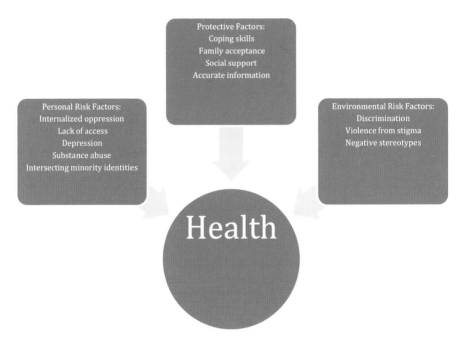

Figure 8.4 – Risk and Protective Factors that Impact LGBTQ People's Health.

Stress can be buffered by the protective factors such as accurate information, family acceptance, social support, and healthy coping strategies. Figure 8.4 depicts the possible relationships among these protective and risk factors—living in the cultural soup of negative stereotypes which create stigma, the LGBTQ individual can have external environmental risk factors such as stigma and negative stereotypes, and personal risk factors such as internalized oppression and stigma consciousness (a heightened sensitivity to stigma), that facilitate the development of physical and mental health problems. Theoretically, if the protective factors outnumber the risk factors, the individual may have strong boundaries to defend against stigma and stay healthy. It is important to keep in mind that many LGBTQ people have strong layers of protection and inner strength that keep them healthy. We do not want to imply that all or even most suffer from physical or mental health problems related to stigma. It is equally important to keep in mind that minority stress and stigma might have impact on the health of family members such as parents, who worry about their LGBTQ children or fear negative repercussions from their communities if their children's identities are known. Minority stress models might also apply to the heterosexual children of LGBTQ parents, or to siblings and other family members of LGBTQ individuals, although little research has focused on these groups.

LGBTQ People's Experiences with Healthcare

This section deals with four main issues that are created by minority stress: disclosure of one's sexual orientation and/or gender identity to a healthcare professional, the reaction that healthcare provider has to the disclosure, treatment received in healthcare settings, and treatment of partners/family in healthcare settings. All of these factors make accessing health care challenging and stressful for LGBTQ people.

Disclosure Decisions

"… I told him that I was gay because if there was a problem I'd rather know right away than build a relationship with a physician and then find out that it was going to be a problem" (Beehler, 2001, p. 140).

"… in kind of the introductory notetaking that the doctor does when they ask you about your medical history, pregnancies, are you on birth control, anything kind of hormonally related. And there's usually some question that I just, you know, around pregnancies and stuff and the use of birth control that I usually say I'm in a lesbian relationship so that's not applicable. And I do that proactively, to put them on notice that I'm out about my sexuality and we can deal with this like adults. So I usually make a kind of proactive move somewhere in that interview process, work it into the conversation" (Boehmer & Case, 2004, p. 1886).

A recent study of the likelihood of disclosing one's sexuality to a healthcare provider showed that gay (90%) and lesbian (87%) individuals were more likely to disclose than bisexual men (61%) or women (67%) (Durso & Meyer, 2013), reflecting the greater levels of biphobia and lack of knowledge of bisexual health issues among healthcare professionals. Decisions to disclose one's sexuality to a healthcare professional are rather complex, and may vary according to generation, educational levels, immigration status, race/ethnicity, couple status, gender, degree of connectedness to LGBT community, location (rural/urban), and reason for seeking care (Austin, 2013; Bernstein et al., 2008; Durso & Meyer, 2013). Some people have greater mistrust of healthcare professionals than others and withhold information about sexuality until they feel comfortable, and others disclose on the first visit. Eliason and Schope (2001) studied disclosure experiences of highly educated lesbian, gay, and bisexual individuals from one Midwestern city. They proposed that disclosure was not a simple yes or no situation, and instead, identified four types of disclosure to healthcare providers:

- Active disclosure: The patients directly told a healthcare professional that they were LGB.
- Passive disclosure: Patients indirectly informed the professional via naming a same-sex partner, wearing a t-shirt or button that proclaims one's sexuality and assumed that the provider would pick up the clue.
- Active nondisclosure: A few patients actively lied about their sexuality to avoid negative consequences.
- Passive nondisclosure: The majority experienced a "don't ask, don't tell" situation, where the provider did not ask, so the patient did not tell.

There were differences in both the types of disclosure and other experiences with health care by gender, with women being more likely to actively disclose (43% compared to men 29%). Women used more protective strategies while in healthcare settings, such as bringing someone along for support, closely monitoring the healthcare provider's behavior, scanning the environment for clues of acceptance, and controlling

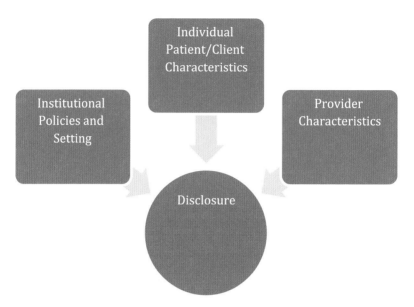

Figure 8.5 – Factors that Influence Disclosure Decisions.

information until feeling safe, than did men. It was suggested that women are more vigilant for two reasons—they are operating under at least two oppressive systems, sexism and heterosexism. The White gay men in this study at least had White and male privilege, if not heterosexual privilege.

Figure 8.5 depicts a model for understanding the factors related to disclosure. On the level of the individual client or patient, age, gender, racial/ethnic identity, religion, educational level, sexual orientation identity label, comfort with own sexuality, comfort with own gender, degree of internalized homophobia, past experience with health care, type of presenting problem (one might be less likely to disclose for an acute problem and more likely for a problem that involves ongoing care), and whether the individual has a partner (whether there is someone who needs to be involved in healthcare decision-making or not). At the provider level, personal characteristics such as age and gender might be important. Some studies suggest that LGBTQ people are more likely to choose female physicians/healthcare professionals because women tend to be more accepting of diverse sexual identities; some perceive younger healthcare professionals to be more likely to be accepting than older ones. Other considerations are body language, verbal language, reputation in the community, and whether the healthcare professional provides an opportunity for patients/clients to disclose. At the institutional level are the policies and procedures such as nondiscrimination policies, staff training, whether benefits are extended to domestic partners of same-sex couples, the written language on the forms, the atmosphere of the waiting room/reception areas, and so on. Which of these factors could you modify in your own work settings?

The research on the percent of LGBTQ people who disclose their sexual and gender identities to healthcare professionals ranges widely, because the overall numbers do not reflect the complexity of the question. Most of the recent research suggests that more than three-fourths of LGB people disclose (less is known about transgender individuals), but this figure may be quite misleading. The LGBTQ people who volunteer to complete surveys about health are probably more "out" in many realms than people who refuse to participate, or are never reached through the sampling procedures. People who label themselves as heterosexual but have significant same-sex experiences have not been studied in terms of healthcare experiences, but are probably less likely to disclose because of the enormous stigma attached to their behavior. They would not be identified unless a healthcare professional asked directly about both sexual identity and same-sex behaviors.

Reactions/Responses from Health Care Providers

In the study by Eliason and Schope (2001), most respondents reported that they had a positive (over 50%) or neutral response from their disclosure to a healthcare professional. However, some reported anger, hostility, discomfort, disgust, embarrassment, fear, and shock on the part of the provider. Some note that when healthcare providers are merely silent after their disclosure, they leave the visit uncertain and concerned that the reaction may have been negative. It is important for care providers to acknowledge the disclosure. A simple statement such as "Thank you for sharing that information" or "Is it ok if I record that information in your medical record?" are neutral ways of acknowledging the disclosure. Those who are comfortable can ask follow-up questions, such as "Do you have a partner?" or "How long have you been out?"

Several studies have gathered the stories of negative experiences. Some of these are recounted below. This first quote indicates an experience with a microaggression rather than any overt discrimination.

> *"When one doctor asked me if I was sexually active (yes) and about what kind of birth control I used, I responded that I didn't use any since I was a lesbian. The attending nurse burst into giggles and flew from the room and the doctor and I finished the exam in silence. This wasn't malicious of course, but did little for my sense of comfort with being open with my healthcare providers (lesbian, age 43)"* (Eliason & Schope, 2001, p. 130).

A respondent in another study experienced judgments about sexual behavior, and the care provider infantilized the patient, and the second one had a care provider who also focused on the stereotype that being a gay man was all about HIV/AIDS:

> *"What I got from him was this judgmental statement like, well, if you should wind up HIV-positive … And he started going into all this stuff like scare tactics, you know. I felt like a thirteen-year-old being lectured about smoking … it took me aback"* (Beehler, 2001, p. 138)

> *"One doctor I just transferred from interpreted every illness in terms of my being gay. Not overtly anti-gay but came not to trust him or feel comfortable discussing my health with me (gay man, age 52)"* (Eliason & Schope, 2001, p. 130).

Finally, one respondent in another study of LGBTQ people in rural areas encountered a referral for reparative therapy based on religion when the patient sought grief therapy:

"Following an episode of … 'weird' behavior, his family took him to an American Indian charismatic healer who identified 'devil possession' … told Leroy that 'homosexuality is wrong … and set up a time for an exorcism" This gay man had sought help for his grief over losing a family member (Willging, Salvador, & Kano, 2006).

LGBTQ People's Treatment in Healthcare Settings

A national LGBTQ advocacy group, Lambda Legal, surveyed LGBTQ people in 2010 about healthcare experiences (Lambda Legal, 2010). Overall, far too many LGBTQ people had experienced poor treatment such as being blamed for their own illnesses (11% LGB and 20% trans people), receiving rough treatment (5% LGB and 8% trans), hearing harsh language from care providers (11% LGB and 21% trans), and even in 2010, 8% of LGB and 26% of trans people had been refused care in a healthcare setting. When the sample was examined by race/ethnicity, the disparities were even more pronounced, with LGBTQ people of color about twice as likely to experience physically rough or abusive treatment from healthcare providers as White LGBTQ people. These are overt acts of discrimination and unconscionable, however, LGBTQ people face even more challenges than these overt acts. Microaggressions are also common in healthcare settings and they increase the level of stress. For example, most healthcare settings are heterosexist—they do not recognize LGBTQ people at all, or if they do, they have no framework for dealing with LGBTQ patients (Röndahl, Bruhner, & Lindhe, 2009; Röndahl, Innala, & Carlsson, 2006).

Treatment of Partners and Family

Another stressor related to health care is how and when the partner or family will be involved in care, and how they will be treated. In areas with no recognition of same-sex relationships, partners without power of attorney (see Chapter 13) may have no legal recourse and may be denied access to their loved ones and have difficulty receiving information about their progress.

"In my experience as both patient and close relative, it's been worse to be the relative—as a patient, they pretty much have to take care of me, but as a relative they can ignore me—like my being there makes the patient homosexual—if I weren't there, she would just be another patient in the lot. But since she had me with her—she suddenly became something else—and it's probably easier to just close your eyes and pretend I'm not there—but I can really only interpret it as if they didn't accept that we had a homosexual relationship—they would much rather talk to our parents, even though we are adults (woman, 30 years)" (Röndahl et al., 2009, p. 378).

"Dr. X on the other hand, had a problem and he asked [my partner] to wait outside. I said you know what? I'm not talking to you without her here. He said, well, we can only talk to a spouse or you know, a family member. I said well, she's both. She's my wife and she's my family. She's my next of kin. I said you know, my mind is not clear and I'm not hearing half the things that are

being said. I want her present. I want her here. So he called her in. But when we were talking … He would only look at me and he would only talk to me." (Boehmer & Case, 2004, p. 1887).

"As soon as I said I was a lesbian, the nurses started giving me disgusting looks. They were nasty to my partner." (Stevens & Hall, 1988, p. 72).

Accessing Healthcare Services

In spite of the stresses of disclosure, and the actual negative experiences of many LGBTQ people, some recent research shows that LGBTQ people use healthcare services at an equivalent or even higher rate than the general population. For example, Bakker et al. (2006) found that gay men were 2.17 times more likely to see a medical specialist than heterosexual men, and 1.6 times more likely to see a mental health professional. Lesbians were 2.06 times more likely to see a mental health provider, but equivalent to heterosexual women in seeing medical specialists (see also Tjepkema, 2008). On the other hand, some research suggests that LGBTQ people might be more likely to use alternative and complementary therapies because of discrimination or mistrust of mainstream healthcare. Matthews, Hughes, Osterman, and Kodl (2005) found that 42% of lesbians had experienced discrimination in health care compared to 35% of heterosexual women, and the lesbians were more likely to use meditation/visualization, chiropractic services, massage, and mental health support groups than were heterosexual women. Similarly, Tjepkema (2008) found that LGB people in Canada were more likely to use alternative care providers than heterosexual people. Chapter 10 deals more with accessing routine care and recommended health screening tests.

There is some inconsistency in this literature on accessing health care. Lewis, Derlega, Clarke, and Kuang (2006) noted that sexual minority individuals often expect to encounter discrimination and prejudice when they access services and as a result, may delay, not access services, or not disclose or feel reluctant to talk about their experiences as LGBTQ to healthcare professionals. More research is needed to address whether those individuals who accessed services more often actually disclosed their sexual or gender identities to the healthcare professional.

Conclusions

Stigma, operating through minority stress, is the major contributor to the elevated risk for physical and mental health disorders in LGBTQ people, working in complex and interactive ways to increase health problems and to decrease access to quality healthcare. The stress of stigma also exacerbates underlying health problems stemming from other causes, making them more debilitating. The burden of stigma-related health disorders can be reduced somewhat by welcoming and inclusive healthcare environments, but interventions are needed at all levels of society to truly improve the health of LGBTQ individuals. Minority stress related to heterosexism, gender normativity, racism, classism, and other forms of oppression need to be reduced via education (such as individual empowerment for clients and culturally appropriate care training for healthcare professionals), healthcare agency policy change, and broader societal change. Chapter 13 addresses institutional factors such as agency climate and policies and procedures.

References

Amadio, D. (2006). Internalized heterosexism, alcohol use, and alcohol-related problems among lesbians and gay men. *Addictive Behaviors, 31*, 1153–1162.

Austin, E. L. (2013). Sexual orientation disclosure to health care providers among urban and non-urban southern lesbians. *Women & Health, 53*(1), 41–55. Retrieved from http://doi.org/10.1080/03630242.2012.743497

Badenes-Ribera, L., Bonilla-Campos, A., Frias-Navarro, D., Pons-Salvador, G., & Monterde-I-Bort, H. (2015). Intimate partner violence in self-identified Lesbians: A systematic review of its prevalence and correlates. *Trauma, Violence & Abuse*. Retrieved from http://doi.org/10.1177/1524838015584363

Bakker, F. C., Sandfort, T. G. M., Wanwesenbeeck, I., van Lindert, H., & Westert, G. P. (2006). Do homosexual persons use health care services more frequently than heterosexual persons: Findings from a Dutch population study. *Social Science & Medicine, 63*, 2022–2030.

Balsam, K. F., Beauchaine, T. P., Mickey, R. M., & Rothblum, E. D. (2005). Mental health of lesbian, gay, bisexual, and heterosexual siblings: Effects of gender, sexual orientation, and family. *Journal of Abnormal Psychology, 114*, 471–476. Retrieved from http://doi.org/10.1037/0021–843X.114.3.471

Beehler, G. P. (2001). Confronting the culture of medicine: gay men's experiences with primary care physicians. *Journal of the Gay and Lesbian Medical Association, 5*(4), 135–141.

Bernstein, K. T., Liu, K. L., Begier, E. M., Koblin, B., Karpati, A., & Murrill, C. (2008). Same-sex attraction disclosure to health care providers among New York City men who have sex with men: Implications for HIV testing approaches. *Archives of Internal Medicine, 168*(13), 1458–1464. Retrieved from http://doi.org/10.1001/archinte.168.13.1458

Boehmer, U., & Case, P. (2004). Physicians don't ask, sometimes patients tell. *Cancer, 101*(8), 1882–1889. Retrieved from http://doi.org/10.1002/cncr.20563

Calton, J. M., Cattaneo, L. B., & Gebhard, K. T. (2015). Barriers to help seeking for lesbian, gay, bisexual, transgender, and queer survivors of intimate partner violence. *Trauma, Violence & Abuse*. Retrieved from http://doi.org/10.1177/1524838015585318

Cochran, S. D., & Mays, V. M. (2007). Physical health complaints among lesbians, gay men, and bisexual and homosexually experienced heterosexual individuals: Results from the California Quality of Life Survey. *American Journal of Public Health, 97*, 2048–2055. Retrieved from http://doi.org/10.2105/AJPH.2006.087254

Duncan, D. T., & Hatzenbuehler, M. L. (2014). Lesbian, gay, bisexual, and transgender hate crimes and suicidality among a population-based sample of sexual-minority adolescents in Boston. *American Journal of Public Health, 104*(2), 272–278. Retrieved from http://doi.org/10.2105/AJPH.2013.301424

Durso, L. E., & Meyer, I. H. (2013). Patterns and predictors of disclosure of sexual orientation to healthcare providers among lesbians, gay men, and bisexuals. *Sexuality Research & Social Policy: Journal of NSRC: SR & SP, 10*(1), 35–42. Retrieved from http://doi.org/10.1007/s13178–012–0105–2

Eliason, M. J., & Schope, R. (2001). Does "Don't Ask, Don't Tell" apply to health care? Lesbian, gay, and bisexual people's disclosure to health care providers. *Journal of the Gay and Lesbian Medical Association, 5*, 125–134.

Erhardt, V. (2006). *Head over heels: Wives who stay with cross-dressers and transsexuals*. New York: Routledge.

Erzen, T. (2006). *Straight to Jesus: Sexual and Christian conversions in the ex-gay movement*. Berkeley, CA: University of California Press.

Frost, D. M., Lehavot, K., & Meyer, I. H. (2015). Minority stress and physical health among sexual minority individuals. *Journal of Behavioral Medicine, 38*(1), 1–8. Retrieved from http://doi.org/10.1007/s10865–013–9523–8

Goffman, E. (1963). *Stigma: Notes on the management of spoiled identity*. Englewood Cliffs, NJ: Prentice-Hall.

Greenwood, G. L., Relf, M. V., Huang, B., Pollack, L. M., Canchola, J. A., & Catania, J. A. (2002). Battering victimization among a probability-based sample of men who have sex with men. *American Journal of Public Health, 92*(12), 1964–1969.

Gruskin, E. P., Byrne, K., Kools, S., & Altschuler, A. (2006). Consequences of frequenting the lesbian bar. *Women & Health, 44*(2), 103–120.

Hatzenbuehler, M. L., Bellatorre, A., & Muennig, P. (2014). Anti-gay prejudice and all-cause mortality among heterosexuals in the United States. *American Journal of Public Health, 104*(2), 332–337. Retrieved from http:doi.org10.2105AJPH.2013.301678

Hatzenbuehler, M. L., Birkett, M., Van Wagenen, A., & Meyer, I. H. (2014). Protective school climates and reduced risk for suicide ideation in sexual minority youths. *American Journal of Public Health, 104*(2), 279–286. Retrieved from http://doi.org/10.2105/AJPH.2013.301508

Hatzenbuehler, M. L., Jun, H.J., Corliss, H. L., & Bryn Austin, S. (2015). Structural stigma and sexual orientation disparities in adolescent drug use. *Addictive Behaviors, 46*, 14–18. Retrieved from http://doi.org/10.1016/j.addbeh.2015.02.017

Hatzenbuehler, M. L., Slopen, N., & McLaughlin, K. A. (2014). Stressful life events, sexual orientation, and cardiometabolic risk among young adults in the United States. *Health Psychology: Official Journal of the Division of Health Psychology, American Psychological Association, 33*(10), 1185–1194. Retrieved from http://doi.org/10.1037/hea0000126

Hedges, C. (2008). *American fascists: The Christian right and the war on America*. New York: Simon and Schuster.

Hitchcock, J. M., & Wilson, H. S. (1992). Personal risking: Lesbian self-disclosure of sexual orientation to professional health care providers. *Nursing Research, 41*(3), 178–183.

Jordan-Young, R. M. (2010). *Brain storm: The flaws in the science of sex differences*. Cambridge, MA: Harvard University Press.

Krieger, N. (2001). Theories for social epidemiology in the 21st century: An ecosocial perspective. *International Journal of Epidemiology, 30*(4), 668–677.

Langenderfer-Magruder, L., Whitfield, D. L., Walls, N. E., Kattari, S. K., & Ramos, D. (2014). Experiences of intimate partner violence and subsequent police reporting among lesbian, gay, bisexual, transgender, and queer adults in Colorado: Comparing rates of cisgender and transgender victimization. *Journal of Interpersonal Violence*. Retrieved from http:doi.org10.11770886260514556767

Lambda Legal. (2010). When health care isn't caring: Lambda Legal's survey of discrimination against LGBT people and -people with HIV. Retrieved May 29, 2015, from http://www.lambdalegal.org/publications/when-health-care-isnt-caring

Lewis, R. J., Derlega, V. J., Clarke, E. G., & Kuang, J. C. (2006). Stigma consciousness, social constraints, and lesbian well-being. *Journal of Counseling Psychology, 53*(1), 48.

Lewis, R. J., Padilla, M. A., Milletich, R. J., Kelley, M. L., Winstead, B. A., Lau-Barraco, C., & Mason, T. B. (2015). Emotional distress, alcohol use, and bidirectional partner violence among lesbian women. *Violence against Women*. Retrieved from http://doi.org/10.1177/1077801215589375

Matthews, A. K., Hughes, T. L., Osterman, G. P., & Kodl, M. M. (2005). Complementary medicine practices in a community-based sample of lesbian and heterosexual women. *Health Care for Women International, 26*(5), 430–447. Retrieved from http://doi.org/10.1080/07399330590933962

Mays, V. M., & Cochran, S. D. (2001). Mental health correlates of perceived discrimination among lesbian, gay, and bisexual adults in the United States. *American Journal of Public Health, 91*(11), 1869–1876.

McKirnan, D. J., & Peterson, P. L. (1989). Alcohol and drug use among homosexual men and women: Epidemiology and population characteristics. *Addictive Behaviors, 14*(5), 545–553. Retrieved from http://doi.org/10.1016/0306–4603(89)90075–0

Meyer, I. H. (2007). Prejudice and discrimination as social stressors. In I. H. Meyer & M. E. Northridge (Eds.), *The health of sexual minorities: Public health perspectives on lesbian, gay, bisexual, and transgender populations* (pp. 242–267). New York: Springer. Retrieved from http://doi.org/10.1007/978–0–387–31334–4_10

Meyer, I. H. (2013). Prejudice, social stress, and mental health in lesbian, gay, and bisexual populations: Conceptual issues and research evidence. *Psychology of Sexual Orientation and Gender Diversity, 1-S,* 3–26. Retrieved from http://doi.org/ http://dx.doi.org/10.1037/2329–0382.1.S.3

Miller, M., Andre, A., Ebin, J., & Bessonova, L. (2007). *Bisexual health: An introduction and model practices for HIV/STI prevention programming.* New York: National Gay & Lesbian Task Force Policy Institute, Fenway Institute, and BiNetUSA.

Mottet, L., & Ohle, J. (2003). *Transitioning our shelters: A guide to making homeless shelters safe for transgender people.* New York: The National Coalition for the Homeless and the National Gay and Lesbian Task Force Policy Institute.

National Coalition of Anti-Violence Programs (NCAVP). (2013). 2012 Report on lesbian, gay, bisexual, transgender, queer, and HIV-affected hate violence. Retrieved July 5, 2015, from http://www.avp.org/resources/avp-resources/248

Oldenburg, C. E., Perez-Brumer, A. G., Hatzenbuehler, M. L., Krakower, D., Novak, D. S., Mimiaga, M. J., & Mayer, K. H. (2015). State-level structural sexual stigma and HIV prevention in a national online sample of HIV-uninfected MSM in the United States. *AIDS, 29*(7), 837–845. Retrieved from http://doi.org/10.1097/QAD.0000000000000622

Pachankis, J. E. (2007). The psychological implications of concealing a stigma: A cognitive-affective-behavioral model. *Psychological Bulletin, 133*(2), 328–345. Retrieved from http://doi.org/10.1037/0033–2909.133.2.328

Pachankis, J. E., Hatzenbuehler, M. L., Hickson, F., Weatherburn, P., Berg, R. C., Marcus, U., & Schmidt, A. J. (2015). Hidden from health: Structural stigma, sexual orientation concealment, and HIV across 38 countries in the European MSM Internet Survey. *AIDS, 29*(10), 1239–1246. Retrieved from http://doi.org/10.1097/QAD.0000000000000724

Pitt, E., & Dolan-Soto, D. (2001). Clinical considerations in working with victims of same-sex domestic violence. *Journal of the Gay and Lesbian Medical Association,* 5:163.

Reback, C. J., Simon, P. A., Bemis, C. C., & Gatson, B. (2001). The Los Angeles transgender health study: Community report. Retrieved July 26, 2015, from http://friendscommunitycenter.org/documents/LA_Transgender_Health_Study.pdf

Reilly, A., & Rudd, N. A. (2007). Stress and dress: Investigating the relationship between social anxiety and appearance management among gay and straight men. *Journal of Homosexuality, 52*(3–4), 151–166. Retrieved from http://doi.org/10.1300/J082v52n03_07

Röndahl, G., Bruhner, E., & Lindhe, J. (2009). Heteronormative communication with lesbian families in antenatal care, childbirth and postnatal care. *Journal of Advanced Nursing, 65*(11), 2337–2344. Retrieved from http://doi.org/10.1111/j.1365–2648.2009.05092.x

Röndahl, G., Innala, S., & Carlsson, M. (2006). Heterosexual assumptions in verbal and non-verbal communication in nursing. *Journal of Advanced Nursing, 56*(4), 373–381. Retrieved from http://doi.org/10.1111/j.1365–2648.2006.04018.x

Sandfort, T. G. M., Bakker, F., Schellevis, F., & Vanwesenbeeck, I. (2009). Coping styles as mediator of sexual orientation- related health differences. *Archives of Sexual Behavior, 38*(2), 253–263. Retrieved from http://doi.org/10.1007/s10508–007–9233–9

Shidlo, A., Schroeder, M., & Drescher, J. (2002). *Sexual conversion therapy: Ethical, clinical and research perspectives.* New York: Haworth.

Stevens, P. E. (1994). Protective strategies of lesbian clients in health care environments. *Research in Nursing & Health, 17*(3), 217–229.

Stevens, P. E., & Hall, J. M. (1988). Stigma, health beliefs and experiences with health care in lesbian women. *Image–The Journal of Nursing Scholarship, 20*(2), 69–73.

Tjaden, P., Thoennes, N., & Allison, C. J. (1999). Comparing violence over the life span in samples of same-sex and opposite-sex cohabitants. *Violence and Victims, 14*(4), 413–425.

Tjaden, P., Thoennes, N., & Allison, C. J. (2000). Comparing stalking victimization from legal and victim perspectives. *Violence and Victims, 15*(1), 7–22.

Tjepkema, M. (2008). Health care use among gay, lesbian and bisexual Canadians. *Health Reports/Statistics Canada, Canadian Centre for Health Information = Rapports Sur La Sante/Statistique Canada, Centre Canadien D'information Sur La Sante, 19*(1), 53–64.

Walters, M. L., Chen, J., & Breiding, M. J. (2013). The National Intimate Partner and Sexual Violence Survey: 2010 findings on victimization by sexual orientation. Retrieved June 27, 2015, from http://www.cdc.gov/violenceprevention/pdf/nisvs_sofindings.pdf

Ward, B. W., Dahlhamer, J. M., Galinsky, A. M., & Joestl, S. S. (2014). Sexual orientation and health among U.S. adults: National health interview survey, 2013. *National Health Statistics Reports*, (77), 1–10.

Warner, J., McKeown, E., Griffin, M., Johnson, K., Ramsay, A., Cort, C., & King, M. (2004). Rates and predictors of mental illness in gay men, lesbians and bisexual men and women: Results from a survey based in England and Wales. *The British Journal of Psychiatry: The Journal of Mental Science, 185*, 479–485. Retrieved from http://doi.org/10.1192/bjp.185.6.479

Willging, C. E., Salvador, M., & Kano, M. (2006). Brief reports: Unequal treatment: mental health care for sexual and gender minority groups in a rural state. *Psychiatric Services, 57*(6), 867–870. Retrieved from http://doi.org/10.1176/appi.ps.57.6.867

Xavier, J., Honnold, J. A., & Bradford, J. B. (2007). *The health, health-related needs, and life-course experiences of transgender Virginians*. Richmond, VA: VA Department of Health.

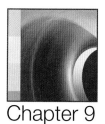

Chapter 9

Substance Abuse and Mental Health

"Everyone's at bars … It's a really small town and there's bars everywhere and everybody, all everyone is doing is drinking. Even in the cafes they're drinking." (Respondent in Condit, Kitaji, Drabble, & Trocki, 2011, p. 351)

As suggested by the quote above, for many young LGBTQ people who came out in a bar context, there is a perception that all LGBTQ people drink. Of course, this is not true, and most LGBTQ people are moderate, light, or nondrinkers, but there is a disproportionate number of LGBTQ people who develop problems with substances. The emphasis on bars is certainly one, but not the only or most important factor in higher rates of substance use. Mental health disorders and substance use are often linked: people use substances to self-medicate painful emotions and/or long-term substance use creates mental health problems. Minority stress plays a role in creating and perpetuating these problems that affect the quality of life of LGBTQ individuals, families, and communities.

Old literature from the late 1800s up to the 1970s tended to link homosexuality with alcoholism and mental disorders, and it was not until there were many years of research to dispel this myth and remove homosexuality from DSM, that there was more thoughtful research on the reasons for higher substance use and mental health disorders (Hughes, 2011). Instead of something inherent in the person, the cause is associated with minority stress and stigma, and at least three sets of factors predict higher rates of both mental health and substance use disorders among LGBTQ individuals. These three factors include (1) living in a hostile unwelcoming climate, such as states or local regions with no legal protections for LGBT people (Hatzenbuehler, McLaughlin, Keyes, & Hasin, 2010) or schools without any LGBTQ friendly groups or policies (e.g., Heck et al., 2014); (2) experiences of discrimination and harassment (e.g., Bostwick, Boyd, Hughes, West, & McCabe, 2014; Nuttbrock et al., 2014); and (3) higher rates of adverse childhood experiences (Blosnich & Andersen, 2014; Friedman et al., 2011; Schneeberger, Dietl, Muenzenmaier, Huber, & Lang, 2014). This chapter begins with a discussion of substance use, including alcohol, drugs, and tobacco, and then discusses common Axis I mental health disorders: depression, anxiety, and suicide.

Substance Abuse

Alcohol Use and Abuse

Several studies have identified higher rates of alcohol-related problems in LGBTQ persons (Bloomfield, 1993; Cochran, Keenan, Schober, & Mays, 2000; Crosby, Stall, Paul, & Barrett, 1998; Dibble, Roberts, Robertson, & Paul, 2002; Drabble & Trocki, 2005;

Table 9.1 – Heavy Drinking and Alcohol Dependence in the Past Year (Data Derived From McCabe et al., 2009)		
	Past Year Heavy Drinking	**Past Year Alcohol Dependence**
Women		
Lesbian	20%	13%
Bisexual	25%	16%
Heterosexual	8%	3%
Men		
Gay	18%	17%
Bisexual	16%	20%
Heterosexual	14%	6%

Garofalo, Mustanski, McKirnan, Herrick, & Donenberg, 2007; Halkitis, Palamar, & Mukherjee, 2007; Hughes, 2003; Hughes et al., 2006; McKirnan & Peterson, 1989; Skinner & Otis, 1996), although the research on rates of current heavy or problematic drinking is less clear. Table 9.1 shows data for heavy drinking and past year alcohol dependence from a large national study (McCabe, Hughes, Bostwick, West, & Boyd, 2009).

LGBTQ people who are in their young adulthood years may drink at comparable rates to their peers as late adolescence and young adulthood tend to be the highest drinking years of the lifespan, whereas older LGBTQ people may drink at higher rates (McKirnan & Peterson, 1989; Skinner & Otis, 1996). In the general population, most adults "mature out" of heavy drinking that occurs mostly in late adolescence and young adulthood. As people marry, have children, and get established in their careers, they go to bars less often and in general, party less. A subset of LGBTQ people who do not (or could not in the past) marry, do not have children, and/or live in neighborhoods or communities where bars or parties with alcohol are readily available, may continue to drink at higher rates through their midlife and elder years, especially if they have found their partners and close friends through these drinking circles. For a more detailed discussion of risk and protective factors for substance abuse, see Hughes and Eliason (2002). Alcohol use and abuse are complex issues, and differing constellations of identities may result in different patterns of use. For example, Mereish and Bradford (2014) found the odds of having a substance use disorder were higher for lesbian and bisexual women compared to heterosexual women (AOR = 2.24) and for gay/bisexual men compared to heterosexual men (AOR = 1.54), but when studied by race, the picture was more complex. White gay and bisexual men had higher rates of substance use disorders than gay/bisexual men of color; but the opposite was true for women, where lesbian/bisexual women of color had higher rates of substance abuse than White lesbian/bisexual women.

Drug Abuse

There is also evidence of higher lifetime and current use of illicit drugs in LGBTQ populations (Cochran, Ackerman, Mays, & Ross, 2004; Drabble & Trocki, 2005; McKirnan

Table 9.2 – Past Year Drug Use and Dependence (Data Derived From McCabe et al., 2009)			
	Marijuana	**Other Drug**	**Drug Dependence**
Women			
Lesbian	17%	13%	8%
Bisexual	22%	14%	3%
Heterosexual	3%	3%	1%
Men			
Gay	25%	17%	4%
Bisexual	13%	18%	6%
Heterosexual	6%	5%	1%

& Peterson, 1989; Skinner & Otis, 1996). Table 9.2 shows data from a national study on marijuana use, other drug use, and diagnoses of drug dependence (combining marijuana and other drug dependence). With changing social norms (and laws) regarding marijuana use, the differences between sexual minority and heterosexual populations may decrease in the future.

Many studies have found different patterns of drug use in lesbians and gay men. Drabble and Trocki (2005) found that lesbians were almost five times more likely and bisexual women six times more likely than heterosexual women to report past year marijuana use. Other illegal substances (e.g., cocaine, methamphetamine, heroin) are used at low frequencies among lesbians as well as heterosexual women. Gay men often use a constellation of substances that differs from lesbians and from heterosexual men. They are more likely to use stimulant drugs as sexual enhancers, such as "club drugs" like ecstasy, poppers, and methamphetamine (Halkitis, Green, & Mourgues, 2005; Koblin et al., 2003; Stall et al., 2001). These drugs, particularly methamphetamine, enhance both the emotional and physical pleasure of sex and prolong sexual encounters, which also increases the risk for sexually transmitted infections such as HIV and hepatitis. The drug and sexual activities may become linked, so that after treatment/abstinence from the drug, sex itself may be a relapse trigger for drug use (Diaz, Heckert, & Sanchez, 2005; Halkitis, Green, & Mourgues, 2005; Semple, Zians, Grant, & Patterson, 2006).

Transgender women, particularly those who are sex workers, have high lifetime rates of illicit drug use. A study in San Francisco reported the following lifetime rates: marijuana, 90%; cocaine, 66%; speed, 57%; LSD, 52%; poppers, 50%; crack, 48%; and heroin, 24% (Clements-Nolle, Marx, Guzman, & Katz, 2001). For many sex workers, drugs are used to cope with the stigma, and drug use/dealing and sex work often go hand in hand. In addition, some transgender women inject silicone or other oils (including liquid paraffin, petroleum jelly, lanolin, flax oil, olive oil, tire sealant, automotive transmission fluid) to give them "curves" that allow them to better pass as women, thus be safer on the street. Variously called "contouring," "fillers," or "getting pumped," these materials are used in lieu of cosmetic surgeries in those who cannot afford surgery (Wilson, Rapues, Jin, & Raymond, 2014). In some urban areas, rates of injecting some substance for cosmetic reasons may be as high as 25% to 33% (Shoptaw, Reback, & Freese, 2002; Xavier, Bobbin, Singer, & Budd, 2005). Often done under unsanitary conditions, with dirty or shared needles, and drugs obtained from the street (with unknown purity), the practice carries risk of HIV and hepatitis, systemic illness, disfigurement, and even death, if the material enters the bloodstream. Over time, silicone and other oils succumb to gravity and settle. It is important for healthcare professionals to assist transgender individuals in identifying safe medical access to hormones and cosmetic procedures, and provide accurate information about the dangers of fillers. Hormones, such as estrogen and testosterone, can also be obtained on the street, and therefore carry risks related to unknown purity and dosage. One study found that trans women who got good transition-related medical services had lower injection drug use (and also lower rates of suicide thoughts and binge drinking) than women without access to transition services (Wilson, Chen, Arayasirikul, Wenzel, & Fisher Raymond, 2014), suggesting that culturally sensitive services lead to better overall health. The motto of the Tom Waddell Clinic in San Francisco, serving transgender populations, is "they came for the hormones; they stayed for the health care." Healthcare professionals who are knowledgeable about transition care may inspire more confidence in their trans patients, and lead to better care overall.

In general, injection drug use carries the highest physical health risks of any substance use. One-third of transgender individuals in San Francisco reported lifetime use of IV drugs (Zevin, 2000) and 22% had a steady sex partner who injected drugs (Nemoto, Luke, Mamo, Ching, & Patria, 1999). Injection drug use among gay men and lesbians is lower than alcohol and noninjection drug use, but still significantly higher than for heterosexual samples. One study of lesbian and bisexual women from low income households found a lifetime rate of injection drug use at 22% compared to 3% for heterosexual women (Scheer, Parks, et al., 2002; Scheer, Peterson, et al., 2002). For gay men (or MSM in general), incidence of injection drug use varies. In one study of young MSM in New York City, nonhomeless MSM had very low rates of current injection drug use (0.3%), homeless youth had higher rates (6%), and MSM who were regular speed users had the highest rates, at 11.9% (Clatts, Goldsamt, & Yi, 2005; Kipke, Weiss, & Wong, 2007; Kral et al., 2005).

Treatment for Alcohol and Drug Problems

There are only a handful of LGBTQ-specific treatment programs in the United States, so most LGBTQ people must seek treatment in mainstream programs, some of which have culturally sensitive programs or counselors. Unfortunately, many substance abuse treatment counselors are not knowledgeable or inclusive of LGBTQ people. There are over 500 Alcoholics Anonymous or Narcotics Anonymous groups specifically for LGBTQ people, but most LGBTQ people attend self-help groups that are designed for heterosexual people. In these programs and self-help groups, LGBTQ people face the same prejudices and discrimination from staff and other clients as they do in everyday life, but at a time when they are even more vulnerable and need support (Cochran, Peavy, & Cauce, 2007; Eliason, 2000; Eliason & Hughes, 2004). Some studies find that LGBTQ people enter treatment with more severe drug and mental health issues than do heterosexuals (Klein & Ross, 2014) but few studies have examined whether the mainstream substance abuse treatment modalities are successful for LGBTQ patients

(Shoptaw et al., 2005, 2008). Because of the higher prevalence of mental health disorders among LGBTQ people, including and especially those with substance use disorders as well, the road to recovery is often more challenging (Lipsky et al., 2012).

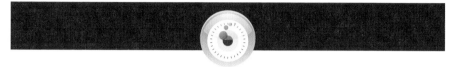

Watch This 9.1

Recovery programs dedicated to the specific challenges of LGBTQ addiction are still rare, but they do exist, and many mainstream programs and groups are becoming increasingly responsive to the unique challenges that LGBTQ people face. Here is a hour-long video with stories told by LGBTQ people about their experiences of recovery.
https://goo.gl/KYxUwW

One effect of external sources of minority stress is that gay bars became one of the central institutions for social support, and one of the few safe spaces where LGBTQ people can congregate and be themselves (Warwick, Douglas, Aggleton, & Boyce, 2003). Smoking and drinking are the primary activities in a bar, and if one meets friends and partners in bars, they are more likely to develop social networks of smokers and drinkers (Weinberg, Williams, & Pryor, 1994). This emphasis on a bar culture may lead to more permissive social norms about alcohol and drug use (Cochran, Grella, & Mays, 2012). Some LGBTQ people, particularly those from racial/ethnic or religious backgrounds that are more negative about same-sex behaviors and those who engage in same-sex behaviors but do not label themselves as LGBTQ, may use substances to overcome shame and guilt about sexual activities (Amadio, 2006; Semple, Patterson, & Grant, 2002) or to offer an excuse for same-sex behaviors ("I was drunk and didn't know what I was doing"). When an LGBTQ person becomes clean and sober, they may need to find new social outlets that serve the same social, emotional, and material forms of social support that gay bars did in the past. This can be challenging in many communities that lack other resources.

Among youth, two major sources of stress that may lead to substance use disorders come from family rejection and hostile school climates. LGBTQ youth who attend schools with gay-straight alliances have a lower risk for use of illicit drugs and misuse of ADHD meds (Heck et al., 2014), showing that even small efforts at school may be very beneficial. Family rejection is all too common even today, and some studies report that bisexual and transgender youth are even more likely to experience parental rejection than gay and lesbian youth. Family rejection is a risk factor for homelessness, a state that puts youth at very high risk for drug use (Anderson, 2009).

Smoking

Smoking is the number one cause of preventable death in the world, contributing to the morbidity and mortality statistics by underlying heart disease, cancer, stroke, and a myriad of lung diseases and other physical health consequences. Of the studies that

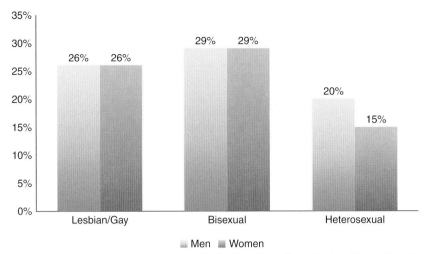

Figure 9.1 – Current Smoking Among U.S. Adults, 2013 (Data Derived From **Ward et al., 2014**).

have gathered information about smoking rates among LGBTQ people, nearly all of them report higher rates than the general population or heterosexual comparison groups (Greenwood & Gruskin, 2007; Tang et al., 2004). Theoretically, nicotine is the ideal drug for stress relief—it is highly portable, widely available, legal, and quick acting, so it is not surprising that people with high levels of stress might be more likely to smoke (Newcomb, Heinz, Birkett, & Mustanski, 2014). The disparity of smoking rates between people in same-sex relationships and people in other-sex relationships is illustrated in Figure 9.1 from a random national survey of people in the United States (Ward, Dahlhamer, Galinsky, & Joestl, 2014).

One study drew a sample from the National Tobacco Survey (Fallin, Goodin, Lee, & Bennett, 2015) and reported that bisexual women had fewer quit attempts, a younger age of onset of smoking, and a higher rate of nicotine dependence than heterosexual or lesbian women. Bisexual men did not differ from gay or heterosexual men. Even if nonsmokers, LGB people are more likely to be exposed to secondhand smoke. In one study, lesbians were more likely to be exposed to smoke in the workplace (21%) than bisexual (7%) or heterosexual (7%) women, and bisexual women were more likely to be exposed to smoke in their households (17%) than lesbian (3%) or heterosexual women (6%). There were no differences among men (Cochran, Bandiera, & Mays, 2013).

Transgender people have not been well-studied in regards to smoking, although one study from the state of Virginia identified even higher rates of smoking than in LGB individuals, with 62% of transgender men and 55% of transgender women reporting current smoking (Xavier, Honnold, & Bradford, 2007). Conron, Mimiaga, and Landers (2010) study of trans people in Massachusetts reported current smoking rates of 36% for trans respondents compared to 17% of nontrans respondents.

LGBTQ people smoke for many of the same reasons as a heterosexual person, but also have higher rates of mood and anxiety disorders than are reported in the general population (Cochran & Mays, 2000a; King et al., 2008). Minority stress (Meyer, 2003) or "gay-related stress" (Rosario, Rotheram-Borus, & Reid, 1996) results from societal stigma, experiences of discrimination, and internalized negative stereotypes about LGBT people (Eliason & Drabble, 2010). One study found that smoking increased the experience of stress, resulting in even greater anxiety, depression, and conduct problems in LGB youth who smoked compared to those who did not (Rosario, Schrimshaw, & Hunter, 2011). Another study found that smoking, sensation-seeking, and impulsivity were related in LGB people (Trocki, Drabble, & Midanik, 2009).

In the general population, mental health problems like depression have been associated with smoking relapse. In one study, Gruskin, Byrne, Altschuler, and Dibble (2008) compared 35 lesbian smokers to 35 heterosexual women smokers; all had a recent failed attempt to quit. Respondents thought that their smoking was related to regulation of negative emotions, stress management, and enhancement of social relationships, but for each category, lesbians reported experiences that were related to sexual orientation stigma. This suggests that stigma related to sexual orientation or gender identity may be a key relapse risk factor for smoking.

Another factor in LGBT smoking is targeted marketing by the tobacco industry. From Project SCUM (an RJ Reynolds plan to market products to gay men in San Francisco), to giveaways at gay bars, funding of LGBTQ organizations and events, and advertising and nontobacco ads and photos that feature tobacco products in LGBTQ publications, the tobacco industry has been engaging in LGBTQ-specific marketing since the mid 1990s (Smith, Offen, & Malone, 2005; Stevens, Carlson, & Hinman, 2004). Stigmatized groups that do not see themselves positively reflected in the mainstream media may be more susceptible to this targeted marketing. In 2006, the cover photo of an LGBT news magazine, The Advocate, featured an actress from the popular Showtime series, The L Word. The scantily clad actress was holding a cigarette and blowing smoke across the top of the page, ironically over text that stated "health matters." Public health advocates were outraged by this depiction of smoking as sexy. Finally, because of the historic and current importance of gay bars in the coming out and social lives of many LGBTQ people and the targeted advertising by alcohol and tobacco companies, drinking and smoking have become "normalized" in many LGBTQ communities, and a libertarian attitude often interferes with public health messages.

Smoking Cessation Programs

It is difficult to address drinking, drug use, and smoking separately, as they so often go hand-in-hand. However, people who seek treatment for their alcohol and drug problems often are not counseled about tobacco use, so rates of smoking remain high even after recovery from alcohol and drug abuse (Eliason & Worthington, 2004). Substance abuse treatment facilities and LGBTQ alcohol and drug-related support groups or self-help groups would be an ideal place for smoking cessation counseling and interventions, as this is the highest risk group for smoking.

One study examined treatment experiences of LGBTQ smokers (Bye, Gruskin, Greenwood, Albright, & Krotski, 2005). This study was a random digit dial survey of Californians, and LGBTQ people were compared to the general population. Overall, LGBTQs were similar to the general population in terms of quit attempts—that is, LGBT people were just as likely to want to quit smoking and just as likely to attempt to quit as heterosexuals (63% of LGBTQ smokers tried to quit in the past year). Of the methods used to quit smoking, 25% of the LGBT sample had used nicotine replacement therapy compared to 16% of general population who used NRT. Unfortunately, fewer LGBTQ people visiting a healthcare professional were advised to quit than heterosexuals. Regarding prevention issues, 37% felt that antismoking campaigns ignore LGBTQ people, and only 32% of men and 20% of women thought that smoking was a bigger problem for LGBTQs than for heterosexuals. Some research indicates that LGB adults are as likely as heterosexuals to desire to quit smoking (Burkhalter, Warren, Shuk, Primavera, & Ostroff, 2009; Pizacani et al., 2009), but among youth, LGB may be less likely to want to quit than heterosexual youth (Remafedi, Jurek, & Oakes, 2008).

One study (Covey, Weissman, LoDuca, & Duan, 2009) compared outcomes for 54 gay/bisexual and 243 heterosexual men in an 8-week intervention with nicotine patch, bupropion and counseling, finding that abstinence rates at the end of the intervention were nearly identical. The authors suggested that generic treatment interventions are effective in the short-term for gay/bisexual participants, but no follow-up data were reported. Other studies have also identified similar success rates with mainstream, non-LGBT tailored smoking cessation programs (Grady et al., 2014).

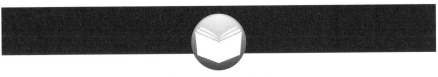

Read This 9.1

The American Lung Association published a free downloadable health disparity report titled "Smoking Out a Deadly Threat: Tobacco Use in the LGBT Community" that is a valuable resource for providers. Here is the Web site that summarizes the report and gives a download link for the report itself: **https://goo.gl/Jp3eQE**

There are a few LGBTQ-specific smoking prevention and intervention campaigns. The public awareness "Gay American Smoke-Out" campaign was introduced in 1994 by the San Jose, California Billy DeFrank Lesbian and Gay Community Center to coincide with the American Cancer Society's "Great American Smoke-Out," typically held the third week in November.

In California and spreading to some other locations, is a curriculum called, *The Last Drag*, which is a group intervention for LGBTQ smokers. It appears to be as successful as any other smoking cessation activity or program, and because it is culturally specific for LGBTQ smokers, may be more attractive than mainstream programs (http://www.lastdrag.org/). In one study, participants of The Last Drag were followed for 6 months after finishing the smoking cessation program (Eliason, Dibble, Gordon, & Soliz, 2012). The Last Drag is a seven session program modeled after the American Lung Association program, but centered in LGBTQ experience and run by LGBTQ facilitators. In the worst case scenario (if all missing data were from participants who had returned to smoking), 36% stopped smoking and were still not smoking at 6 months. In the best case scenario, the success rate was

50%–either result is comparable to mainstream smoking cessation programs. Other culturally tailored smoking cessation programs for LGBTQ smokers have also been found to be successful (Matthews, Li, Kuhns, Tasker, & Cesario, 2013).

A study of transgender women and smoking found that experiencing discrimination was linked to not wanting to quit as well as to less successful quit attempts, demonstrating the positive link between stigma and smoking behaviors (Gamarel et al., 2015).

Finally, structural level interventions to reduce tobacco use such as increased prices and taxes and public efforts to educate the population about tobacco benefit LGBTQ people. Hatzenbuehler, Birkett, Van Wagenen, and Meyer (2014) found a smaller discrepancy in smoking rates by sexual orientation in states with more restrictive tobacco control measures.

Mental Health

Depression and Anxiety

Mental health disorders are biopsychosocial entities, and some are more influenced by genetics and biological factors whereas others have a firmer foundation in social and environmental circumstances that create stress. It is likely that LGBTQ people have about the same rate as heterosexual people of the more biologically based disorders such as schizophrenia and bipolar disorder, but higher rates of disorders that are more directly affected by stress and stigma. Indeed, LGBTQ individuals report higher rates of depression and anxiety disorders than the general population (Bostwick, Boyd, Hughes, & McCabe, 2010; Cochran & Mays, 2000a; Cochran et al., 2001; Gilman et al., 2001; Mills et al., 2004; Warner et al., 2004). Figures 9.2 and 9.3 below show these rates of mood and anxiety disorders by gender and sexual identity.

LGBTQ people of color have even higher rates of depression and anxiety than White LGBTQ people (Cochran & Mays, 1994; Cochran, Sullivan, & Mays, 2003;

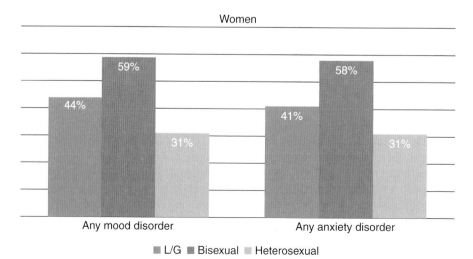

Figure 9.2 – Mood and Anxiety Disorders by Sexual Orientation Among Women (Data Derived From **Bostwick et al., 2010**).

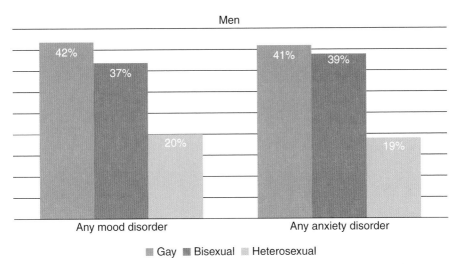

Figure 9.3 – Mood and Anxiety Disorders by Sexual Orientation Among Men (Data Derived From **Bostwick et al., 2010**).

Gilman et al., 2001; Greene, 1997), supporting the idea that multiple sources of stigma adds more minority stress to life. Jorm, Korten, Rodgers, Jacomb, and Christensen (2002) reported that bisexual people had the poorest mental health of any of the sexual identity groups in their study, reflecting the even greater stigma attached to bisexual identity than to gay or lesbian identity.

Transgender individuals fight an additional battle along with the mental health effects of enormous societal stigma—their very identities are still pathologized by the inclusion of Gender Dysphoria in the DSM-V. In addition, the amount of discrimination, harassment, and threatened or actual violence that they experience is a source of constant stress. Many clinics and hospitals that provide hormone therapy and/or perform gender reassignment surgeries require that transgender individuals undergo extensive counseling and receive clearance from a mental health professional before they can have surgery. Finding mental health providers with an expertise in transgender counseling is difficult at best, and putting the mental health provider in a "gate-keeper" role may be a barrier to a productive, therapeutic relationship (Hale, 2007). The need to get clearance from a mental health provider also puts an additional financial burden on transgender individuals. Few insurance plans cover any of the costs of transition.

Suicide

Along with the higher rates of depression are higher rates of suicidal ideation and attempts (Safren & Heimberg, 1999). Among transgender individuals, rates of suicidal ideation are as high as 64%, with the rate of lifetime suicide attempts at 16% to 37% (Grossman & D'Augelli, 2007; Mottet & Ohle, 2003). Cochran and Mays (2000b) reported that among MSM, 19.3% had a lifetime suicide attempt, compared to 3.6% of heterosexual men. Lhomond and Saurel-Cubizolles (2006) examined French women and found that 10.4% of WSW reported a lifetime suicide attempt compared to 3.9%

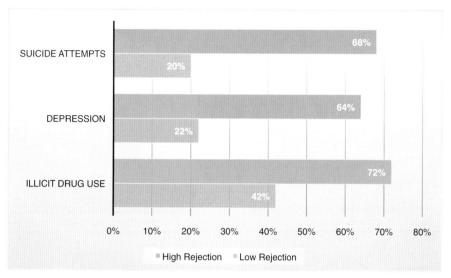

Figure 9.4 – The Relationship Between Parental Rejection and Health Outcomes (Data Derived From **Ryan et al., 2009**).

of exclusively heterosexual women. Nearly every study conducted on suicide attempts and suicide ideation has found higher rates among LGBTQ people (Haas et al., 2011).

Studies of suicide behaviors show a few consistent findings. The attempts that LGBTQ people make are more severe and more likely to result in hospitalizations, suggesting that they are not an attempt to get attention but a true desire to take one's own life (Plöderl et al., 2013). We know little about completed suicide because coroner's reports and psychological autopsy studies have rarely assessed the sexual or gender identity of the deceased (Haas et al., 2011). Suicide attempts may peak during the months or years before coming out (disclosing one's sexual or gender identity), so other people in the deceased person's life may not be aware of the inner turmoil that led to the suicide (Meyer, 2003).

Among LGBTQ youth, family rejection and school bullying are predictors of suicide attempts (as well as depression and substance abuse). Ryan, Huebner, Diaz, and Sanchez (2009) studied how family rejections of children coming out as LGB or T, impacts health outcomes. When the sample was divided into youth who had experienced low versus high rejection from parents, the results were startling. Figure 9.4 shows just how much parental rejection impacts mental health outcomes.

Having support at school is another factor in reducing suicide risks (and other risks as well). Data from the Youth Behavioral Risk Factors Survey from eight states and cities found that LGB students living in locations with protective school climates had fewer thoughts of suicide than LGB students in more hostile school climates (Hatzenbuehler, Birkett, Van Wagenen, & Meyer, 2014).

Body Image

Lesbians appear to be less affected by cultural imperatives for women to be thin, and have higher body self-esteem than heterosexual women (French, Story, Remafedi,

Resnick, & Blum, 1996; Share & Mintz, 2002). Some authors suggest that relating to other women sexually can lead lesbian and bisexual women to appreciate and know their own bodies more thoroughly, and become more confident about their sexual attractiveness, thus the cultural standards about women's bodies lose some of their power (Beren, Hayden, Wilfley, & Grilo, 1996). Being freed from unrealistic standards of physical size and shape may allow stress from stigma to trigger dysfunctional over-eating or binge eating, increasing the risk for obesity. The majority of studies that compare women by weight or BMI have found lesbian/bisexual women to be more likely to fall into categories of overweight or obese than heterosexual women (Bowen, Balsam, & Ender, 2008; Eliason et al., 2015), but the consequences of larger body size have not yet been adequately studied among sexual minority women (Eliason et al., 2015). As will be shown in Chapter 10, there is little evidence for an increase in rates of disorders usually associated with obesity among sexual minority women (Eliason, 2014).

Gay and bisexual men have different pressures—to be lean and muscular (a desire shared by many heterosexual men as well). They are more likely to experience body dissatisfaction than heterosexual men. As heterosexual men's bodies are increasingly objectified in the media, as women's bodies have been for years, men's body images have been suffering. Gay male culture has a long history of objectifying men's bodies in print and in videos, and tends to place strong emphasis on physical attractiveness and youthfulness, particularly in a hypermasculine body (Brand, Rothblum, & Solomon, 1992)—a concept that one commentator called "body fascism." This cultural critic, Michael Signorile noted, "I think it's because we were all insecure, we all feel inferior … gay men are made to feel effeminate, and that's seen as being bad. One way to feel superior is to overcompensate in being macho" (Mann, 1998, p. 348).

Body image problems may be associated with higher risk for eating disorders. Gay and bisexual men are more prone to eating disorders such as anorexia and bulimia than heterosexual men (Carlat, Camargo, & Herzog, 1997; Martins, Tiggemann, & Kirkbride, 2007), and lesbian/bisexual women are more prone to binge eating than heterosexual women (Austin et al., 2009; Bradford, Ryan, & Rothblum, 1994; Mason & Lewis, 2015). The link between minority stress, body image, and eating disorders deserves more attention.

Body image problems are a major component of the transition process for transgender individuals, although the extent to which any individual experiences body dissatisfaction will vary widely. On one extreme, a few transgender individuals are so dissatisfied with their bodies that they mutilate their genitals, and perhaps as many as 1 in 18 have thought about self-mutilation (Israel & Tarver, 1997). Others inject silicone or other oils to appear more feminized, or take excessive amounts of testosterone to masculinize their appearance. Some transgender individuals are not unhappy with their bodies, but change their names, clothing, hairstyles or other outward trappings to match their image of themselves. The common theme is aligning outward appearance with an internal image of oneself. For those who need to align their physical bodies, genital reconstructions, mastectomies, facial reconstructions, and other cosmetic surgical interventions may be necessary. The vast majority of those who have surgical interventions are satisfied with the results—one study of 218 postoperative transgender individuals 4 to 24 years after surgery found that only 3.8% regretted their decision later (Landen, Wålinder, Hambert, & Lundström, 1998). Another study reported high levels of body satisfaction and self-confidence in postoperative transgender men and women (Kraemer, Delsignore, Schnyder, & Hepp, 2008). Hormone therapies are also effective in creating some of the changes that align the physical body with the psychological image, and speech training, gender coaching, and fashion advice may also help (Kirk & Kulkarni, 2006; Lawrence, 2007). Consult with the World Professional Association for Transgender Health (WPATH) for specific healthcare issues related to transition.

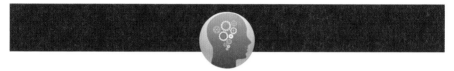

Think About It 9.1

Many people in the press and on talk shows have questioned the "sanity" of genital reconstruction because they are permanent. However, rarely do we question the sanity of a person having a face lift, nose job, or botox injection, procedures which are also relatively permanent and carry risk. Why do we put genitals in a different category than other body parts?

Treatment of Mental Health Issues

More LGB people attend self-help groups than heterosexual individuals—this may represent a cost and time-effective mode of treatment that is acceptable to LGB persons (Grella, Cochran, Greenwell, & Mays, 2011; Jessup & Dibble, 2012). Tjepkema (2008) also found higher use of self-help groups among LGBs in Canada. Some LGBTQ people, especially White lesbians, value therapy as a means of improving the quality of life, but finding mental health providers with a good understanding of the impact of stigma based on sexual and gender identifications can be a challenge (Jones & Gabriel, 1999; Page, 2004). Focusing only on individual level factors in therapy, and ignoring the sociopolitical basis of stigma, can be victim-blaming and counterproductive to improvements in mental health (Kitzinger & Perkins, 1993). Page (2004) surveyed bisexual individuals about their experiences with mental health providers, and found that 10% reported having a provider who was moderately or extremely unaccepting of their bisexuality, and felt that these providers invalidated or pathologized their identities. Similarly, a survey of lesbians and gay men found that 25% had experienced a therapist who was "unreceptive … judgmental, discouraging, or dismissive" of their sexuality issues (Jones & Gabriel, 1999, p. 214).

Conclusions

A consistent finding in the research literature on LGBTQ peoples' responses to minority stress and stigma is that there are higher rates of alcohol, drug, and tobacco use and Axis I mental health disorders, especially depression and anxiety disorders. Some authors relate that the uncomfortable emotions related to internalized oppression (shame, guilt) and the stress induced by discrimination and harassment lead to self-medication with substances as well as leading to mental health disorders. A major challenge for an LGBTQ person with substance use or mood disorders is finding an

LGBTQ competent therapist. Primary healthcare providers can provide a useful service by knowing what resources are available for referrals in their communities.

References

Amadio, D. (2006). Internalized heterosexism, alcohol use, and alcohol-related problems among lesbians and gay men. *Addictive Behaviors, 31*, 1153–1162.

Anderson, S. C. (2009). *Substance use disorders in lesbian, gay, bisexual, and transgender clients: Assessment and treatment.* Columbia University Press. Retrieved from https://books.google.com/books?id / uT1LAAAAQBAJ&dq / Substance%2Buse%2Bdisorders%2Bin%-2Blesbian,%2Bgay,%2Bbisexual%2Band%2Btransgender%2Bclients:%2BAssessment%2Band%2Btreatment&lr /

Austin, S. B., Ziyadeh, N. J., Corliss, H. L., Rosario, M., Wypij, D., Haines, J., … Field, A. E. (2009). Sexual orientation disparities in purging and binge eating from early to late adolescence. *The Journal of Adolescent Health: Official Publication of the Society for Adolescent Medicine, 45*(3), 238–245. Retrieved from http://doi.org/10.1016/j.jadohealth.2009.02.001

Beren, S. E., Hayden, H. A., Wilfley, D. E., & Grilo, C. M. (1996). The influence of sexual orientation on body dissatisfaction in adult men and women. *The International Journal of Eating Disorders, 20*, 135–141. Retrieved from http://doi.org/10.1002/(SICI)1098–108X(199609)20:23.0.CO;2-H

Bloomfield, K. (1993). A comparison of alcohol consumption between lesbians and heterosexual women in an urban population. *Drug and Alcohol Dependence, 33*, 257–269.

Blosnich, J. R., & Andersen, J. P. (2014). Thursday's child: The role of adverse childhood experiences in explaining mental health disparities among lesbian, gay, and bisexual US adults. *Social Psychiatry and Psychiatric Epidemiology, 50*(2), 335–338. Retrieved from http://doi.org/10.1007/s00127–014–0955–4

Bostwick, W. B., Boyd, C. J., Hughes, T. L., & McCabe, S. E. (2010). Dimensions of sexual orientation and the prevalence of mood and anxiety disorders in the United States. *American Journal of Public Health, 100*(3), 468–475. Retrieved from http://doi.org/10.2105/AJPH.2008.152942

Bostwick, W. B., Boyd, C. J., Hughes, T. L., West, B. T., & McCabe, S. E. (2014). Discrimination and mental health among lesbian, gay, and bisexual adults in the United States. *The American Journal of Orthopsychiatry, 84*(1), 35–45. Retrieved from http://doi.org/10.1037/h0098851

Bowen, D. J., Balsam, K. F., & Ender, S. R. (2008). A review of obesity issues in sexual minority women. *Obesity, 16*(2), 221–228. Retrieved from http://doi.org/10.1038/oby.2007.34

Bradford, J. B., Ryan, C., & Rothblum, E. D. (1994). National lesbian health care survey: Implications for mental health care. *Journal of Consulting and Clinical Psychology, 62*, 228–242.

Brand, P., Rothblum, E. D., & Solomon, L. J. (1992). A comparison of lesbians, gay men, and heterosexuals on weight and restrained eating. *The International Journal of Eating Disorders, 11*, 253–259.

Burkhalter, J. E., Warren, B., Shuk, E., Primavera, L., & Ostroff, J. S. (2009). Intention to quit smoking among lesbian, gay, bisexual, and transgender smokers. *Nicotine & Tobacco Research: Official Journal of the Society for Research on Nicotine and Tobacco, 11*(11), 1312–1320. Retrieved from http://doi.org/10.1093/ntr/ntp140

Bye, L., Gruskin, E. P., Greenwood, G., Albright, V., & Krotski, K. (2005). California lesbians, gays, bisexuals, and transgender (LGBT) tobacco use survey—2004. Retrieved July 26, 2015, from https://www.cdph.ca.gov/programs/tobacco/Documents/Resources/Publications/CTCP-LGBTTobaccoStudy.pdf.

Carlat, D. J., Camargo, C. A., Jr., & Herzog, D. B. (1997). Eating disorders in males: A report on 135 patients. *The American Journal of Psychiatry, 154*, 1127–1132.

Clatts, M. C., Goldsamt, L. A., & Yi, H. (2005). An emerging HIV risk environment: A preliminary epidemiological profile of an MSM POZ Party in New York City. *Sexually Transmitted Infections*, *81*, 373–376. Retrieved from http://doi.org/10.1136/sti.2005.014894

Clements-Nolle, K., Marx, R., Guzman, R., & Katz, M. (2001). HIV prevalence, risk behaviors, health care use, and mental health status of transgender persons. *American Journal of Public Health*, *91*(6), 915–921.

Cochran, B. N., Peavy, K. M., & Cauce, A. M. (2007). Substance abuse treatment providers' explicit and implicit attitudes regarding sexual minorities. *Journal of Homosexuality*, *53*(3), 181–207. Retrieved from http://doi.org/10.1300/J082v53n03_10

Cochran, S. D., Ackerman, D., Mays, V. M., & Ross, M. W. (2004). Prevalence of non-medical drug use and dependence among homosexually active men and women in the US population. *Addiction*, *99*(8), 989–998. Retrieved from http://doi.org/10.1111/j.1360–0443.2004.00759.x

Cochran, S. D., Bandiera, F. C., & Mays, V. M. (2013). Sexual orientation–related differences in tobacco use and secondhand smoke exposure among US adults aged 20 to 59 years: 2003–2010 National Health and Nutrition Examination Surveys. *American Journal of Public Health*, *103*(10), 1837–1844. Retrieved from http://doi.org/10.2105/AJPH.2013.301423

Cochran, S. D., Grella, C. E., & Mays, V. M. (2012). Do substance use norms and perceived drug availability mediate sexual orientation differences in patterns of substance use? Results from the California Quality of Life Survey II. *Journal of Studies on Alcohol and Drugs*, *73*(4), 675–685. Retrieved from http://doi.org/10.15288/jsad.2012.73.675

Cochran, S. D., Keenan, C., Schober, C., & Mays, V. M. (2000). Estimates of alcohol use and clinical treatment needs among homosexually active men and women in the U.S. population. *Journal of Consulting and Clinical Psychology*, *68*(6), 1062–1071. Retrieved from http://doi.org/10.1037//0022–006x.68.6.1062

Cochran, S. D., & Mays, V. M. (1994). Depressive distress among homosexually active African American men and women. *The American Journal of Psychiatry*, *151*, 524–529.

Cochran, S. D., & Mays, V. M. (2000a). Lifetime prevalence of suicide symptoms and affective disorders among men reporting same-sex sexual partners: Results from NHANES III. *Journal of Consulting and Clinical Psychology*, *90*, 573–578.

Cochran, S. D., & Mays, V. M. (2000b). Relation between psychiatric syndromes and behaviorally defined sexual orientation in a sample of the US population. *American Journal of Epidemiology*, *151*, 516–523.

Cochran, S. D., Mays, V. M., Bowen, D. J., Gage, S., Bybee, D., Roberts, S. J., … White, J. (2001). Cancer-related risk indicators and preventive screening behaviors among lesbians and bisexual women. *American Journal of Public Health*, *91*, 591–597.

Cochran, S. D., Sullivan, J. G., & Mays, V. M. (2003). Prevalence of mental disorders, psychological distress, and mental health services use among lesbian, gay, and bisexual adults in the United States. *Journal of Consulting and Clinical Psychology*, *71*, 53–61.

Condit, M., Kitaji, K., Drabble, L., & Trocki, K. (2011). Sexual minority women and alcohol: Intersections between drinking, relational contexts, stress and coping. *Journal of Gay & Lesbian Social Services*, *23*(3), 351–375. Retrieved from http://doi.org/10.1080/10538720.2011.588930

Conron, K. J., Mimiaga, M. J., & Landers, S. J. (2010). A population-based study of sexual orientation identity and gender differences in adult health. *American Journal of Public Health*, *100*(10), 1953–1960. Retrieved from http://doi.org/10.2105/AJPH.2009.174169.

Covey, L. S., Weissman, J., LoDuca, C., & Duan, N. (2009). A comparison of abstinence outcomes among gay/bisexual and heterosexual male smokers in an intensive, non-tailored smoking cessation study. *Nicotine & Tobacco Research: Official Journal of the Society for Research on Nicotine and Tobacco*, *11*(11), 1374–1377. Retrieved from http://doi.org/10.1093/ntr/ntp137

Crosby, G. M., Stall, R. D., Paul, J. P., & Barrett, D. C. (1998). Alcohol and drug use patterns have declined between generations of younger gay–bisexual men in San Francisco. *Drug and Alcohol Dependence, 52*(3), 177–182. Retrieved from http://doi.org/10.1016/S0376–8716(98)00093–3

Diaz, R. M., Heckert, A. L., & Sanchez, F. J. (2005). Reasons for stimulant use among Latino gay men in San Francisco: A comparison between methamphetamine and cocaine users. *Journal of Urban Health: Bulletin of the New York Academy of Medicine, 82*, i71–i78.

Dibble, S. L., Roberts, S. A., Robertson, P. A., & Paul, S. M. (2002). Risk factors for ovarian cancer: Lesbian and heterosexual women. *Oncology Nursing Forum, 29*, E1–E7. Retrieved from http://doi.org/10.1188/02.ONF.E1-E7

Drabble, L., & Trocki, K. (2005). Alcohol consumption, alcohol-related problems, and other substance use among lesbian and bisexual women. *Journal of Lesbian Studies, 9*, 19–30.

Eliason, M. J. (2000). Substance abuse counselor's attitudes regarding lesbian, gay, bisexual, and transgendered clients. *Journal of Substance Abuse, 12*(4), 311–328. Retrieved from http://doi.org/10.1016/S0899–3289(01)00055–4

Eliason, M. J. (2014). Chronic physical health problems in sexual minority women: A review of the literature. *LGBT Health, 1*, 259–268.

Eliason, M. J., Dibble, S. L., Gordon, R., & Soliz, G. (2012). The last drag: A smoking cessation group intervention for lesbian, gay, bisexual, and transgender individuals. *Journal of Homosexuality, 59*, 864–878.

Eliason, M. J., & Drabble, L. (2010). Got a light? Lesbians and smoking. In S. L. Dibble & P. A. Robertson (Eds.), *Lesbian Health 101* (pp. 125–140). San Francisco, CA: UCSF Nursing Press.

Eliason, M. J., & Hughes, T. L. (2004). Substance abuse counselor's attitudes about lesbian, gay, bisexual, and transgender -clients: Urban versus rural counselors. *Substance Use & Misuse, 39*, 625–644.

Eliason, M. J., Ingraham, N., Fogel, S. C., McElroy, J. A., Lorvick, J., Mauery, D. R., & Haynes, S. (2015). A systematic review of the literature on weight in sexual minority women. *Women's Health Issues: Official Publication of the Jacobs Institute of Women's Health, 25*(2), 162–175. Retrieved from http://doi.org/10.1016/j.whi.2014.12.001

Eliason, M. J., & Worthington, L. (2004). Smoking and alcohol/drug use in participants at a smoke-free gay pride celebration. Unpublished Paper. Department of Health Education, San Francisco State University.

Fallin, A., Goodin, A., Lee, Y. O., & Bennett, K. (2015). Smoking characteristics among lesbian, gay, and bisexual adults. *Preventive Medicine, 74*, 123–130. Retrieved from http://doi.org/10.1016/j.ypmed.2014.11.026

French, S. A., Story, M., Remafedi, G., Resnick, M. D., & Blum, R. W. (1996). Sexual orientation and prevalence of body dissatisfaction and eating disordered behaviors: A population-based study of adolescents. *The International Journal of Eating Disorders, 19*(2), 119–126. Retrieved from http://doi.org/10.1002/(SICI)1098–108X(199603)19:23.0.CO;2-Q

Friedman, M. S., Marshal, M. P., Guadamuz, T. E., Wei, C., Wong, C. F., Saewyc, E. M., & Stall, R. (2011). A meta-analysis of disparities in childhood sexual abuse, parental physical abuse, and peer victimization among sexual minority and sexual nonminority individuals. *American Journal of Public Health, 101*(8), 1481–1494. Retrieved from http://doi.org/10.2105/AJPH.2009.190009

Gamarel, K. E., Mereish, E. H., Manning, D., Iwamoto, M., Operario, D., & Nemoto, T. (2015). Minority stress, smoking patterns, and cessation attempts: Findings from a community-sample of transgender women in the San Francisco bay area. *Nicotine & Tobacco Research: Official Journal of the Society for Research on Nicotine and Tobacco, 18*(3), 306–313. Retrieved from http://doi.org/10.1093/ntr/ntv066

Garofalo, R., Mustanski, B. S., McKirnan, D. J., Herrick, A., & Donenberg, G. R. (2007). Methamphetamine and young men who have sex with men: Understanding patterns and correlates of use and the association with HIV-related sexual risk. *Archives of Pediatrics & Adolescent Medicine*, *161*(6), 591–596. Retrieved from http://doi.org/10.1001/archpedi.161.6.591

Gilman, S. E., Cochran, S. D., Mays, V. M., Hughes, M., Ostrow, D., & Kessler, R. C. (2001). Risk of psychiatric disorders among individuals reporting same-sex sexual partners in the National Comorbidity Survey. *American Journal of Public Health*, *91*(6), 933–939.

Grady, E. S., Humfleet, G. L., Delucchi, K. L., Reus, V. I., Muñoz, R. F., & Hall, S. M. (2014). Smoking cessation outcomes among sexual and gender minority and nonminority smokers in extended smoking treatments. *Nicotine & Tobacco Research: Official Journal of the Society for Research on Nicotine and Tobacco*, *16*(9), 1207–1215. Retrieved from http://doi.org/10.1093/ntr/ntu050

Greene, B. (1997). Ethnic minority lesbians and gay men: Mental health and treatment issues. In B. Greene (Ed.), *Ethnic and cultural diversity among lesbians and gay men*. Thousand Oaks, CA: Sage Publications, Inc.

Greenwood, G. L., & Gruskin, E. P. (2007). LGBT Tobacco and Alcohol Disparities. In I. H. Meyer & M. E. Northridge (Eds.), *The health of sexual minorities* (pp. 566–583). New York: Springer. Retrieved from http://doi.org/10.1007/978–0–387–31334–4_23

Grella, C. E., Cochran, S. D., Greenwell, L., & Mays, V. M. (2011). Effects of sexual orientation and gender on perceived need for treatment by persons with and without mental disorders. *Psychiatric Services*, *62*(4), 404–410. Retrieved from http://doi.org/10.1176/appi.ps.62.4.404

Grossman, A. H., & D'Augelli, A. R. (2007). Transgender youth and life-threatening behaviors. *Suicide & Life-Threatening Behavior*, *37*(5), 527–537. Retrieved from http://doi.org/10.1521/suli.2007.37.5.527

Gruskin, E. P., Byrne, K. M., Altschuler, A., & Dibble, S. L. (2008). Smoking it all away: Influences of stress, negative emotions, and stigma on lesbian tobacco use. *Journal of LGBT Health Research*, *4*(4), 167–179.

Haas, A. P., Eliason, M. J., Mays, V. M., Mathy, R. M., Cochran, S. D., D'Augelli, A. R., … Clayton, P. J. (2011). Suicide and suicide risk in lesbian, gay, bisexual, and transgender populations: Review and recommendations. *Journal of Homosexuality*, *58*(1), 10–51. Retrieved from http://doi.org/10.1080/00918369.2011.534038

Hale, C. J. (2007). Ethical problems with the mental health evaluation standards of care for adult gender variant prospective patients. *Perspectives in Biology and Medicine*, *50*(4), 491–505. Retrieved from http://doi.org/10.1353/pbm.2007.0047

Halkitis, P. N., Green, K. A., & Mourgues, P. (2005). Longitudinal investigation of methamphetamine use among gay and bisexual men in New York City: findings from Project BUMPS. *Journal of Urban Health: Bulletin of the New York Academy of Medicine*, *82*(1 Suppl 1), i18–i25. Retrieved from http://doi.org/10.1093/jurban/jti020

Halkitis, P. N., Palamar, J. J., & Mukherjee, P. P. (2007). Poly-club-drug use among gay and bisexual men: A longitudinal analysis. *Drug and Alcohol Dependence*, *89*(2–3), 153–160. Retrieved from http://doi.org/10.1016/j.drugalcdep.2006.12.028

Hatzenbuehler, M. L., Birkett, M., Van Wagenen, A., & Meyer, I. H. (2014). Protective school climates and reduced risk for suicide ideation in sexual minority youths. *American Journal of Public Health*, *104*(2), 279–286. Retrieved from http://doi.org/10.2105/AJPH.2013.301508

Hatzenbuehler, M. L., McLaughlin, K. A., Keyes, K. M., & Hasin, D. S. (2010). The impact of institutional discrimination on psychiatric disorders in lesbian, gay, and bisexual populations: A prospective study. *American Journal of Public Health*, *100*(3), 452–459. Retrieved from http://doi.org/10.2105/AJPH.2009.168815

Heck, N. C., Livingston, N. A., Flentje, A., Oost, K., Stewart, B. T., & Cochran, B. N. (2014). Reducing risk for illicit drug use and prescription drug misuse: High school gay-straight alliances and lesbian, gay, bisexual, and transgender youth. *Addictive Behaviors*, *39*(4), 824–828. Retrieved from http://doi.org/10.1016/j.addbeh.2014.01.007

Hughes, T. L. (2003). Lesbians' drinking patterns: Beyond the data. *Substance Use & Misuse*, *38*(11–13), 1739–1758.

Hughes, T. L., & Eliason, M. J. (2002). Substance Use and Abuse in Lesbian, Gay, Bisexual and Transgender Populations. *The Journal of Primary Prevention*, *22*(3), 263–298. Retrieved from http://doi.org/10.1023/A:1013669705086

Hughes, T. L. (2011). Alcohol-related problems among sexual minority women. *Alcoholism Treatment Quarterly*, *29*(4), 403–435. Retrieved from http://doi.org/10.1080/07347324.2011.608336

Hughes, T. L., Wilsnack, S. C., Szalacha, L. A., Johnson, T., Bostwick, W. B., Seymour, R., … Kinnison, K. E. (2006). Age and racial/ethnic differences in drinking and drinking-related problems in a community sample of lesbians. *Journal of Studies on Alcohol*, *67*(4), 579–590. Retrieved from http://doi.org/10.15288/jsa.2006.67.579

Israel, G. E., & Tarver, D. E. (1997). *Transgender care: Recommended guidelines, practical information, and personal accounts*. Philadelphia, PA: Temple University Press.

Jessup, M. A., & Dibble, S. L. (2012). Unmet mental health and substance abuse treatment needs of sexual minority elders. *Journal of Homosexuality*, *59*(5), 656–674. Retrieved from http://doi.org/10.1080/00918369.2012.665674

Jones, M. A., & Gabriel, M. A. (1999). Utilization of psychotherapy by lesbians, gay men, and bisexuals: Findings from a nationwide survey. *The American Journal of Orthopsychiatry*, *69*(2), 209–219.

Jorm, A. F., Korten, A. E., Rodgers, B., Jacomb, P. A., & Christensen, H. (2002). Sexual orientation and mental health: Results from a community survey of young and middle-aged adults. *The British Journal of Psychiatry: The Journal of Mental Science*, *180*, 423–427.

King, M., Semlyen, J., Tai, S. S., Killaspy, H., Osborn, D., Popelyuk, D., & Nazareth, I. (2008). A systematic review of mental disorder, suicide, and deliberate self harm in lesbian, gay and bisexual people. BMC Psychiatry, 8, 70. Retrieved from http://doi.org/10.1186/1471-244X-8-70

Kipke, M. D., Weiss, G., & Wong, C. F. (2007). Residential status as a risk factor for drug use and HIV risk among young men who have sex with men. *AIDS and Behavior*, *11*(6 Suppl), 56–69. Retrieved from http://doi.org/10.1007/s10461-006-9204-5

Kirk, S. C., & Kulkarni, C. (2006). The whole person: A paradigm for integrating the mental and physical health of trans clients. In M. Shankle (Ed.), The handbook of lesbian, gay, bisexual, and transgender public health: A practitioners guide to service (pp. 145–174). New York: Haworth.

Kitzinger, C., & Perkins, R. (1993). *Changing our minds: Lesbian feminism and psychology*. NYU Press.

Klein, A. A., & Ross, B. L. (2014). Substance use and mental health severity among LGBTQ individuals attending Minnesota model-based residential treatment. *Journal of Gay & Lesbian Social Services, 26*(3), 303–317. Retrieved from http://doi.org/10.1080/10538720.2014.924459

Koblin, B. A., Chesney, M. A., Husnik, M. J., Bozeman, S., Celum, C. L., Buchbinder, S., … Coates TJ; EXPLORE Study Team. (2003). High-risk behaviors among men who have sex with men in 6 US cities: Baseline data from the EXPLORE Study. *American Journal of Public Health*, *93*(6), 926–932.

Kraemer, B., Delsignore, A., Schnyder, U., & Hepp, U. (2008). Body image and transsexualism. *Psychopathology*, *41*(2), 96–100. Retrieved from http://doi.org/10.1159/000111554

Kral, A. H., Lorvick, J., Ciccarone, D., Wenger, L., Gee, L., Martinez, A., & Edlin, B. R. (2005). HIV prevalence and risk behaviors among men who have sex with men and inject drugs in San Francisco. *Journal of Urban Health: Bulletin of the New York Academy of Medicine*, *82*(1 Suppl 1), i43–i50. Retrieved from http://doi.org/10.1093/jurban/jti023

Landen, M., Wålinder, J., Hambert, G., & Lundström, B. (1998). Factors predictive of regret in sex reassignment. *Acta Psychiatrica Scandinavica*, *97*(4), 284–289.

Lawrence, A. A. (2007). Transgender health concerns. In I. H. Meyer & M. E. Northridge (Eds.), *The Health of Sexual Minorities: Public health perspectives on lesbian, gay, bisexual, and transgender populations* (pp. 473–505). New York: Springer. Retrieved from http://doi.org/10.1007/978-0-387-31334-4_19

Lhomond, B., & Saurel-Cubizolles, M.-J. (2006). Violence against women and suicide risk: The neglected impact of same-sex sexual behaviour. *Social Science & Medicine*, *62*(8), 2002–2013. Retrieved from http://doi.org/10.1016/j.socscimed.2005.08.026

Lipsky, S., Krupski, A., Roy-Byrne, P., Huber, A., Lucenko, B. A., & Mancuso, D. (2012). Impact of sexual orientation and co-occurring disorders on chemical dependency treatment outcomes. *Journal of Studies on Alcohol and Drugs*, *73*(3), 401–412. Retrieved from http://doi.org/10.15288/jsad.2012.73.401

Mann, W. J. (1998). *The men from the boys*. New York: Penguin.

Martins, Y., Tiggemann, M., & Kirkbride, A. (2007). Those speedos become them: The role of self-objectification in gay and heterosexual men's body image. *Personality & Social Psychology Bulletin*, *33*(5), 634–647. Retrieved from http://doi.org/10.1177/0146167206297403

Mason, T. B., & Lewis, R. J. (2015). Minority stress and binge eating among lesbian and bisexual women. *Journal of Homosexuality*, *62*(7), 971–992. Retrieved from http://doi.org/10.1080/00918369.2015.1008285

Matthews, A. K., Li, C.-C., Kuhns, L. M., Tasker, T. B., & Cesario, J. A. (2013). Results from a community-based smoking cessation treatment program for LGBT smokers. *Journal of Environmental and Public Health*, *2013*, 984508. Retrieved from http://doi.org/10.1155/2013/984508

McCabe, S. E., Hughes, T. L., Bostwick, W. B., West, B. T., & Boyd, C. J. (2009). Sexual orientation, substance use behaviors and substance dependence in the United States. *Addiction*, *104*(8), 1333–1345. Retrieved from http://doi.org/10.1111/j.1360-0443.2009.02596.

McKirnan, D. J., & Peterson, P. L. (1989). Alcohol and drug use among homosexual men and women: Epidemiology and population characteristics. *Addictive Behaviors*, *14*(5), 545–553. Retrieved from http://doi.org/10.1016/0306-4603(89)90075-0

Mereish, E. H., & Bradford, J. B. (2014). Intersecting identities and substance use problems: Sexual orientation, gender, race, and lifetime substance use problems. *Journal of Studies on Alcohol and Drugs*, *75*(1), 179–188. Retrieved from http://doi.org/10.15288/jsad.2014.75.179

Meyer, I. H. (2003). Prejudice, social stress, and mental health in lesbian, gay, and bisexual populations: Conceptual issues and research evidence. *Psychological Bulletin*, *129*(5), 674–697. Retrieved from http://doi.org/10.1037/0033-2909.129.5.674

Mills, T. C., Paul, J., Stall, R., Pollack, L., Canchola, J., Chang, Y. J., … Catania, J. A. (2004). Distress and depression in men who have sex with men: The urban men's health study. *The American Journal of Psychiatry*, *161*(2), 278–285. Retrieved from http://doi.org/10.1176/appi.ajp.161.2.278

Mottet, L., & Ohle, J. (2003). *Transitioning our shelters: A guide to making homeless shelters safe for transgender people. New York: The National Coalition for the Homeless and the National Gay and Lesbian Task Force Policy Institute.* New York: National Gay and Lesbian Task Force Policy Institute.

Nemoto, T., Luke, D., Mamo, L., Ching, A., & Patria, J. (1999). HIV risk behaviours among male-to-female transgenders in comparison with homosexual or bisexual males and heterosexual females. *AIDS Care*, *11*(3), 297–312. Retrieved from http://doi.org/10.1080/09540129947938

Newcomb, M. E., Heinz, A. J., Birkett, M., & Mustanski, B. (2014). A longitudinal examination of risk and protective factors for cigarette smoking among lesbian, gay, bisexual, and transgender youth. *The Journal of Adolescent Health: Official Publication of the*

Society for Adolescent Medicine, *54*(5), 558–564. Retrieved from http://doi.org/10.1016/j.jadohealth.2013.10.208

Nuttbrock, L., Bockting, W., Rosenblum, A., Hwahng, S., Mason, M., Macri, M., & Becker, J. (2014). Gender abuse and incident HIV/STI among transgender women in New York City: Buffering effect of involvement in a transgender community. *AIDS and Behavior*. Retrieved from http://doi.org/10.1007/s10461–014–0977–7

Page, E. H. (2004). Mental health services experiences of bisexual women and bisexual men. Journal of Bisexuality, 4(1–2), 137–160. Retrieved from http://doi.org/10.1300/J159v04n01_11

Pizacani, B. A., Rohde, K., Bushore, C., Stark, M. J., Maher, J. E., Dilley, J. A., & Boysun, M. J. (2009). Smoking-related knowledge, attitudes and behaviors in the lesbian, gay and bisexual community: A population-based study from the U.S. Pacific Northwest. *Preventive Medicine*, *48*(6), 555–561. Retrieved from http://doi.org/10.1016/j.ypmed.2009.03.013

Plöderl, M., Wagenmakers, E.-J., Tremblay, P., Ramsay, R., Kralovec, K., Fartacek, C., & Fartacek, R. (2013). Suicide risk and sexual orientation: A critical review. *Archives of Sexual Behavior*, *42*(5), 715–727. Retrieved from http://doi.org/10.1007/s10508–012–0056-y

Remafedi, G., Jurek, A. M., & Oakes, J. M. (2008). Sexual identity and tobacco use in a venue-based sample of adolescents and young adults. *American Journal of Preventive Medicine*, *35*(6 Suppl), S463–S4670. Retrieved from http://doi.org/10.1016/j.amepre.2008.09.002

Rosario, M., Rotheram-Borus, M. J., & Reid, H. (1996). Gay-related stress and its correlates among gay and bisexual male adolescents of predominantly Black and Hispanic background. *Journal of Community Psychology*, *24*(2), 136–159.

Rosario, M., Schrimshaw, E. W., & Hunter, J. (2011). Cigarette smoking as a coping strategy: Negative implications for subsequent psychological distress among lesbian, gay, and bisexual youths. *Journal of Pediatric Psychology*, *36*(7), 731–742. Retrieved from http://doi.org/10.1093/jpepsy/jsp141

Ryan, C., Huebner, D., Diaz, R. M., & Sanchez, J. (2009). Family rejection as a predictor of negative health outcomes in white and Latino lesbian, gay, and bisexual young adults. *Pediatrics*, *123*(1), 346–352. Retrieved from http://doi.org/10.1542/peds.2007–3524

Safren, S. A., & Heimberg, R. G. (1999). Depression, hopelessness, suicidality, and related factors in sexual minority and heterosexual adolescents. *Journal of Consulting and Clinical Psychology*, *67*(6), 859–866.

Scheer, S., Parks, C. A., McFarland, W., Page-Shafer, K., Delgado, V., Ruiz, J. D., … Klausner, J. D. (2002). Self-reported sexual identity, sexual behaviors and health risks: Examples from a population-based survey of young women. *Journal of Lesbian Studies*, *7*(1), 69–83.

Scheer, S., Peterson, I., Page-Shafer, K., Delgado, V., Gleghorn, A., Ruiz, J., … Klausner, J.; Young Women's Survey Team. (2002). Sexual and drug use behavior among women who have sex with both women and men: Results of a population-based survey. *American Journal of Public Health*, *92*(7), 1110–1112.

Schneeberger, A. R., Dietl, M. F., Muenzenmaier, K. H., Huber, C. G., & Lang, U. E. (2014). Stressful childhood experiences and health outcomes in sexual minority populations: A systematic review. *Social Psychiatry and Psychiatric Epidemiology*, *49*(9), 1427–1445. Retrieved from http://doi.org/10.1007/s00127–014–0854–8

Semple, S. J., Patterson, T. L., & Grant, I. (2002). Motivations associated with methamphetamine use among HIV+ men who have sex with men. *Journal of Substance Abuse Treatment*, *22*(3), 149–156.

Semple, S. J., Zians, J., Grant, I., & Patterson, T. L. (2006). Methamphetamine use, impulsivity, and sexual risk behavior among HIV-positive men who have sex with men. *Journal of Addictive Diseases*, *25*(4), 105–114. Retrieved from http://doi.org/10.1300/J069v25n04_10

Share, T. L., & Mintz, L. B. (2002). Differences between lesbians and heterosexual women in disordered eating and related attitudes. *Journal of Homosexuality*, *42*(4), 89–106. Retrieved from http://doi.org/10.1300/J082v42n04_06

Shoptaw, S., Reback, C. J., & Freese, T. E. (2002). Patient characteristics, HIV serostatus, and risk behaviors among gay and bisexual males seeking treatment for methamphetamine abuse and dependence in Los Angeles. *Journal of Addictive Diseases*, *21*(1), 91–105.

Shoptaw, S., Reback, C. J., Larkins, S., Wang, P.C., Rotheram-Fuller, E., Dang, J., & Yang, X. (2008). Outcomes using two tailored behavioral treatments for substance abuse in urban gay and bisexual men. *Journal of Substance Abuse Treatment*, *35*(3), 285–293. Retrieved from http://doi.org/10.1016/j.jsat.2007.11.004

Shoptaw, S., Reback, C. J., Peck, J. A., Yang, X., Rotheram-Fuller, E., Larkins, S., … Hucks-Ortiz, C. (2005). Behavioral treatment approaches for methamphetamine dependence and HIV-related sexual risk behaviors among urban gay and bisexual men. *Drug and Alcohol Dependence*, *78*(2), 125–134. Retrieved from http://doi.org/10.1016/j.drugalcdep.2004.10.004

Skinner, W. F., & Otis, M. D. (1996). Drug and alcohol use among lesbian and gay people in a southern U.S. sample: Epidemiological, comparative, and methodological findings from the Trilogy Project. *Journal of Homosexuality*, *30*(3), 59–92. Retrieved from http://doi.org/10.1300/J082v30n03_04

Smith, E. A., Offen, N., & Malone, R. E. (2005). What makes an ad a cigarette ad? Commercial tobacco imagery in the lesbian, gay, and bisexual press. *Journal of Epidemiology and Community Health*, *59*(12), 1086–1091. Retrieved from http://doi.org/10.1136/jech.2005.038760

Stall, R., Paul, J. P., Greenwood, G., Pollack, L. M., Bein, E., Crosby, G. M., … Catania, J. A. (2001). Alcohol use, drug use and alcohol-related problems among men who have sex with men: the Urban Men's Health Study. *Addiction*, *96*(11), 1589–1601. Retrieved from http://doi.org/10.1080/09652140120080723

Stevens, P., Carlson, L. M., & Hinman, J. M. (2004). An analysis of tobacco industry marketing to lesbian, gay, bisexual, and transgender (LGBT) populations: Strategies for mainstream tobacco control and prevention. *Health Promotion Practice*, *5*(3 Suppl), 129S–134S. Retrieved from http://doi.org/10.1177/1524839904264617

Tang, H., Greenwood, G. L., Cowling, D. W., Lloyd, J. C., Roeseler, A. G., & Bal, D. G. (2004). Cigarette smoking among lesbians, gays, and bisexuals: How serious a problem? (United States). *Cancer Causes & Control: CCC*, *15*(8), 797–803. Retrieved from http://doi.org/10.1023/B:CACO.0000043430.32410.69

Tjepkema, M. (2008). Health care use among gay, lesbian and bisexual Canadians. *Health Reports/Statistics Canada, Canadian Centre for Health Information = Rapports Sur La Sante/Statistique Canada, Centre Canadien D'information Sur La Sante*, *19*(1), 53–64.

Trocki, K. F., Drabble, L. A., & Midanik, L. T. (2009). Tobacco, marijuana, and sensation seeking: comparisons across gay, lesbian, bisexual, and heterosexual groups. *Psychology of Addictive Behaviors: Journal of the Society of Psychologists in Addictive Behaviors*, *23*(4), 620–631. Retrieved from http://doi.org/10.1037/a0017334

Ward, B. W., Dahlhamer, J. M., Galinsky, A. M., & Joestl, S. S. (2014). Sexual orientation and health among U.S. adults: National health interview survey, 2013. *National Health Statistics Reports*, (*77*), 1–10.

Warner, J., McKeown, E., Griffin, M., Johnson, K., Ramsay, A., Cort, C., & King, M. (2004). Rates and predictors of mental illness in gay men, lesbians and bisexual men and women: Results from a survey based in England and Wales. *The British Journal of Psychiatry: The Journal of Mental Science*, *185*, 479–485. Retrieved from http://doi.org/10.1192/bjp.185.6.479

Warwick, I., Douglas, N., Aggleton, P., & Boyce, P. (2003). Context matters: The educational potential of gay bars revisited. *AIDS Education and Prevention: Official Publication of the International Society for AIDS Education*, *15*(4), 320–333.

Weinberg, M. S., Williams, C. J., & Pryor, D. W. (1994). *Dual attraction: Understanding bisexuality.* Oxford: Oxford University Press.

Wilson, E. C., Chen, Y.-H., Arayasirikul, S., Wenzel, C., & Fisher Raymond, H. (2014). Connecting the dots: Examining transgender women's utilization of transition-related medical care and associations with mental health, substance use, and HIV. *Journal of Urban Health: Bulletin of the New York Academy of Medicine, 92*(1), 182–192. Retrieved from http://doi.org/10.1007/s11524-014-9921-4

Wilson, E., Rapues, J., Jin, H., & Raymond, H. F. (2014). The use and correlates of illicit silicone or "fillers" in a population-based sample of transwomen, San Francisco, 2013. *The Journal of Sexual Medicine, 11*(7), 1717–1724. Retrieved from http://doi.org/10.1111/jsm.12558

Xavier, J. M., Bobbin, M., Singer, B., & Budd, E. (2005). A needs assessment of transgendered people of color living in Washington, DC. *International Journal of Transgenderism, 8*(2–3), 31–47. Retrieved from http://doi.org/10.1300/J485v08n02_04

Xavier, J., Honnold, J. A., & Bradford, J. B. (2007). The health, health-related needs, and life-course experiences of transgender Virginians. Richmond, VA: VA Department of Health.

Zevin, B. (2000). Demographics of the transgender clinic at San Francisco's Tom Waddell Health Center. In *Proceedings of the transgender care conference*, San Francisco, CA.

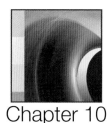

Chapter 10

Physical Health Disorders

"Dr [X]... had a problem and he asked her to wait outside. I said ... I'm not talking to you without her here. He said, well, we can only talk to a spouse or you know, a family member. I said well, she's both. She's my wife and she's my family. She's my next of kin. I said you know, my mind is not clear and I'm not hearing half of the things that are being said. I want her present"—woman with breast cancer (Boehmer & Case, 2006, p. 51).

Until recently, most LGBTQ health research focused almost entirely on HIV/AIDS and other sexually transmitted infections (STIs), mental health, and substance abuse (Coulter, Kenst, Bowen, & Scout, 2014). It was not until large health surveillance questionnaires started adding sexual orientation questions that we could begin to compare LGB people to comparable heterosexual people on other health outcomes. Few studies have added questions about gender identity, so we know much less about transgender people's health. As we overcome this lack of data, there is growing evidence of physical health challenges that occur in LGBTQ communities, related to minority stress and stigma.

Sell (2015, http://www.lgbtdata.com/) collects information on the state and national survey tools that include sexual orientation questions. Some of these include the Behavioral Risk Factors Surveillance Survey (BRFSS) used to track health in each state of the United States (eight states as of early 2015 had sexual orientation questions), the National Health Interview Survey (NHIS), the National Health and Nutrition Examination Survey, the National Study of Family Growth, and the National Alcohol Study. Most of these surveys have been used for more than 25 years, but the sexual orientation questions were not added until after the year 2000. These surveys with careful methodologies to collect representative samples from the population will give us much better health information about LGBTQ populations when they all include questions on sexual orientation and gender identity.

Minority stress theory would predict that ongoing exposure to stress would lead to more unhealthy behaviors that affect health (such as smoking, drinking, unhealthy eating); limit access to preventative health screenings (mammogram, prostate screening, pap test, colonoscopy); and ultimately the effects of the chronic stress would damage organ systems and lead to chronic physical health problems such as heart disease or diabetes. This chapter addresses these three major topics: health risk behavior and screening, actual rates of some of the more common chronic physical health conditions, and finally, a short section on HIV/AIDS. But it is important to keep in mind the quote that starts this chapter, and remember that any increase in illness that puts

LGBTQ people in greater contact with healthcare systems and providers, puts them at risk for encountering stressful situations.

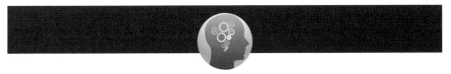

Think About It 10.1

In addition to the scientific rationale for obtaining accurate and reliable information related to LGBTQ physical health, doing so is a matter of biomedical ethics. To neglect these populations in scientific research is a violation of basic human rights. Read this Introduction (**https://goo.gl/KKMxcU**) to the Hastings Center September 2014 report on LGBT Bioethics, in which the Editors of this special issue explain the ethical responsibility to be inclusive of LGBT populations.

Risk Behavior and Health Screening Behaviors

Chapter 9 already addressed the higher rates of alcohol, drug, and tobacco use among LGBTQ people and proposed that one reason for higher use of substances is to relieve stress. These substance use behaviors carry elevated risk for physical health conditions such as cancer, liver diseases, lung disorders, a host of infections, and lowered immunity to disease in general. In this section of the chapter, we will focus on health screening behaviors. Do LGBTQ people get the recommended health screenings for their age and gender? The population based surveys like the Behavioral Risk Factor Surveillance System (BRFSS) ask questions about such screening and give us some insight, however the data are rather limited at this point. Most of these studies have a very wide age range, and do not report intersectional data. That is, perhaps socioeconomic status, age, race/ethnicity and other factors are as, or more important, than sexual orientation as predictors for health screenings, and there is very little data that explores interactions between and among these important traits of identity. Only a few of the studies reported in this section had questions about gender identity.

Exercise is one component of good health. The National Health Interview Survey (NHIS) data (Ward, Dahlhamer, Galinsky, & Joestl, 2014) found no differences by sexual orientation and gender for meeting federal guidelines for aerobic activity (nor did Blosnich, Farmer, Lee, Silenzio, & Bowen, 2014). Boehmer, Miao, Linkletter, & Clark (2012) found no differences for men but lesbians (42%) got more vigorous activity than heterosexual (31%) or bisexual women (38%). A few studies reported on physical activity levels of transgender individual with quite diverse findings: 23% to 55% did not get adequate exercise (Conron, Scott, Stowell, & Landers, 2012; Fredriksen-Goldsen, Kim, Barkan, Muraco, & Hoy-Ellis, 2013; Reisner, Gamarel, Dunham, Hopwood, & Hwahng, 2013). The data are too scant to draw many conclusions about physical activity among LGBT people, pointing toward an important area for future research. It may be that gyms, recreation centers, and other venues for exercise may be not welcoming of LGBTQ people and may affect rates of physical activity, or that neighborhood level issues, such as crime rates and safety concerns are important factors in limiting exercise.

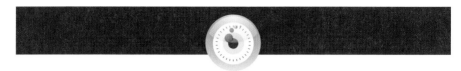

Watch This 10.1

One of biggest challenges for LGBTQ people who are living with various health challenges is finding meaningful support and encouragement in dealing with their issues. Watch this inspiring video showing a group of older lesbians who participated in a DIFO (Doing It For Ourselves) group that provided education and support focused on body size and other health issues common to many (**https://vimeo.com/97944423**).

A few studies reported no differences in rates of colonoscopy (Boehmer et al., 2012; Conron, Mimiaga, & Landers, 2010), although one study found gay and bisexual men were more likely to get colonoscopies than heterosexual men (Blosnich et al., 2014). In one interesting, but isolated finding, heterosexual men (49%) and lesbian/bisexual women (47%) in North Carolina (Matthews & Lee, 2014) were much more likely to have a firearm in the house than gay/bisexual men (20%) or heterosexual women (35%). More gay and bisexual men received flu shots than heterosexual men (Fredriksen-Goldsen et al., 2013; Ward et al., 2014) but fewer lesbian/bisexual women or the same number as heterosexual women got flu shots (Blosnich et al., 2014; Fredriksen-Goldsen et al., 2013).

At least three studies reported PSA testing (a screening test for prostate cancer). One of those found gay men less likely than heterosexual or bisexual men to be screened (Conron et al., 2010) and two found gay and bisexual men to be less likely than heterosexual men to be screened (Blosnich et al., 2014; Fredriksen-Goldsen et al., 2013). Transgender women still have a prostate and need screening for PSA levels, but there appears to be little research on this.

Important forms of screening tests for women are mammograms and pap tests. The data on this is muddy. Older studies were fairly consistent in finding that lesbian and bisexual women were less likely to obtain these screenings (Cochran et al., 2001; Diamant, Schuster, & Lever, 2000; Koh, 2000; Rankow & Tessaro, 1998; Valanis et al., 2000; White & Dull, 1997), but more recent data are mixed. One study reported that lesbians had a higher rate of mammography (65%) than heterosexual (59%) or bisexual (56%) women (Conron et al., 2010). Most studies find lesbian/bisexual women less likely to get regular pap tests than heterosexual women. Predictors of getting a pap test include higher income, having health insurance coverage, disclosing one's sexual orientation to the healthcare provider, having providers who recommend screening to the patient, and having an abnormal cervical cancer test result in the past (Agénor, Krieger, Austin, Haneuse, & Gottlieb, 2014; Charlton et al., 2011; Fish & Anthony, 2005; Tracy, Schluterman, & Greenberg, 2013). Some factors that predict not getting a Pap test include fear of discrimination, not disclosing sexual orientation to the provider, being less knowledgeable about screening guidelines, and having no sexual partners (Matthews, Brandenburg, Johnson, & Hughes, 2004; Tracy, Lydecker, & Ireland, 2010; Tracy et al., 2013). Transgender men still have a cervix and therefore need pap tests, but one study reported that they were less likely than cisgender women to be up-to-date on pap tests (Peitzmeier, Khullar, Reisner, & Potter, 2014).

There do seem to be some small differences in accessing routine care in general. In response to a question about having a health checkup in the past year, one national population study found that lesbian/bisexual women were less likely to have had a checkup than heterosexual women. Gay/bisexual men, on the other hand, seemed to have routine care as often as heterosexual men (Ward et al., 2014). Among participants who were age 18 to 44, more gay and bisexual men (74% and 75%, respectively) than heterosexual men (69%) reported having a usual place to receive medical care. Among women, lesbian (66%) and bisexual (70%) women were less likely to have a medical home than heterosexual women (81%).

Chronic Physical Health Disorders

Given all the elevated risk behaviors related to smoking, drinking, drug use, and stress, we might assume that LGBTQ people will have much higher rates of chronic physical conditions that are related to stress. But the data are not really clear about this yet. Almost all of these population surveys have a simple question about self-perceived overall health. We will examine one of those studies here: The National Health Interview Survey (NHIS).

Ward et al. (2014) reported the number of participants who said that their health was excellent or very good. Table 10.1 shows this data by gender and sexual orientation. There are more differences among women than men, and among men, gay men actually were more likely to report excellent/very good health than heterosexual men, a finding also reported by Jesdale and Mitchell (2012). It appears that the majority of LGBTQ people perceive themselves as healthy. Unfortunately, this study did not report the numbers who reported fair or poor health, but a few other studies have done that,

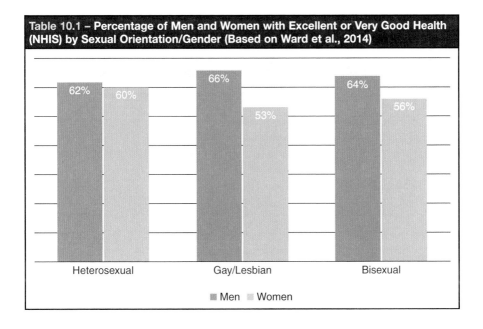

Table 10.1 – Percentage of Men and Women with Excellent or Very Good Health (NHIS) by Sexual Orientation/Gender (Based on Ward et al., 2014)

and several find higher rates of fair/poor health among LGB respondents (Thomeer, 2013). These findings may suggest a greater range of health status among LGB people, with more people at the extremes. Conron et al. (2012) reported that transgender respondents were no more likely than cisgender respondents to report fair/poor health.

Next, we will look at the data for some of the most common chronic illnesses in the population today: diabetes, heart disease, hypertension, asthma, disability, and cancer. What do the population studies tell us about actual rates of disorder? As you will see, there is not a lot of convincing evidence for differences in rates of most of these disorders, although the data available still have some significant limitations.

Diabetes

Tables 10.2 and 10.3 show data from six population-based studies that asked people whether they had ever been diagnosed with diabetes. Table 10.2 shows data for women and Table 10.3 for men. This is particularly interesting when the majority of studies find that lesbian and bisexual women are more likely to fit into categories of obese than heterosexual women, a finding often assumed to be associated with higher risk for diabetes (Eliason, Ingraham, et al., 2015). In fact, several studies find higher rates of diabetes in heterosexual men and women. There is no clear health disparity related to diabetes in LGB people, men or women. Only one study reported diabetes rates in transgender respondents, and found no differences compared to cisgender respondents (Conron, Scott, Stowell, & Landers, 2012). Most studies rely on self-report, limiting the reliability of this information. One study that examined HbA1c levels of young adults (just under age 30), found that gay and bisexual men had a lower HBA1c than heterosexual men and lesbian/bisexual women did not differ from heterosexual women (Hatzenbuehler, McLaughlin, & Slopen, 2013). Since diabetes is age-related, this does not adequately address prevalence of diabetes across the lifespan.

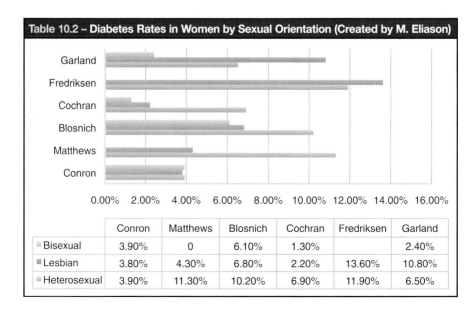

Table 10.2 – Diabetes Rates in Women by Sexual Orientation (Created by M. Eliason)

	Conron	Matthews	Blosnich	Cochran	Fredriksen	Garland
Bisexual	3.90%	0	6.10%	1.30%		2.40%
Lesbian	3.80%	4.30%	6.80%	2.20%	13.60%	10.80%
Heterosexual	3.90%	11.30%	10.20%	6.90%	11.90%	6.50%

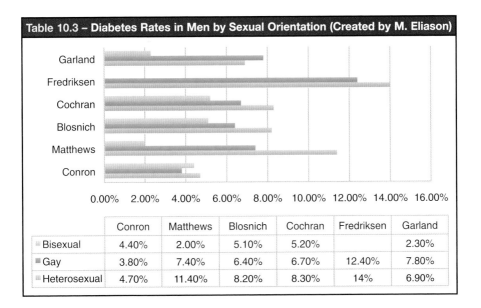

Table 10.3 – Diabetes Rates in Men by Sexual Orientation (Created by M. Eliason)

	Conron	Matthews	Blosnich	Cochran	Fredriksen	Garland
Bisexual	4.40%	2.00%	5.10%	5.20%		2.30%
Gay	3.80%	7.40%	6.40%	6.70%	12.40%	7.80%
Heterosexual	4.70%	11.40%	8.20%	8.30%	14%	6.90%

Heart Disease

Most studies in this section reported on just one simple indicator of heart disease, such as a lifetime diagnosis of any type of heart disease, so the literature provides only a crude self-report measure. Most of the studies do not report striking differences by sexual orientation, although a couple of studies are suggestive in pointing to higher risk for bisexual men (Blosnich et al., 2014; Garland-Forshee, Fiala, Ngo, & Moseley, 2014). None of the recent data found differences in self-reported heart disease among women by sexual orientation (Blosnich et al., 2014; Cochran & Mays, 2007; Cochran, Mays, Alegria, Ortega, & Takeuchi, 2007; Conron et al., 2010; Fredriksen-Goldsen et al., 2014; Garland-Forshee et al., 2014; Matthews & Lee, 2014). Nor did the one population-based study of transgender people find any differences in rates of heart disease (Conron et al., 2012). Tables 10.4 and 10.5 show rates of heart disease for women and men, respectively.

One precursor of heart disease is hypertension. Most of the studies found no difference, or higher rates of hypertension among heterosexual men and women compared to LGB people (Cochran & Mays, 2007; Matthews & Lee, 2014). Similar data are found for reports of high cholesterol, with no consistent findings of elevations among LGB people (Garland-Forshee et al., 2014; Matthews & Lee, 2014). A series of studies using lab data from the National Longitudinal Study of Adolescent Health examined risk factors for cardiovascular disease. In one study, gay and bisexual men had slightly higher diastolic blood pressure and faster pulse rates than heterosexual men, but lesbian and bisexual women did not differ from heterosexual women on any of the measures (Hatzenbuehler et al., 2013). Another study found that gay men had roughly twice the rate of hypertension as heterosexual men, even when controlling for minority stress, smoking, alcohol and drug use, BMI, and physical activity. There were no differences between women by sexual orientation (Everett & Mollborn, 2013). Finally, a study of inflammation and immune functioning found that gay and bisexual men had higher levels of C-reactive protein and Epstein–Barr virus than heterosexual men, but lesbians had lower

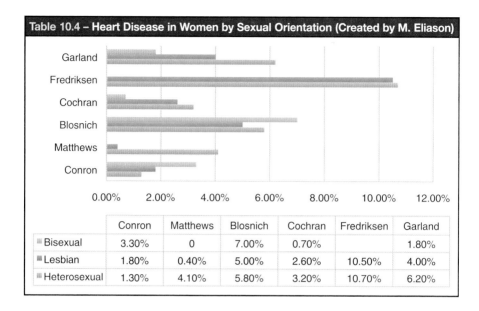

Table 10.4 – Heart Disease in Women by Sexual Orientation (Created by M. Eliason)

	Conron	Matthews	Blosnich	Cochran	Fredriksen	Garland
■ Bisexual	3.30%	0	7.00%	0.70%		1.80%
■ Lesbian	1.80%	0.40%	5.00%	2.60%	10.50%	4.00%
■ Heterosexual	1.30%	4.10%	5.80%	3.20%	10.70%	6.20%

levels of CRP than heterosexual women and no difference on EBV (Everett, Rosario, McLaughlin, & Austin, 2014). The participants in these studies were young adults, but the findings do suggest a differential risk for heart disease for gay and bisexual men.

Asthma

One fairly reliable difference between LGBT and heterosexual respondents in many studies is for asthma prevalence. Whether national samples, state health surveillance, or local samples, asthma rates appear to be elevated (Blosnich, Lee, Bossarte, &

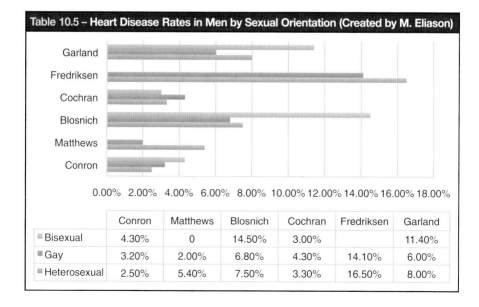

Table 10.5 – Heart Disease Rates in Men by Sexual Orientation (Created by M. Eliason)

	Conron	Matthews	Blosnich	Cochran	Fredriksen	Garland
■ Bisexual	4.30%	0	14.50%	3.00%		11.40%
■ Gay	3.20%	2.00%	6.80%	4.30%	14.10%	6.00%
■ Heterosexual	2.50%	5.40%	7.50%	3.30%	16.50%	8.00%

Asthma	Other-Sex Couples Men	Same-Sex Male Couples	Other-Sex Couples Women	Same-Sex Female Couples
Lifetime	11%	17%	15%	26%
Current	6%	12%	10%	21%

Table 10.6 – Lifetime and Current Asthma Diagnoses in a U.S. National Study (Based on Blosnich et al., 2013)

Silenzio, 2013; Fredriksen-Goldsen et al., 2013; Heck & Jacobson, 2006), although the rates seem to differ more for women than men by sexual orientation (Matthews & Lee, 2014). To illustrate these differences, Table 10.6 shows rates from a national study where participants were asked about the gender of their sexual partners. Both men and women in same-sex relationships had higher rates of asthma, and in a logistic regression, younger age, lower income, and being overweight or obese were associated with asthma. When controlling for these other factors, being in a same-sex relationship was also a powerful correlate of asthma. Curiously, having ever smoked was a factor in women's reports of asthma, but not men's (Blosnich, Bossarte, Silver, & Silenzio, 2013; Blosnich et al., 2013).

Disability

Another area that needs more exploration is the prevalence of disability. Questions about disability are asked in quite diverse ways, so it is challenging to compare across the studies. Some surveys ask about any disability that affects activities of daily living and other surveys are more specific in asking about physical limitations or need for special equipment. For example, Cochran and Mays (2007) found few disparities when asking about major physical disabilities (for men, 3% of heterosexual, 2% of gay men, and 4% of bisexual men responded yes; for women, 3% of heterosexual, 2% of lesbians, and 1% of bisexual women), however, there were bigger differences when asked if they had any functional health limitations (for men: 19% heterosexual, 24% gay, 31% bisexual; for women: 21% heterosexual, 31% lesbian, 38% bisexual). Many studies provide some evidence that overall disability rates are higher among LGB people, but do not provide information on specific types or severity of disability (Eliason, Martinson, & Carabez, 2015). Because of the higher frequency of mental health and substance use disorders of many types among LGBTQ people, prevalence of disability may be increased. Rates of physical disability may be comparable to heterosexual populations.

Cancer

Cancer risks have been discussed in some studies. Cancer burden is not distributed equally in the population, and most racial/ethnic minority groups have lower survival rates from cancer (American Cancer Society, 2011), suggesting that stigma creates health disparities around access to screening, early diagnosis, and cancer treatment. Only a few studies have examined cancer risk and cancer incidence among LGBTQ people, primarily because cancer registries do not yet include questions about sexual or gender identities, thus it is challenging to study cancer disparities. Because of the high prevalence of cancers that differentially affect women and men, the rest of this section considers those gender differences.

• Cancer and Women

By far the most studied cancer among women is breast cancer. Most of the research has focused on breast cancer *risk factors* (not the actual occurrence), and proposes that the risks may be higher for lesbians/bisexual women than for heterosexual women because lesbian/bi women are less likely to bear children, more likely to be overweight, and more likely to be current or past smokers and heavy drinkers (Cochran et al., 2001; Dibble, Roberts, Robertson, & Paul, 2002; Dibble, Roberts, Robertson, & Paul, 2004; Roberts & Sorensen, 1999). In addition, some studies have reported that lesbians are less likely to get pap tests and mammograms (Cochran et al., 2001; Diamant et al., 2000; Koh, 2000; Rankow & Tessaro, 1998; Valanis et al., 2000; White & Dull, 1997), therefore, cancers may not be identified as early.

One small-scale convenience sample study found higher rates of breast cancer among lesbians than heterosexual women (Dibble, Vanoni, & Miaskowski, 1997), but several other studies have not found sexual orientation differences in reports of breast cancer among women (Austin et al., 2012; Cochran & Mays, 2007; Fredriksen-Goldsen, Kim, & Barkan, 2012; Frisch, Smith, Grulich, & Johansen, 2003; Mays, Yancey, Cochran, Weber, & Fielding, 2002). A review of longitudinal NHIS data from 1997 to 2003 found no difference in the overall mortality rate for women, but a higher mortality rate from breast cancer in women in same-sex relationships compared to women in relationships with men (Cochran & Mays, 2012).

In regards to other forms of cancers, one study found lesbian and heterosexual women had comparable prevalence of cervical cancer, lesbians had slightly higher prevalence of uterine cancer, and bisexual women had significantly higher reports of cervical cancer. However, when the data were adjusted for age, race, education, income, and nativity, the sexual orientation differences disappeared, suggesting that factors other than sexual identity were more important (Boehmer, Miao, & Ozonoff, 2011; Mattocks et al., 2013). Mattocks et al. (2013) studied female veterans and found no difference in rates of cervical, ovarian, or uterine cancers by sexual identity. One study of young women in Australia who reported any cancer in the past 3 years did not find differences by sexual orientation (McNair, Szalacha, & Hughes, 2011). Boehmer et al. (2011) found no difference by sexual orientation on reports of any cancer in adulthood in California women. In another California state dataset, colon cancer was reported by 2.8% of heterosexual and 4.5% of lesbian women (not significant) and the rate of "other" cancers approached significance, but with heterosexual women reporting more cancers (41%) than lesbian (31%) or bisexual women (26%). A risk-prediction model using data from a large cohort of U.S. women and adjusting for confounding variables, found no difference in risk for colon cancer by sexual orientation (Austin et al., 2012).

• Cancer and Men

Literature on cancer among gay and bisexual men has focused primarily on anal cancer and cancers related to HIV status. Men who engage in anal sex should have annual anal pap tests to screen for cancer (Margolies & Goeren, 2009) as some data suggests MSM are at higher risk. There are high rates of HPV infection among MSM, which may be associated with higher rates of anal cancer (Frisch et al., 2003). Rates of anal cancer in the general population are about two cases per 100,000 people, but one study suggested rates in MSM might be 20 times higher among those who are HIV negative and 40 times higher among those who are HIV positive (Margolies & Goeren, 2009). People who are HIV positive must be monitored closely for a wide variety of cancers that are associated with HIV, such as Kaposi sarcoma, lymphoma, anal cancer, and lung cancer (Engels, 2007; Martró et al., 2007; Robbins et al., 2015).

Cochran and Mays (2007) found that among men, those who called themselves heterosexual but had same-sex experiences had higher rates of cancer diagnoses (4.3%) than heterosexual (1.1%), gay (0.8%), or bisexual men (0). Blosnich et al. (2014) reported higher rates of prostate cancer among bisexual men (7.8%) compared to gay men (3.4%) or heterosexual men (4.3%), but Boehmer et al. (2011) found lower rates of prostate cancer but higher rates of colon cancer among gay and bisexual men than heterosexual men.

• *Cancer and Transgender People*

Little is known about cancer risks among transgender individuals. There is growing evidence that about half of trans men, many of whom still have a uterus and cervix, do not get regular pap tests because the trans men themselves or the healthcare providers are uncomfortable with physical examinations (Peitzmeier et al., 2014; Rachlin, Green, & Lombardi, 2008). There has been some concern raised in the literature about the risk for breast cancer related to long-term cross-sex hormone use, but a large study of transgender veterans found no evidence of an increase in breast cancer (Brown & Jones, 2015).

• *Risk Factors for Cancer*

The higher smoking rate among LGBTQ people warrants more attention to rates of lung cancer as well. Thus far, there have not been focused studies on the long-term health effects of smoking among LGBTQ people, but it is likely that there are higher rates of COPD and lung cancer among older LGBTQ individuals. In addition, heavy drinking may be associated with certain types of cancer. The lack of findings of increased cancer rates in the studies cited above may have to do with the age of the respondents, as cancer rates increase with age.

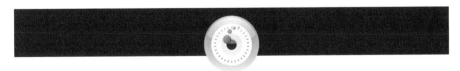

Think About It 10.2

Sexually transmitted disease (STD) or sexually transmitted infection (STI)? What's in a word? Many specialists are using the more accurate term STI to describe acute illnesses that are transmitted sexually. We do not refer to a cold or the flu as diseases, but as acute illnesses or infections. Most of the STIs are also acute, thus the less stigmatizing term is warranted.

HIV/AIDS

Sexual orientation and gender identity are not risk factors for HIV/AIDS or STIs. Instead, specific sexual behaviors that can be performed by any person, or combination of persons, carry risk only if one of the partners is infected. Sexual activities, outside of heterosexual married missionary vaginal sex, are often stigmatized in our society, and in spite of the proliferation of sexual images in the media, most of the culture is rather sex phobic. Therefore, stigma often leads to judgments about whether women should express that they like sex, about how many partners, and what kind of partners are appropriate, and what behaviors are acceptable forms of sex and which are not. The number of sexual partners or the types of sexual activities are not in and of themselves risk factors—they are only risky if the partner has HIV or an STI.

Some activities are more likely to transmit an STI than others, if one partner is infected. Where stigma increases the risks for LGBTQ people to contract STIs is the lack of adequate sex education about how to have sex safely. One could argue that heterosexuals are equally lacking in adequate sex education as youth, but there are many sources of accurate information available once heterosexuals become late adolescents or young adults. Some LGBTQ communities have focused safer sex education campaigns, but on the whole, LGBTQ people do not get comprehensive, LGBTQ-focused sexuality education from school, home, or healthcare professionals unless they seek out services from HIV prevention programs.

HIV still disproportionately affects men who have sex with men (MSM). Table 10.7 shows the exposure categories recorded by the CDC for HIV disease. Male to male sexual contact still leads the list for men. By the end of 2011, of all people who had died of AIDS in the United States, 47% were gay or bisexual men. Nationwide, about 18% of MSM are HIV positive, and even today, many are not aware of their status. But not all MSM are equally affected; rates are highest among young African-American and Latino MSM (Center for Disease Control and Prevention, 2015). Regular testing for sexually active MSM is essential in both prevention and getting affected individuals into treatment as early as possible.

Transgender individuals, particularly MTF, have among the highest rates of HIV infection of any group (Herbst et al., 2008). Baral et al. (2013) studied the global epidemic of HIV and reported that trans women had a 48.8 times higher odds of being HIV positive than adults in the general population. The elevated rates are related to the very high number of transgender women who cannot find safe employment and must engage in sex work to survive (Poteat, Reisner, & Radix, 2014). Transgender women of color are at particular risk (Nemoto, Operario, & Keatley, 2005, 2006; Sausa, Keatley, & Operario, 2007), and HIV/STI stemming from gender abuse by sexual partners increases their risks (Nuttbrock et al., 2014).

Table 10.7 – New HIV Diagnoses in 2013 by Transmission Type (Based on Center for Disease Control and Prevention, 2013)		
Transmission	Men	Women
MSM	30, 689	Na
Injection drug use	1942	1154
MSM plus IDU	1270	Na
Heterosexual sex	3887	8031
Other	99	93

Table 10.8 – Risks for Acquiring HIV (Based on Smith et al., 2005)	
Risk Exposure Behavior	**Risk per 10,000 Exposures to an Infected Source**
Blood transfusion	9,000
Needle-sharing drug use	67
Receptive anal sex	50
Receptive penile-vaginal sex	10
Insertive anal sex	6.5
Insertive penile-vaginal sex	5
Receptive oral sex with a man	1
Insertive oral sex with a man	0.5

Table 10.8 shows the risk of acquiring HIV by the different risk exposure categories, suggesting that blood-sharing activities are much more potent transmitters of HIV than are sexual activities, yet same-sex sexual behaviors are even more stigmatized in society than injection drug use.

For more information on STIs and HIV/AIDS, see the CDC website for extensive information. Transmission of many STIs and HIV can be reduced dramatically by consistent use of condoms or other barrier methods, and there are two prevention medication strategies currently available: PrEp (pre-exposure prophylaxis) is taken daily by individuals at high risk for HIV, and PEP (postexposure prophylaxis) is started within 72 hours of a potential exposure event and is taken for 28 days. HIV treatment options are more complex, ever-evolving and beyond the scope of this book.

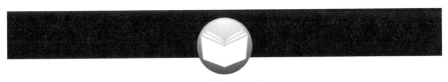

Read This 10.1

The U.S. Substance Abuse and Mental Health Services Administration (SAMHSA) published a report in 2013 that summarizes what are currently recognized as the top health issues for each LGB and T population. Go to **https://goo.gl/voz3qb** to download and read this valuable resource.

Conclusions

In summary, HIV/STI rates continue to be relatively high among men who have sex with men and transgender women. With better treatment options now, AIDS has become a chronic illness, not an immediate threat to life. Prevention activities are still critically needed to reduce rates of new infection, particularly among men of color. In regards to other chronic health disorders, however, there are not striking differences in prevalence rates of many of the most common disorders that affect the adult population. Paradoxically, in spite of more risk factors and less frequent screening, LGBTQ people do not seem to have higher rates of diabetes, heart disease, or most cancers. Perhaps the LGBTQ people who respond to the population-based survey interviews are healthier than the general population of LGBTQ people. We really have no way of knowing what a representative sample of LGBTQ people looks like. But the studies we have available to us at this time suggest that minority stress may have greater impact on mental health and substance use than on the development of chronic physical health disorders. Even if LGBTQ people have approximately the same rate of chronic physical illnesses as heterosexual people, their experiences in the clinic and hospital may still differ because of encountering uneducated or even hostile healthcare providers and systems that render them invisible.

References

Agénor, M., Krieger, N., Austin, S. B., Haneuse, S., & Gottlieb, B. R. (2014). Sexual orientation disparities in Papanicolaou test use among US Women: The role of sexual and reproductive health services. *American Journal of Public Health, 104*(2), e68–e73. Retrieved from http://doi.org/10.2105/AJPH.2013.301548

American Cancer Society. (2011). Cancer facts & figures for African Americans 2011. Retrieved June 16, 2015, from http://www.cancer.org/acs/groups/content/@epidemiologysurveilance/documents/document/acspc-027765.pdf

Austin, S. B., Pazaris, M. J., Rosner, B., Bowen, D. J., Rich-Edwards, J., & Spiegelman, D. (2012). Application of the Rosner-Colditz risk prediction model to estimate sexual orientation group disparities in breast cancer risk in a US cohort of premenopausal women. *Cancer Epidemiology, Biomarkers & Prevention, 21*(12), 2201–2208. Retrieved from http://cebp.aacrjournals.org/content/21/12/2201.short

Baral, S. D., Poteat, T., Strömdahl, S., Wirtz, A. L., Guadamuz, T. E., & Beyrer, C. (2013). Worldwide burden of HIV in transgender women: A systematic review and meta-analysis. *The Lancet Infectious Diseases, 13*(3), 214–222. Retrieved from http://doi.org/10.1016/S1473-3099(12)70315-8

Blosnich, J. R., Bossarte, R., Silver, E., & Silenzio, V. (2013). Health care utilization and health indicators among a national sample of U.S. veterans in same-sex partnerships. *Military Medicine, 178*(2), 207–212.

Blosnich, J. R., Farmer, G. W., Lee, J. G., Silenzio, V. M., & Bowen, D. J. (2014). Health inequalities among sexual minority adults: Evidence from Ten U.S. states, 2010. *American Journal of Preventive Medicine, 46*(4), 337–349. Retrieved from http://doi.org/10.1016/j.amepre.2013.11.010

Blosnich, J. R., Lee, J. G., Bossarte, R., & Silenzio, V. M. (2013). Asthma disparities and within-group differences in a national, probability sample of same-sex partnered adults. *American Journal of Public Health, 103*(9), e83–e87. Retrieved from http://doi.org/10.2105/AJPH.2013.301217

Boehmer, U., & Case, P. (2006). Sexual minority women's interactions with breast cancer providers. *Women & Health, 44*(2), 41–58.

Boehmer, U., Miao, X., & Ozonoff, A. (2011). Cancer survivorship and sexual orientation. *Cancer, 117*(16), 3796–3804. Retrieved from http://doi.org/10.1002/cncr.25950

Boehmer, U., Miao, X., Linkletter, C., & Clark, M. A. (2012). Adult health behaviors over the life course by sexual orientation. *American Journal of Public Health, 102*(2), 292–300. Retrieved from http://doi.org/10.2105/AJPH.2011.300334

Brown, G. R., & Jones, K. T. (2015). Incidence of breast cancer in a cohort of 5,135 transgender veterans. *Breast Cancer Research and Treatment, 149*(1), 191–198. Retrieved from http://doi.org/10.1007/s10549–014–3213–2

Center for Disease Control and Prevention. (2015). CDC-facts sheet-HIV among African American gay and bisexual men-HIV among African Americans-Risk-HIV/AIDS. Retrieved June 10, 2015, from http://www.cdc.gov/hiv/risk/racialethnic/bmsm/facts/index.html

Charlton, B. M., Corliss, H. L., Missmer, S. A., Frazier, A. L., Rosario, M., Kahn, J. A., & Austin, S. B. (2011). Reproductive health screening disparities and sexual orientation in a cohort study of U.S. adolescent and young adult females. *The Journal of Adolescent Health, 49*(5), 505–510. Retrieved from http://doi.org/10.1016/j.jadohealth.2011.03.013

Cochran, S. D., & Mays, V. M. (2007). Physical health complaints among lesbians, gay men, and bisexual and homosexually experienced heterosexual individuals: Results from the California Quality of Life Survey. *American Journal of Public Health, 97*, 2048–2055. Retrieved from http://doi.org/10.2105/AJPH.2006.087254

Cochran, S. D., & Mays, V. M. (2012). Risk of breast cancer mortality among women cohabiting with same sex partners: Findings from the National Health Interview Survey, 1997–2003. *Journal of Women's Health, 21*(5), 528–533. Retrieved from http://doi.org/10.1089/jwh.2011.3134

Cochran, S. D., Mays, V. M., Alegria, M., Ortega, A. N., & Takeuchi, D. (2007). Mental health and substance use disorders among Latino and Asian American lesbian, gay, and bisexual adults. *Journal of Consulting and Clinical Psychology, 75*, 785–794.

Cochran, S. D., Mays, V. M., Bowen, D. J., Gage, S., Bybee, D., Roberts, S. J., … White, J. (2001). Cancer-related risk indicators and preventive screening behaviors among lesbians and bisexual women. *American Journal of Public Health, 91*, 591–597.

Conron, K. J., Mimiaga, M. J., & Landers, S. J. (2010). A population-based study of sexual orientation identity and gender differences in adult health. *American Journal of Public Health, 100*(10), 1953–1960. Retrieved from http://doi.org/10.2105/AJPH.2009.174169

Conron, K. J., Scott, G., Stowell, G. S., & Landers, S. J. (2012). Transgender health in Massachusetts: Results from a household probability sample of adults. *American Journal of Public Health, 102*(1), 118–122. Retrieved from http://doi.org/10.2105/AJPH.2011.300315

Coulter, R. W., Kenst, K. S., Bowen, D. J., & Scout. (2014). Research funded by the National Institutes of Health on the health of lesbian, gay, bisexual, and transgender populations. *American Journal of Public Health, 104*(2), e105–e112. Retrieved from http://doi.org/10.2105/AJPH.2013.301501

Diamant, A. L., Schuster, M. A., & Lever, J. (2000). Receipt of preventive health care services by lesbians. *American Journal of Preventive Medicine, 19*, 141–148.

Dibble, S. L., Roberts, S. A., Robertson, P. A., & Paul, S. M. (2002). Risk factors for ovarian cancer: Lesbian and heterosexual women. *Oncology Nursing Forum, 29*, E1–E7. Retrieved from http://doi.org/10.1188/02.ONF.E1-E7

Dibble, S. L., Roberts, S. A., Robertson, P. A., & Paul, S. M. (2004). Breast cancer risk profiles between lesbians and their heterosexual sisters. *Women's Health Issues, 14*, 60–68.

Dibble, S. L., Vanoni, J. M., & Miaskowski, C. (1997). Women's attitudes toward breast cancer screening procedures: Differences by ethnicity. *Women's Health Issues: Official Publication of the Jacobs Institute of Women's Health, 7*, 47–54.

Eliason, M. J., Ingraham, N., Fogel, S. C., McElroy, J. A., Lorvick, J., Mauery, D. R., & Haynes, S. (2015). A systematic review of the literature on weight in sexual minority women. *Women's Health Issues, 25*(2), 162–175. Retrieved from http://doi.org/10.1016/j.whi.2014.12.001

Eliason, M. J., Martinson, M., & Carabez, R. (2015). Disability among sexual minority women: Descriptive data from an invisible population. *Journal of LGBT Health research*, LGBT Health, *2*(2), 113–120. Retrieved from http://doi.org/10.1089/lgbt.2014.009

Engels, E. A. (2007). Infectious agents as causes of non-Hodgkin lymphoma. *Cancer Epidemiology, Biomarkers & Prevention*, *16*, 401–404. Retrieved from http://doi.org/10.1158/1055–9965.EPI-06–1056

Everett, B., & Mollborn, S. (2013). Differences in hypertension by sexual orientation among U.S. young adults. *Journal of Community Health*, *38*(3), 588–596. Retrieved from http://doi.org/10.1007/s10900–013–9655–3

Everett, B. G., Rosario, M., McLaughlin, K. A., & Austin, S. B. (2014). Sexual orientation and gender differences in markers of inflammation and immune functioning. *Annals of Behavioral Medicine*, *47*(1), 57–70. Retrieved from http://doi.org/10.1007/s12160–013–9567–6

Fish, J., & Anthony, D. (2005). UK national lesbians and health care survey. *Women & Health*, *41*(3), 27–45. Retrieved from http://doi.org/10.1300/J013v41n03_02

Fredriksen-Goldsen, K. I., Cook-Daniels, L., Kim, H.-J., Erosheva, E. A., Emlet, C. A., Hoy-Ellis, C. P., … Muraco, A. (2014). Physical and mental health of transgender older adults: An at-risk and underserved population. *The Gerontologist*, *54*(3), 488–500. Retrieved from http://doi.org/10.1093/geront/gnt021

Fredriksen-Goldsen, K., Kim, H., & Barkan, S. (2012). Disability among lesbian, gay, and bisexual adults: Disparities in prevalence and risk. *American Journal of Public Health*, *102*, 16–21.

Fredriksen-Goldsen, K. I., Kim, H. J., Barkan, S. E., Muraco, A., & Hoy-Ellis, C. P. (2013). Health disparities among lesbian, gay, and bisexual older adults: Results from a population-based study. *American Journal of Public Health*, *103*, 1802–1809. Retrieved from http://doi.org/10.2105/AJPH.2012.301110

Frisch, M., Smith, E., Grulich, A., & Johansen, C. (2003). Cancer in a population-based cohort of men and women in registered homosexual partnerships. *American Journal of Epidemiology*, *157*(11), 966–972. Retrieved from http://doi.org/10.1093/aje/kwg067

Garland-Forshee, R. Y., Fiala, S. C., Ngo, D. L., & Moseley, K. (2014). Sexual orientation and sex differences in adult chronic conditions, health risk factors, and protective health practices, Oregon, 2005–2008. *Preventing Chronic Disease*, *11*, E136. Retrieved from http://doi.org/10.5888/pcd11.140126

Hatzenbuehler, M. L., McLaughlin, K. A., & Slopen, N. (2013). Sexual orientation disparities in cardiovascular biomarkers among young adults. *American Journal of Preventive Medicine*, *44*(6), 612–621. Retrieved from http://doi.org/10.1016/j.amepre.2013.01.027

Heck, J. E., & Jacobson, J. S. (2006). Asthma diagnosis among individuals in same-sex relationships. *The Journal of Asthma: Official Journal of the Association for the Care of Asthma*, *43*(8), 579–584. Retrieved from http://doi.org/10. 1080/02770900600878289

Herbst, J. H., Jacobs, E. D., Finlayson, T. J., McKleroy, V. S., Neumann, M. S., Crepaz, N., & HIV/AIDS Prevention Research Synthesis Team. (2008). Estimating HIV prevalence and risk behaviors of transgender persons in the United States: A systematic review. *AIDS and Behavior, 12*(1), 1–17. Retrieved from http://doi.org/10.1007/s10461–007–9299–3

Jesdale, B. M., & Mitchell, J. W. (2012). Reported excellent health among men in same-sex and mixed-sex couples: Behavioral Risk Factor Surveillance System, 1993–2010. *Journal of Homosexuality*, *59*(6), 788–807. Retrieved from http://doi.org/10.1080/00918369.2012.694755

Koh, A. S. (2000). Use of preventive health behaviors by lesbian, bisexual, and heterosexual women: Questionnaire survey. *The Western Journal of Medicine*, *172*(6), 379–384.

Margolies, L., & Goeren, B. (2009). *Anal cancer, HIV, and gay/bisexual men. Gay Men's Health Crisis Treatment Issues*. New York, NY.

Martró, E., Esteve, A., Schulz, T. F., Sheldon, J., Gambús, G., Muñoz, R., … Casabona, J. (2007). Risk factors for human Herpesvirus 8 infection and AIDS-associated Kaposi's sarcoma among men who have sex with men in a European multicentre study. *International Journal of Cancer*, *120*(5), 1129–1135.

Matthews, A. K., Brandenburg, D. L., Johnson, T. P., & Hughes, T. L. (2004). Correlates of underutilization of gynecological cancer screening among lesbian and heterosexual women. *Preventive Medicine, 38*(1), 105–113.

Matthews, D. D., & Lee, J. G. L. (2014). A profile of North Carolina lesbian, gay, and bisexual health disparities, 2011. *American Journal of Public Health, 104*(6), e98–e105. Retrieved from http://doi.org/10.2105/AJPH.2013.301751

Mattocks, K. M., Sadler, A., Yano, E. M., Krebs, E. E., Zephyrin, L., Brandt, C., ... Haskell, S. (2013). Sexual victimization, health status, and VA healthcare utilization among lesbian and bisexual OEF/OIF veterans. *Journal of General Internal Medicine, 28*(Suppl 2), S604–S608. Retrieved from http://doi.org/10.1007/s11606–013–2357–9

Mays, V. M., Yancey, A. K., Cochran, S. D., Weber, M., & Fielding, J. E. (2002). Heterogeneity of health disparities among -African American, Hispanic, and Asian American women: Unrecognized influences of sexual orientation. *American Journal of Public Health, 92*(4), 632–639.

McNair, R., Szalacha, L. A., & Hughes, T. L. (2011). Health status, health service use, and satisfaction according to sexual identity of young Australian women. *Women's Health Issues, 21*(1), 40–47. Retrieved from http://doi.org/10.1016/j.whi.2010.08.002

Nemoto, T., Operario, D., & Keatley, J. (2005). Health and social services for male-to-female transgender persons of color in San Francisco. *International Journal of Transgenderism, 8*(2–3), 5–19. Retrieved from http://doi.org/10.1300/J485v08n02_02

Nemoto, T., Operario, D., & Keatley, J. (2006). Health and social services for male-to-female transgender persons of color in San Francisco. In W. O. Bockting & E. Avery (Eds.), *Transgender health and HIV prevention: Needs assessment studies from transgender communities across the United States* (pp. 5–20). Haworth.

Nuttbrock, L., Bockting, W., Rosenblum, A., Hwahng, S., Mason, M., Macri, M., & Becker, J. (2014). Gender abuse and incident HIV/STI among transgender women in New York City: Buffering effect of involvement in a transgender community. *AIDS and Behavior.* Retrieved from http://doi.org/10.1007/s10461–014–0977–7

Peitzmeier, S. M., Khullar, K., Reisner, S. L., & Potter, J. (2014). Pap test use is lower among female-to-male patients than non-transgender women. *American Journal of Preventive Medicine, 47*(6), 808–812. Retrieved from http://doi.org/10.1016/j.amepre.2014.07.031

Poteat, T., Reisner, S. L., & Radix, A. (2014). HIV epidemics among transgender women. *Current Opinion in HIV and AIDS, 9*(2), 168–173. Retrieved from http://doi.org/10.1097/COH.0000000000000030

Rachlin, K., Green, J., & Lombardi, E. (2008). Utilization of health care among female-to-male transgender individuals in the United States. *Journal of Homosexuality, 54*(3), 243–258. Retrieved from http://doi.org/10.1080/00918360801982124

Rankow, E. J., & Tessaro, I. (1998). Cervical cancer risk and Papanicolaou screening in a sample of lesbian and bisexual women. *The Journal of Family Practice, 47*(2), 139–143.

Reisner, S. L., Gamarel, K. E., Dunham, E., Hopwood, R., & Hwahng, S. (2013). Female-to-male transmasculine adult health: A mixed-methods community-based needs assessment. *Journal of the American Psychiatric Nurses Association, 19*(5), 293–303. Retrieved from http://doi.org/10.1177/1078390313500693

Robbins, H. A., Pfeiffer, R. M., Shiels, M. S., Li, J., Hall, H. I., & Engels, E. A. (2015). Excess cancers among HIV-infected people in the United States. *Journal of the National Cancer Institute, 107*(4). Retrieved from http://doi.org/10.1093/jnci/dju503

Roberts, S. J., & Sorensen, L. (1999). Health related behaviors and cancer screening of lesbians: Results from the Boston Lesbian Health Project. *Women & Health, 28*(4), 1–12. Retrieved from http://doi.org/10.1300/J013v28n04_01

Sausa, L. A., Keatley, J., & Operario, D. (2007). Perceived risks and benefits of sex work among transgender women of color in San Francisco. *Archives of Sexual Behavior, 36*(6), 768–777. Retrieved from http://doi.org/10.1007/s10508–007–9210–3

Sell, R. (2015). LGBTData.com. Retrieved June 3, 2015, from http://www.lgbtdata.com/

Smith, D. K., Grohskopf, L. A., Black, R. J., Auerbach, J. D., Veronese, F., Struble, K. A., … Greenberg, A. E; U.S. Department of Health and Human Services. (2005). Antiretroviral postexposure prophylaxis after sexual, injection-drug use, or other nonoccupational exposure to HIV in the United States: recommendations from the US Department of Health and Human Services. *MMWR. Recommendations and Reports: Morbidity and Mortality Weekly Report. Recommendations and Reports/Centers for Disease Control, 54*(RR-2), 1–20. Retrieved from http://francais.cdc.gov/mmwr/preview/mmwrhtml/rr5402a1.htm

Thomeer, M. B. (2013). Sexual minority status and self-rated health: the importance of socioeconomic status, age, and sex. *American Journal of Public Health, 103*, 881–888. Retrieved from http://doi.org/10.2105/AJPH.2012.301040

Tracy, J. K., Lydecker, A. D., & Ireland, L. (2010). Barriers to cervical cancer screening among lesbians. *Journal of Women's Health, 19*(2), 229–237. Retrieved from http://doi.org/10.1089/jwh.2009.1393

Tracy, J. K., Schluterman, N. H., & Greenberg, D. R. (2013). Understanding cervical cancer screening among lesbians: A national survey. *BMC Public Health, 13*, 442. Retrieved from http://doi.org/10.1186/1471–2458–13–442

Valanis, B. G., Bowen, D. J., Bassford, T., Whitlock, E., Charney, P., & Carter, R. A. (2000). Sexual orientation and health: Comparisons in the women's health initiative sample. *Archives of Family Medicine, 9*(9), 843–853.

Ward, B. W., Dahlhamer, J. M., Galinsky, A. M., & Joestl, S. S. (2014). Sexual orientation and health among U.S. adults: National health interview survey, 2013. *National Health Statistics Reports, (77)*, 1–10.

White, J. C., & Dull, V. T. (1997). Health risk factors and health-seeking behavior in lesbians. *Journal of Women's Health/The Official Publication of the Society for the Advancement of Women's Health Research, 6*(1), 103–112.

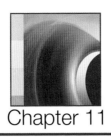

Chapter 11

Provider Attitudes and Knowledge

"It would be very damaging if you got into interactions with healthcare providers in which you were considered deviant … it is like putting your life in someone's hands who really hates you." (respondent in Stevens & Hall, 1988, p. 71)

The fundamental purpose of this book is to provide healthcare professionals with a general introduction to LGBTQ experience in general and to point toward many factors that are related to health disparities for these communities. Healthcare systems are a microcosm of society, where institutionalized heterosexism and gender normativity affect policies, procedures, and even individual provider attitudes. Accessing health care means running a gauntlet of strangers, each potentially negative or ambivalent about LGBTQ people. From the receptionist to the unit nurses and medical students, the physical therapist and the person who delivers the meals, to the social workers and chaplains and unit clerks, patients will come into contact with many providers with differing levels of knowledge and attitudes. So many different people may take a history from the patient (unit clerks, nurses, medical students, attending physicians) and each episode of coming out brings a pang of anxiety about the potential reaction from the provider.

We believe that improving provider attitudes and knowledge are at the heart of any effort to end LGBTQ health and healthcare disparities, but this is much easier said than done. If you are reading this book, you are likely to sincerely want to learn and take steps that are needed to provide better care, but many well-intended healthcare workers still remain unaware of the changes that need to happen. In this chapter, we present evidence of the effects of stigma on provider attitudes and knowledge—evidence that provides the rationale for moving ahead with projects that address the existing gaps in knowledge and attitudes. Negative or uninformed healthcare providers perpetuate the health disparities seen in LGBTQ populations. The chapter ends with recommendations for curriculum changes in health professional student education and in continuing education for providers. In a later chapter, we will address the other system-wide structural changes that need to happen.

Existing Provider Attitudes and Knowledge

It is widely recognized that LGBTQ patients often receive substandard care, even refusal of care, have less access to care because of inadequate medical insurance coverage, and avoid care due in part to negative experiences in the healthcare system (The Joint Commission, 2011). Chapter 8 provided more detail on the types of poor treatment that many LGBTQ people and their partners/families have experienced. This lack of quality care stems from more than a century of stigma in healthcare settings as well as in society as a whole. In spite of depathologizing of homosexuality in the mid 1970s, progress in educating healthcare professionals has been excruciatingly slow, and few providers have received the information they need to provide quality care. In fact, even today a significant minority of providers seek to "treat" homosexuality using damaging tactics generally described as "conversion" or "reparative" therapies (Association of American Medical Colleges [AAMC], 2014), although these strategies have been denounced by all the major healthcare professional organizations. Reparative therapy for minor-aged youth has been legally banned in California, New Jersey, and Oregon as of mid-2015. See Chapter 8 for more detail on reparative therapies. Healthcare professionals who actively try to convert or "cure" LGBTQ people are relatively rare, but the majority of healthcare professionals lack knowledge that is needed to provide the best care.

Significant disparities in LGBTQ health care are perpetrated by providers who
- Harbor unconscious bias and negative attitudes toward people who are LGBTQ, that is, professionals who have not undergone a process of examining attitudes acquired early in life that may have been inaccurate.
- Engage in overtly discriminatory behaviors such as refusing to care for LGBTQ patients or provide less nurturing or respectful care that may affect patient well-being or their likelihood of continuing care;
- Engage in subtle behaviors that perpetuate stereotypes or are dismissive of LGBTQ patients' rights to quality care or fair treatment (microaggressions);
- Fail to recognize signs of minority stress that lead to high-risk behaviors and endanger health status; and/or
- Are not prepared to adequately communicate with LGBTQ individuals and families, resulting in inadequate histories and assessments because of a lack of knowledge of LGBTQ terminology and recognition of the reality of LGBTQ lives.

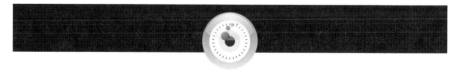

Watch This 11.1

Watch this 10-minute video prepared by the New York City Health and Hospitals Corporation to highlight the importance of understanding LGBTQ experience—not simply a person's diagnosis—to provide effective care. Titled "To Treat Me, You Have to Know Who I Am" the video features a number of LGBTQ people who describe their situations, and what they encountered in the healthcare system when they needed care.
    https://goo.gl/5vVaQR

Historical Overview of Healthcare Provider Attitude Studies

Healthcare providers worldwide do not have a strong record in terms of knowledge and positive attitudes related to LGBTQ health, and even less related to the life experience of LGBTQ people. Tragically, the education provided for entry in to all the healthcare disciplines has almost entirely ignored LGBTQ health, and educators have only recently begun to recognize this as a problem. Over and over again, healthcare providers report having received little or no education or training related to LGBTQ health, and what educational content is reported tends to relate only to HIV/AIDS as a disease, perpetrating many of the harmful myths and stereotypes related to LGBTQ experience. In the following sections, we discuss the limited evidence related to the knowledge and attitudes of nurses, physicians, and providers in other disciplines, then we will address the state of education for healthcare providers as a basis for creating change.

Nursing

One of the earliest studies in the field of nursing that aimed to determine provider attitudes was conducted by Carla Randall, whose master's thesis reported on the findings of a survey of BSN faculty attitudes toward lesbians (Randall, 1987). She described a high prevalence of negative attitudes among nurse educators, including the misguided belief among one-fifth of the 100 respondents that the AIDS virus is commonly transmitted between lesbians. Over half of these educators believed that lesbianism is not a natural expression of human sexuality, and over 25% felt uncomfortable communicating with someone they knew to be a lesbian. Many nurse educators in the 1980s and 90s reported that they were discouraged from conducting research on LGBTQ topics or teaching this content in didactic or clinical courses (Randall & Eliason, 2012).

A Swedish nurse researcher conducted a series of studies about nurses' and nursing students' knowledge and attitudes, finding that 36% of practicing nurses and 26% of nursing students would not care for HIV positive patients if given the option (Röndahl, Innala, & Carlsson, 2004a), nurses who believed that homosexuality was congenital rather than acquired tended to have more positive attitudes (Röndahl, Innala, & Carlsson, 2004b), and 36% of practicing nurses but only 9% of student nurses would refrain from caring for homosexual patients if they could (Röndahl et al., 2004b). These findings are interesting, given the overall longer history of acceptance of LGBTQ people in Scandinavian countries.

Recent studies that have examined both attitudes and knowledge of nurses and nurse educators reflect a general shift toward more positive attitudes, but significant gaps in knowledge about LGBTQ health still exist (Carabez, Pellegrini, Mankovitz, Eliason, & Dariotis, 2015b; Dorsen, 2012; Klotzbaugh & Spencer, 2014; Lim, Johnson, & Eliason, 2015). For example, one study found that 85% of senior nursing students felt they were not prepared by their nursing education to provide quality care to LGBTQ patients, and 1 in 10 thought that their religious values might get in the way of quality care (Carabez et al., 2015b). A study of practicing nurses in the San Francisco Bay Area revealed that 80% of them had received no education or training on LGBTQ issues in nursing school, continuing education, or inservice (Carabez, Pellegrini, Mankovitz, Eliason, Ciano, et al., 2015a). In a study of nurse administrators, nearly 25% considered themselves very religious, and that was a predictor of more negativity about LGBTQ people (Klotzbaugh & Spencer, 2014). A recent study (Sabin, Riskind, & Nosek, 2015) that measured both implicit (unconscious) and explicit (conscious) bias among healthcare workers found that nurses had strong particularly widespread implicit preference for heterosexual people, and heterosexual male nurses had the greatest degree of bias. This implicit bias may affect patient care on a level that the provider is only dimly aware of.

Fewer studies have addressed nurses' attitudes and knowledge of transgender patients (Bauer et al., 2009; Merryfeather & Bruce, 2014). In one study of practicing nurses, many professed to have little understanding of the transgender experience, with some confusing the concepts of sexual orientation and gender identity, and many manifestations of discomfort in even discussing the topic (Carabez, Eliason, & Martinson, 2016). Although many nurses acknowledged that transgender patients may experience high rates of substance abuse and violence, very few related this to stigma. In another study, nurses were asked if their agencies/institutions have gender inclusive questions on forms—questions that could identify transgender patients (Carabez, Pellegrini, Mankowitz, Eliason, & Scott, 2015c). The majority of nurses did not even understand the question.

Much progress has been made in the past decade, and changes in society in general have shifted nurses' attitudes about LGBTQ people and increased their desire to learn about them. Among nurse educators, there is now a strong belief that LGBTQ issues are important to include in the curriculum, but most educators still report a lack of knowledge to be able to incorporate this education (Sirota, 2013). A recent survey of over 1,000 nurse faculty members found that the average time devoted to LGBTQ topics in nursing education was slightly over 2 hours, although 17% reported there was no LGBTQ content at all in their programs (Lim et al., 2015). This lack of inclusion of LGBTQ health was not because of resistance to teaching about these topics, as 70% of respondents indicated that they were willing and ready to teach these topics, and 75% indicated they would be comfortable teaching LGBTQ topics. The challenge now is creating adequate faculty development to prepare nurse educators, and changes in curricula to assure that these issues are addressed adequately.

Medicine

In medicine, a survey of members of the San Diego County Medical Society in 1982 found 58% overall were homophobic, with men having higher homophobia scores than women (Mathews, Booth, Turner, & Kessler, 1986). This survey was repeated in 1999 (Smith & Mathews, 2007), with a sample that was 78% male and 93% heterosexual (the earlier study did not ask about respondents' sexual orientation). Although rates of homophobia had dropped to 19%, the finding that one in five physicians was still overtly homophobic was shocking. On a positive note, the percent of respondents who said that they would not admit a highly qualified gay student to medical school dropped from 29% in 1982 to 3% in 1999.

Chaimowitz (1991) studied staff in one Canadian medical school and found that 26% of psychiatric faculty, 33% of psychiatric residents, and 36% of family practice residents were homophobic, with men showing more homophobia than women. One in four second year medical students in Chicago (Klamen, Grossman, & Kopacz, 1999) believed that homosexuality is immoral and 9% considered it a mental illness, 15 years after homosexuality was removed from the DSM. Another study found that medical students, residents, and physician faculty members witnessed events of "derogatory homophobic discrimination" in their medical colleagues to the same extent as they witnessed gender and racial discrimination (Oancia, Bohm, Carry, Cujec, & Johnson, 2000). In a study of more than 1,000 New Mexican physicians (Ramos, Tellez, Palley, Umland, & Skipper, 1998), 11% stated that they would not refer a patient to an LGBT physician. Similarly, 25% of family practice program directors said that they would not match openly gay residents to their programs (Oriel, Madlon-Kay, Govaker, & Mersy, 1996).

Sanchez, Rabatin, Sanchez, Hubbard, & Kalet (2006) surveyed medical students in clinical rotations and found that fewer than half always interviewed their patients about same-sex behaviors, and the majority said that they rarely or never knew a patient's sexual orientation. More than one-fourth (28%) said that they were uncomfortable meeting an LGBT patient's needs. Finally, Kitts (2010) surveyed residents and attending physicians at one medical school and reported that 23% agreed that same-sex relationships are always or almost always wrong, and only 29% would routinely discuss sexual orientation with adolescent patients. An earlier study (Lena, Wiebe, Ingram, & Jabbour, 2002) had found that 70% of pediatricians said they did not address sexual orientation of their patients because they lacked knowledge to address sexual minority youth if they did ask the questions.

One study in the early 1980s examined attitudes about "transsexual" (the term they used in this study) patients (Franzini & Casinelli, 1986). A random sample of physicians from the AMA and psychologists from the National Register of Health Service Providers were surveyed. Psychologists reported more positive attitudes about transsexual patients than did physicians. Most respondents said that transsexuals would be better off if they gave up their desire for surgery (61%), 54% thought that surgery was harmful to their mental health, and 72% thought that gender reassignment surgery was not advisable. Clearly there is a need for more research on attitudes about transgender patients.

In one recent study, Burke et al. (2015) surveyed nearly 4,500 heterosexual first year medical students from 49 medical schools in the United States. They found high rates of two kinds of bias; 46% of respondents showed explicit bias, or consciously controlled negative attitudes; and shockingly, 74% demonstrated implicit bias, or automatic responses that are outside of conscious awareness. Positive attitudes were associated with greater contact with LGBT people, more favorable experiences with the contact, and greater levels of empathy. This bias may explain the problems with many of the studies cited here, namely, poor response rates. Sabin et al. (2015) also studied implicit bias, finding that although most people had some implicit bias for people of the same sexuality, LGB healthcare providers showed less bias than heterosexual healthcare providers.

In 2008, the American Medical Association (AMA) and GLMA: Health Professionals Advancing LGBT Equality, attempted to survey a random sample of physicians from the AMA database. Other studies conducted by the AMA have resulted in response rates of over 90%, but this one, on physician knowledge, experience, and attitudes about LGBT patients, resulted in only a 11% response rate, too low to yield any reliable findings (Matt Wynia of the American Medical Association, personal communication). This low response rate was in spite of sending out the survey three times and providing incentives for participation.

A study of osteopathic medical students echoed recent findings of nursing students: most had positive attitudes, but lacked sufficient knowledge for quality patient care (Lapinski, Sexton, & Baker, 2014), and the same finding was supported by a large scale survey of medical students from both allopathic and osteopathic schools; they were willing and wanted to learn more about LGBTQ health, but felt unprepared by the medical school curriculum (White et al., 2015). One study reported that U.S. medical schools had a median of about 5 hours of LGBTQ content across the entire curriculum, with 7% indicating no LGBTQ content in pre-clinical courses and 33% having no LGBTQ content in clinical rotations (Obedin-Maliver et al., 2011). Interviews with medical school deans and chief medical officers across the United States (Khalili, Leung, & Diamant, 2015) found that 52% of hospitals had no LGBT training at all, whereas 32% had some limited level of training, and only 16% had comprehensive training. On the other hand, 80% had an interest to do more LGBT training.

Other Health Disciplines

Findings among other disciplines, such as psychology and social work, are very similar, suggesting that while attitudes are gradually changing, there is still a persistent level of homonegativity, gender normativity, and a general lack of knowledge of LGBTQ experience that prevails among a minority of healthcare providers (Harris, Nightengale, & Owen, 1995; Lapinski et al., 2014; More, Whitehead, & Gonthier, 2004; Willging, Salvador, & Kano, 2006). Little research has focused on other healthcare professionals such as physician assistants, dentists, and physical therapists. It is important to study all the healthcare professionals and ancillary staff with whom LGBTQ patients come into contact, including nursing assistants, receptionists, technicians, dieticians, patient navigators, and even housekeepers, as they also affect the overall climate in a healthcare setting. Many studies of negative attitudes about LGBT people have found a very strong link to education. Those with lower levels of education tend to have more negative attitudes; therefore, workers in nonprofessional service jobs may be even more likely than doctors, nurses, and other highly trained professionals, to have negative attitudes that may impact patient care.

Improving Health Professional Education

The lack of LGBTQ content in all healthcare profession curricula is astounding (Corliss, Shankle, & Moyer, 2007; Khalili et al., 2015; Lim et al., 2015; More et al., 2004; Obedin-Maliver et al., 2011; Wallick, Cambre, & Townsend, 1992). The only mention related to LGBTQ health has been, and often still is, the inclusion of content on HIV/AIDS, which in itself perpetuates a host of myths and stereotypes, including the myth that same-sex sexuality itself is dangerous, "contagious," and to be feared.

    Part of the problem lies in the fact that faculty themselves are not prepared and a few are unwilling to address LGBT health issues. Further, many faculty feel overburdened already with the vast scope of content that they are compelled to include, so the mere mention of including yet another curriculum component is beyond comprehension. Nevertheless, there is now widespread recognition that not only is it imperative to address LGBTQ health in professional education, but doing so is feasible and enriches the overall goal of preparing compassionate, knowledgeable, and culturally competent practitioners (Carabez et al., 2016; Kirkpatrick, Esterhuizen, Jesse, & Brown, 2015; Wong, 2014). Several advocacy efforts have been initiated in healthcare disciplines to correct the gaps in knowledge about LGBTQ issues.

Advocacy Efforts with Mainstream Health Organizations/Institutions

Advocacy on behalf of LGBTQ health is one of the most important steps that all health-care providers have at their fingertips. Advocacy happens at all levels—in interactions with individual patients and families, by promoting and making visible a welcoming environment in each healthcare setting, by working with organizational groups to adopt positive LGBTQ policies, and by addressing LGBTQ issues in boardrooms, classrooms, and conferences. By reading and learning the information in this book you are better prepared to advocate for LGBTQ issues in all of these arenas. There are a number of important organizational LGBTQ advocacy actions and policies that have been adopted by a number of professional organizations, and that provide inspiration for future actions.

The IOM 2011 Report titled "The Health of Lesbian, Gay, Bisexual, and Trans-gender People: Building a Foundation for Better Understanding" is one of the most important advocacy statements to appear on behalf of LGBT health. It provides the rationale and guidelines on which a number of new initiatives can be based to improve the quality of LGBTQ health care, and an excellent framework from which to conceptualize curriculum changes that incorporate LGBTQ health (Institute of Medicine, 2011). Table 11.1 shows a model for using the research priorities of the IOM report to create a template for advocacy at all levels, and for LGBTQ-101 training for health-care professional training.

In medicine, the LGBT Advisory Committee of the American Medical Association (http://www.ama-assn.org/ama/pub/about-ama/our-people/member-groups-sections/glbt-advisory-committee.page) has issued a number of policy statements related to LGBTQ patient care, including policies on general discrimination issues, patient-related policies, physician-related policies, and education and structural policies (to review see http://www.ama-assn.org/ama/pub/about-ama/our-people/member-groups-sections/glbt-advisory-committee/ama-policy-regarding-sexual-orientation.page?).

The National Student Nurses Association was among the first nursing organizations to make public policy statements advocating inclusion of LGBTQ information in nursing curricula. Their 2010 paper advocated for culturally competent education (National Student Nurses Association, 2010). Then in 2012, NSNA expanded their position to advocate for implementation of practices based on the Joint Commission Report (National Student Nurses Association, 2012).

The American Academy of Nursing established an LGBTQ Expert Panel in 2011, and has since issued a number of recent policy statements that advocate for LGBTQ health policy issues:

- 2012—support for marriage equality (http://www.aannet.org/pr-71612–2012-marriage-equality)
- 2012—Health Care for Sexual Minority and Gender Diverse Populations—(http://www.aannet.org/assets/lgbtq%20overachstatement%20final%207%2011%2012.pdf)
- February 2015—Health care decision making and hospital visitation (http://www.nursingoutlook.org/article/S0029–6554(14)00295–4/fulltext)

Table 11.1 – Using the IOM Report to Improve Provider Education and LGBTQ Patient Care Advocacy

Priority Area	Implications for Education	Implications for Advocacy
Intersecting demographics	Assure adequate curricular content related to demographics that intersect with sexual orientation and gender identity.	Include characteristics of LGBTQ populations such as age (and age of sexual and gender identity milestones), race/ethnicity, sex/gender, geographic location, education, parental status, relationship status, etc. in standard data collection.
Social influences	Focus on the effects of stigma on income, safety, and health. Teach basic terminology related to sex, gender, and sexuality and assess student's use of appropriate language and knowledge of the needs of and experiences of different subsets of the LGBTQ population.	Assure familiarity with basic terminology related to sex, gender, and sexuality so that providers use appropriate language for different subsets of the LGBTQ population when taking histories, and that they advocate for systems change to collect information about sexuality and gender.
Healthcare inequalities	Assure that students learn the current evidence related to LGBTQ disparities related to mental health, physical health, and access to quality healthcare services.	Apply research evidence on health disparities, especially that coming from population-based health surveillance tools such as NHANES, NHIS, BRFSS, CHIS, NESARC, NHSDA, YRBS, and others.
Intervention research	In educational settings, design and implement student research projects addressing the effectiveness of approaches to care for LGBTQ clients and families.	This is the area most lacking in research to support clinical practice. There are several HIV prevention models and a few substance abuse and mental health interventions, but much more research is needed. Explore whether and when culturally specific treatment models are necessary as opposed to mainstream treatments that are meant to be applicable to all.
Transgender-specific healthcare needs	Since transgender patients have the most unique healthcare needs and are the least familiar to healthcare providers, extra training on terminology, transition care, and respectful treatment is sorely needed.	Assure that all providers and students are familiar with resources such as WPATH (World Professional Association on Transgender Health) and the National Center of Excellence on Transgender Health.

NHANES, National Health and Nutrition Examination Survey; NHIS, National Health Interview Survey; BRFSS, Behavioral Risk Factors Surveillance Survey; CHIS, California Health Interview Survey; NESARC, National Epidemiological Survey on Alcohol and Related Conditions; NHSDA, National Household Survey on Drug Abuse; YRBS, Youth Risk Behavior Survey.

- June 2015—two policy statements—(1) opposition to reparative therapy and (2) opposing employment discrimination based on sexual orientation and/or gender identity (http://www.aannet.org/index.php?option=com_content&view=article&id=851:american-academy-of-nursing-opposes-reparative-therapy-and-employment-discrimination-against-lgbt-individuals&catid=23:news&Itemid=133)

Resources for Improving Practice and Curricular Inclusion

While there is still a long way to go, and there remains a great need for further research on which to base education and practice, it is no longer the case that there is a dearth of resources on which to build adequate LGBTQ-inclusive curricula. There are now a host of resources available that can used in any healthcare discipline for undergraduate, graduate, and continuing education, some of which can be used or adapted for any discipline, and some of which are specific to a discipline. Table 11.2 shows a number of the resources that are currently available.

There are two major issues in any effort to include LGBTQ issues in healthcare educational curricula: content and placement. Ideas for content can be found in Table 11.1, based on the IOM report on LGBT health. Placement is more challenging, but here are some suggestions for where this LGBTQ content might be located, depending on the way the curriculum is currently designed:

- Courses or lectures on lifespan development can include issues of identity development, such as the coming out process and how it differs across the life course.
- Lectures on discrimination, health disparities, and social justice can include the concepts of minority stress, heterosexism, and gender normativity.
- Courses or units that deal with assessment can introduce common terminology and help students practice asking more inclusive questions that might foster disclosures.
- Units on family can discuss the myriad ways that people, including LGBTQ individuals, forge families and urge broadening our definitions of family.
- Units about specific diseases or disorders can include some case studies that depict the issues that an LGBTQ person might experience, such as the difficulties of an FTM transgender person seeking routine gynecological care, or how a gay man might experience recovery from a heart attack, or how a bisexual person is perceived on a psychiatric unit, or how a lesbian seeking fertility treatments to conceive might face additional barriers to conception.
- Gerontology modules might address health disparities and discuss how LGBTQ elders might be treated in institutional settings.
- Sexual health units can include LGBTQ issues that extend beyond HIV and STIs. For example, discussing use of Viagra among gay and bisexual men, treatment of sexual dysfunction resulting from estrogen use in transgender women, or dealing with childhood sexual abuse experiences among lesbian and bisexual women.

Until healthcare training programs commit to inclusive and integrated educational models, there will continue to be a need for separate LGBTQ content. We would recommend that the best placement of the introductory information on LGBTQ issues is within an introduction to clinical care unit or a diversity course rather than the usual

Table 11.2 – Resources for Improving Practice and Curricular Inclusion	
Resource	**Description**
LavenderHealth.org http://lavenderhealth.org/education/	Contains an extensive section on education that includes guidelines for preparation, a sample syllabus, learning resources and activities including case studies, and guidelines for best educational practices. The authors are nurses, but the content is intended to be used by any healthcare discipline. All resources can be freely used with attribution.
GLMA White Paper by Shane Snowdon (2013) titled "Recommendations for Enhancing the Climate for LGBT Students and Employees in Health Professional Schools http://www.glma.org/_data/n_0001/resources/live/Recommendations%20for%20Enhancing%20LGBT%20Climate%20in%20Health%20Professional%20Schools.pdf	Focuses on educational programs and organizations, but outlines important ways to improve the climate of an organization that can be used in any setting to be more inclusive of LGBTQ students and employees, creative ways to advocate for LGBTQ people, and learning activities that can be used in any setting.
Human Rights Campaign http://www.hrc.org/the-hrc-story	One of the most important advocacy groups in the United States. The Healthcare Equality Index (HEI) and the Corporate Equality Index (CEI) provide a tangible way for organizations to demonstrate their progress in achieving basic LGBTQ Equality standards. The website contains a number of resources, and addresses a wide range of topics that intersect with LGBTQ health for people of all ages.
George Washington University LGBT Health Graduate Certificate Program http://lgbt.columbian.gwu.edu/	GW's LGBT Health Policy & Practice Program is the first practice-focused, interdisciplinary graduate certificate in the nation that trains current and future healthcare leaders and policy advocates on issues relating to the health and well-being of the lesbian, gay, bisexual, and transgender community.
The Williams Institute, UCLA http://williamsinstitute.law.ucla.edu/mission/	A national think tank at UCLA Law that conducts rigorous, independent research on sexual orientation and gender identity and public policy. The website contains papers that they have produced based on their work, all of which provide resources for not only those in the legal professions, but for the public at large. Focuses on using the U.S. Census and other large datasets to gain better understanding of the characteristics of LGBTQ individuals and families.
American Medical Association LGBT Advisory Committee http://www.ama-assn.org/ama/pub/about-ama/our-people/member-groups-sections/glbt-advisory-committee/glbt-resources.page?	Provides a web page giving links to important LGBTQ health resources, focusing on articles, podcasts, handouts, and presentations produced by the AMA and other leaders in the LGBT health field.

Table 11.2 – Resources for Improving Practice and Curricular Inclusion (*continued*)	
Resource	**Description**
Fenway Institute National LGBT Health Education Center http://www.lgbthealtheducation.org/	Provides learning modules, on-demand webinars and online resources that can be used in any setting to promote LGBTQ knowledge and awareness. The second edition of the Fenway Guide to Lesbian, Gay, Bisexual and Transgender Health is a leading textbook for LGBTQ health.
Local LGBT Health Centers	It is important to know that these exist, even if they are not located near you. This is not a comprehensive list, but these Centers have existed for a number of years serving their communities, and they offer a number of online resources and information that may be useful for anyone. <ul><li>Lyon Martin Health Services (part of 360 Health) San Francisco, CA—http://lyon-martin.org/</li><li>Los Angeles LGBT Center, Los Angeles, CA—http://www.lalgbtcenter.org/</li><li>Mazzoni Center, Philadelphia, PA—https://mazzonicenter.org/</li><li>Howard Brown Health Center, Chicago, CA—http://www.howardbrown.org/</li><li>Whitman Walker Health, Washington, DC—http://www.whitman-walker.org/</li><li>Callen Lorde Community Health Center, New York City, NY—http://callen-lorde.org/</li><li>Fenway Health, Boston, MA—http://fenwayhealth.org/</li></ul>

first (and often only) mention within human sexuality or HIV/AIDS modules. More advanced information can be placed within each specialty area (reproductive health, diversity, pediatrics, cardiovascular health, etc.).

Training Requirements for Practitioners

Given the history of next to zero LGBTQ education in professional training programs, it is safe to conclude that providers today have very little, if any, formal education. Therefore a dedicated program of LGBTQ continuing education in all settings is urgently needed to skill up practitioners in the field (Hanssmann, Morrison, & Russian, 2008; Stott, 2013). Some states now require that all physicians and nurses receive cultural diversity training on a regular basis. This could become a federal mandate, with a provision that diversity training include sexual orientation and gender identity.

Until that happens, there are many more journal articles and programs appearing that provide continuing education—here are a few examples:

- Caring for transgender patients—an article with continuing education credits available for nurses http://journals.lww.com/nursingmadeincrediblyeasy/pages/articleviewer.aspx?year=2014&issue=11000&article=00006&type =Fulltext (Hein & Levitt, 2014).

- The Fenway Institute's National LGBT Health Education Center (http://www.lgbthealtheducation.org/) provides educational programs, resources and consultation, with continuing education credits for both physicians and nurses.
- The GLMA annual conference (http://glma.org/) provides continuing education credit for most types of healthcare professionals, with a wide range of topics related to LGBTQ patient care, structural issues, and curricular innovations.
- The Substance Abuse and Mental Health Services Administration (SAMHSA) has several training tools: http://www.samhsa.gov/behavioral-health-equity/lgbt/curricula

Conclusions

Heterosexual healthcare professionals have historically not received any education about LGBTQ issues in their training programs, allowing myths and stereotypes learned earlier in life to go unchallenged and affect clinical practice. This chapter has shown that there is a shift in attitudes in the past 10 to 20 years so that now most healthcare providers are open and willing to learn about LGBTQ health issues, but professional training/education programs have lagged behind in providing such education.

References

Association of American Medical Colleges (AAMC). (2014). *Implementing curricular and institutional climate changes to improve health care for individuals who are LGBT, gender non-conforming or born with DSD*. Retrieved July 25, 2015, from https://www.aamc.org/download/414172/data/lgbt.pdf

Bauer, G. R., Hammond, R., Travers, R., Kaay, M., Hohenadel, K. M., & Boyce, M. (2009). "I don't think this is theoretical; this is our lives": How erasure impacts health care for transgender people. *The Journal of the Association of Nurses in AIDS Care: JANAC, 20*(5), 348–361. Retrieved from http://doi.org/10.1016/j.jana.2009.07.004

Burke, S. E., Dovidio, J. F., Przedworski, J. M., Hardeman, R. R., Perry, S. P., Phelan, S. M., … van Ryn, M. (2015). Do contact and empathy mitigate bias against gay and lesbian people among heterosexual first-year medical students? A report from the medical student CHANGE study. *Academic Medicine: Journal of the Association of American Medical Colleges, 90*(5), 645–651. Retrieved from http://doi.org/10.1097/ACM.0000000000000661

Carabez, R., Eliason, M. J., & Martinson, M. (2016). Nurses' knowledge about transgender patient care: A qualitative study. *Advances in Nursing Science, 39*(3), 257–271.

Carabez, R., Pellegrini, M., Mankovitz, A., Eliason, M. J., Ciano, M., & Scott, M. (2015a). "Never in all my years …": Nurses' education about LGBT health. *Journal of Professional Nursing: Official Journal of the American Association of Colleges of Nursing, 31*(4), 323–329. Retrieved from http://doi.org/10.1016/j.profnurs.2015.01.003

Carabez, R., Pellegrini, M., Mankovitz, A., Eliason, M. J., & Dariotis, W. M. (2015b). Nursing students' perceptions of their knowledge of lesbian, gay, bisexual, and transgender Issues: Effectiveness of a multi-purpose assignment in a public health nursing class. *The Journal of Nursing Education, 54*(1), 50–53. Retrieved from http://doi.org/10.3928/01484834–20141228–03

Carabez, R., Pellegrini, M., Mankovitz, A., Eliason, M., & Scott, M. (2015). Does your organization use gender inclusive forms? Nurses' confusion about trans* terminology. *Journal of clinical nursing, 24*(21–22), 3306–3317.

Chaimowitz, G. A. (1991). Homophobia among psychiatric residents, family practice residents and psychiatric faculty. *Canadian Journal of Psychiatry. Revue Canadienne de Psychiatrie, 36*(3), 206–209.

Corliss, H. L., Shankle, M. D., & Moyer, M. B. (2007). Research, curricula, and resources related to lesbian, gay, bisexual, and transgender health in US schools of public health. *American Journal of Public Health, 97,* 1023–1027. Retrieved from http://doi.org/10.2105/AJPH.2006.086157

Dorsen, C. (2012). An integrative review of nurse attitudes towards lesbian, gay, bisexual, and transgender patients. *The Canadian Journal of Nursing Research = Revue Canadienne de Recherche En Sciences Infirmieres, 44,* 18–43.

Franzini, L. R., & Casinelli, D. L. (1986). Health professionals' factual knowledge and changing attitudes toward transsexuals. *Social Science & Medicine, 22*(5), 535–539.

Hanssmann, C., Morrison, D., & Russian, E. (2008). Talking, gawking, or getting it done: Provider trainings to increase cultural and clinical competence for transgender and gender-nonconforming patients and clients. *Sexuality Research & Social Policy: Journal of NSRC: SR & SP, 5,* 5–23.

Harris, M. B., Nightengale, J., & Owen, N. (1995). Health care professionals' experience, knowledge, and attitudes concerning homosexuality. *Journal of Gay & Lesbian Social Services, 2*(2), 91–108. Retrieved from http://doi.org/10.1300/J041v02n02_06

Hein, L. C., & Levitt, N. (2014). Caring for…Transgender patients. *Nursing Made Incredibly Easy!, 12,* 28–36. Retrieved from http://doi.org/10.1097/01.nme.0000454745.49841.76

Institute of Medicine. (2011). *The health of lesbian, gay, bisexual, and transgender people: Building a foundation for better understanding.* Washington, DC: National Academies Press. Retrieved from http://www.iom.edu/Reports/2011/The-Health-of-Lesbian-Gay-Bisexual-and-Transgender-People.aspx

Khalili, J., Leung, L. B., & Diamant, A. L. (2015). Finding the perfect doctor: Identifying lesbian, gay, bisexual, and transgender-competent physicians. *American Journal of Public Health, 105*(6), 1114–1119. Retrieved from http://doi.org/10.2105/AJPH.2014.302448

Kirkpatrick, M. K., Esterhuizen, P., Jesse, E., & Brown, S. T. (2015). Improving self-directed learning/intercultural competencies: Breaking the silence. *Nurse Educator, 40,* 46–50. Retrieved from http://doi.org/10.1097/NNE.0000000000000092

Kitts, R. L. (2010). Barriers to optimal care between physicians and lesbian, gay, bisexual, transgender, and questioning adolescent patients. *Journal of Homosexuality, 57*(6), 730–747. Retrieved from http://doi.org/10.1080/00918369.2010.485872

Klamen, D. L., Grossman, L. S., & Kopacz, D. R. (1999). Medical student homophobia. *Journal of Homosexuality, 37,* 53–63. Retrieved from http://doi.org/10.1300/J082v37n01_04

Klotzbaugh, R., & Spencer, G. (2014). Magnet nurse administrator attitudes and opportunities: Toward improving lesbian, gay, bisexual, or transgender-specific healthcare. *The Journal of Nursing Administration, 44,* 481–486. Retrieved from http://doi.org/10.1097/NNA.0000000000000103

Lapinski, J., Sexton, P., & Baker, L. (2014). Acceptance of lesbian, gay, bisexual, and transgender patients, attitudes about their treatment, and related medical knowledge among osteopathic medical students. *The Journal of the American Osteopathic Association, 114,* 788–796.

Lena, S. M., Wiebe, T., Ingram, S., & Jabbour, M. (2002). Pediatricians' knowledge, perceptions, and attitudes towards providing health care for lesbian, gay, and bisexual adolescents. *Annals, 35*(7), 406–410.

Lim, F., Johnson, M., & Eliason, M. J. (2015). A national survey of faculty knowledge, experience, and readiness for teaching lesbian, gay, bisexual, and transgender health in baccalaureate nursing programs. *Nursing Education Perspectives, 36*(3), 144–152. Retrieved from http://doi.org/10.5480/14–1355

Mathews, W. C., Booth, M. W., Turner, J. D., & Kessler, L. (1986). Physicians' attitudes toward homosexuality–survey of a California County Medical Society. *The Western Journal of Medicine*, *144*(1), 106–110.

Merryfeather, L., & Bruce, A. (2014). The invisibility of gender diversity: Understanding transgender and transsexuality in nursing literature. *Nursing Forum*, *49*(2), 110–123. Retrieved from http://doi.org/10.1111/nuf.12061

More, F. G., Whitehead, A. W., & Gonthier, M. (2004). Strategies for student services for lesbian, gay, bisexual, and transgender students in dental schools. *Journal of Dental Education*, *68*, 623–632.

National Student Nurses Association. (2010). *In support of increasing culturally competent education about gay, lesbian bisexual, transgender (LGBT) individuals.* Retrieved July 26, 2015, from http://www.nsna.org/Portals/0/Skins/NSNA/pdf/Final%20Resolutions%20 2010%20_11.pdf

National Student Nurses Association. (2012). *Resolution: Implementing practices suggested in the joint commission report, "Advancing effective communication, cultural competence, and patient- and family-centered care for the lesbian, gay, bisexual, and transgender (LGBT) community: A field guide".* Retrieved June 29, 2015, from http://www.nsna.org/Portals/0/ Skins/NSNA/pdf/2012%20NSNA%20Resolutions.pdf

Oancia, T., Bohm, C., Carry, T., Cujec, B., & Johnson, D. (2000). The influence of gender and specialty on reporting of abusive and discriminatory behaviour by medical students, residents and physician teachers. *Medical Education*, *34*(4), 250–256. Retrieved from http://doi. org/10.1046/j.1365–2923.2000.00561.x

Obedin-Maliver, J., Goldsmith, E. S., Stewart, L., White, W., Tran, E., Brenman, S., … Lunn, M. R. (2011). Lesbian, gay, bisexual, and transgender-related content in undergraduate medical education. *JAMA: The Journal of the American Medical Association*, *306*(9), 971–977. Retrieved from http://doi.org/10.1001/jama.2011.1255

Oriel, K. A., Madlon-Kay, D. J., Govaker, D., & Mersy, D. J. (1996). Gay and lesbian physicians in training: Family practice program directors' attitudes and students' perceptions of bias. *Family Medicine*, *28*, 720–725.

Ramos, M. M., Tellez, C. M., Palley, T. B., Umland, B. E., & Skipper, B. J. (1998). Attitudes of physicians practicing in New Mexico toward gay men and lesbians in the profession. *Academic Medicine: Journal of the Association of American -Medical Colleges*, *73*, 436–438.

Randall, C. (1987). Lesbian-phobia: A survey of BSN educators. *Cassandra: Radical Feminist Nurses Newsjournal, 5*, 12–14.

Randall, C. E., & Eliason, M. J. (2012). Out lesbians in nursing: What would Florence say? *Journal of Lesbian Studies*, *16*(1), 65–75. Retrieved from http://doi.org/10.1080/10894160 .2011.557644

Röndahl, G., Innala, S., & Carlsson, M. (2004a). Nurses' attitudes towards lesbians and gay men. *Journal of Advanced Nursing*, *47*(4), 386–392. Retrieved from http://doi. org/10.1111/j.1365–2648.2004.03116.x

Röndahl, G., Innala, S., & Carlsson, M. (2004b). Nursing staff and nursing students' emotions towards homosexual patients and their wish to refrain from nursing, if the option existed. *Scandinavian Journal of Caring Sciences*, *18*(1), 19–26.

Sabin, J. A., Riskind, R. G., & Nosek, B. A. (2015). Health care providers' implicit and explicit attitudes toward lesbian women and gay men. *American Journal of Public Health*, e1–e11. Retrieved from http://doi.org/10.2105/AJPH.2015.302631

Sanchez, N. F., Rabatin, J., Sanchez, J. P., Hubbard, S., & Kalet, A. (2006). Medical students' ability to care for lesbian, gay, bisexual, and transgendered patients. *Family Medicine*, *38*, 21–27.

Sirota, T. (2013). Attitudes among nurse educators toward homosexuality. *The Journal of Nursing Education, 52*(4), 219–227. Retrieved from http://doi.org/10.3928/01484834–20130320–01

Smith, D. M., & Mathews, W. C. (2007). Physicians' attitudes toward homosexuality and HIV: Survey of a California Medical Society- revisited (PATHH-II). *Journal of Homosexuality*, 52(3–4), 1–9. Retrieved from http://doi.org/10.1300/J082v52n03_01

Snowdon, S. (2013). Recommendations for enhancing the climate for LGBT students and employees in health professional schools: A GLMA white paper. Retrieved June 29, 2015, from http://www.glma.org/_data/n_0001/resources/live/Recommendations%20for%20Enhancing%20LGBT%20Climate%20in%20Health%20Professional%20Schools.pdf

Stevens, P. E., & Hall, J. M. (1988). Stigma, health beliefs and experiences with health care in lesbian women. *Image–The Journal of Nursing Scholarship*, 20(2), 69–73.

Stott, D. B. (2013). The training needs of general practitioners in the exploration of sexual health matters and providing sexual healthcare to lesbian, gay and bisexual patients. *Medical Teacher*, 35, 752–759. Retrieved from http://doi.org/10.3109/0142159X.2013.801943

The Joint Commission. (2011). *Advancing effective communication, cultural competence, and patient- and family-centered care for the Lesbian, Gay, Bisexual and Transgender (LGBT) community: A field guide.* Retrieved July 26, 2015, from http://www.jointcommission.org/assets/1/18/LGBTFieldGuide.pdf

Wallick, M. M., Cambre, K. M., & Townsend, M. H. (1992). How the topic of homosexuality is taught at U.S. medical schools. *Academic Medicine: Journal of the Association of American Medical Colleges*, 67, 601–603.

White, W., Brenman, S., Paradis, E., Goldsmith, E. S., Lunn, M. R., Obedin-Maliver, J., … Garcia, G. (2015). Lesbian, gay, bisexual, and transgender patient care: Medical students' preparedness and comfort. *Teaching and Learning in Medicine*, 27(3), 254–263. Retrieved from http://doi.org/10.1080/10401334.2015.1044656

Willging, C. E., Salvador, M., & Kano, M. (2006). Brief reports: Unequal treatment: mental health care for sexual and gender minority groups in a rural state. *Psychiatric Services*, 57(6), 867–870. Retrieved from http://doi.org/10.1176/appi.ps.57.6.867

Wong, J. (2014). Medical school hotline: Looking forward and enriching John A. Burns School of Medicine's curriculum: Lesbian, gay, bisexual, and transgender healthcare in medical education. *Hawai'i Journal of Medicine & Public Health: A Journal of Asia Pacific Medicine & Public Health*, 73(10), 329–331.

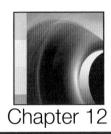

Chapter 12

LGBTQ Healthcare Professionals

"I was team teaching a community health course. I wanted to include LGBT health issues. The other faculty member was adamant about not doing this. This person was also a friend of mine. I felt very betrayed ... She would not have tolerated this exclusion if it was a religious, ethnic, or racial group ... I was the only out LGBT person, others were not going to risk their standing by being out." —(Participant in study by Eliason, DeJoseph, Dibble, Deevey, & Chinn, 2011)

Some research suggests that LGBTQ people, because of their experiences of alienation and discrimination, are more likely to choose health and human services careers, determined to make life better for future generations (Baumle, Compton, & Poston, 2009). Yet, we know little about how they fare in these careers, and what the effects of working within heterosexist and gender normative settings are on the health and well-being of the employees. Some studies have been done of the workplace environment in corporate America (Fidas, Cooper, & Raspanti, 2014) and some research has surveyed hospitals for inclusive policies (Hanneman, 2014), but only a handful of studies have examined the impact of workplace climate on LGBTQ healthcare professionals. As one study of Canadian physicians in training put it, "considerable energy and emotions are spent by gay and lesbian medical students and residents navigating training programs, which may be, at best, indifferent, and at worst, hostile" (Risdon, Cook, & Willms, 2000, p. 331).

Like racism and other attitudes that sustain barriers between people, negative attitudes in healthcare settings toward LGBTQ employees have far-reaching negative effects. These attitudes also negatively influence the education of all healthcare professionals, and ultimately, both the quality of health care for patients/clients, and the general climate of the healthcare setting. Unfortunately, there has been little empirical research on the experiences of openly LGBTQ healthcare providers, and most of this has focused on gay men and lesbians who are relatively "out." There is virtually no knowledge about how closeted LGBTQ healthcare professionals negotiate the workplace, the price exacted by being closeted in a healthcare setting, or the experiences of bisexual and transgender healthcare professionals. The little research on this topic suggests that the personal consequences for those affected by hostile or unwelcoming workplaces limit their ability to practice to their fullest, just as they are limited in their ability to live life to the fullest.

In the next few sections, we review the limited research on LGBTQ employees in the various healthcare professions. Most of the existing work has been done with

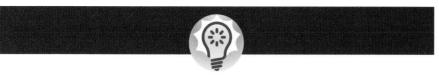

Imagine This 12.1

Imagine that you are one of the faculty members in this situation, and also a close friend of Jane, a long-time faculty member and full Professor, who was appointed as the dean of the School of Nursing, and highly respected among the faculty. She provided leadership for the start of a new PhD program in nursing, taught at all levels in the School, and served on many University committees throughout her years of service. Her appointment as Dean came about in part because of faculty support. Jane had always been a closeted lesbian, thinking that no one guessed about her sexual identity. She assumed that by living a very strict double life, and even making frequent derogatory jokes about nurse faculty who might be seen as lesbians ("they live together but claim to have separate bedrooms — ha ha"), that her own identity was well concealed. About a year into her deanship, she was suddenly fired, with no explanation from the University administrators. People closest to her urged her to fight back, knowing that the action came about because of "leaks" to the University administrators that she was a lesbian. Her performance as dean had been highly respected and in one short year she had accomplished many things on behalf of the School. Jane refused to fight back, and instead removed herself from all contact with friends, moved far away to another city, and was not able to reconnect with nursing for several years.

Imagine how you, as Jane's friend, might have reacted in this situation, and what could have made the situation different?

physicians and nurses (both students and practicing professionals). We supplement the empirical research with comments and stories from LGBTQ healthcare professionals, such as this one from a transgender-identified nurse:

> *"despite declaring their comfort with my transition, most of my coworkers have a very difficult time with pronouns, now 9 months later. I 'pass' as a male with strangers, have facial hair and a deep voice, and yet my coworkers very often refer to me as 'she' or try to do without pronouns altogether. The hard part is playing pronoun police and their embarrassed reactions to me drawing attention to their misuse."* (Eliason, DeJoseph, et al., 2011, p. 242)

Think about how you would respond in this situation where you knew a coworker as one sex/gender and then they become another. Why is it so hard for many of us to use the pronouns and names that our colleagues choose?

Physicians and Medical Schools

> *"... in a single day, a gay doctor might find himself 'passing' to avoid homophobia but also revealing his homosexual identity to show affinity with a gay patient or as a desexualization strategy to resolve problems in examining a woman patient ... This movement between different personas can generate real tensions, as, for example, professionals ponder what will*

happen if attempts to 'pass' are undermined by the subsequent discovery of sexual[ity]." (Hughes, 2004, p. 1211)

There is a small body of research on LGBTQ students and physicians' experiences within medical schools and medical settings. In one of the earliest studies, Schatz and O'Hanlan (1994) surveyed the members of the American Association of Physicians for Human Rights, an LGBT healthcare association (now called GLMA: Health Professionals Advancing LGBT Equality, and open to healthcare professionals from all disciplines). Of 1,311 members at the time, 711 completed the surveys, representing 46 states, and over 50 medical subspecialties. These respondents represented the continuum of "outness" with about 24% saying that more than 90% of their colleagues knew of their sexuality, and 22% saying that less than 10% of their colleagues knew. Only about 20% were out to their patients. The authors found that:

- 17% of LGBT physicians had been refused privileges or denied promotion or employment based on their sexuality;
- 34% had experienced verbal harassment from their professional colleagues; and
- 37% had been socially ostracized.

Shockingly, 88% had heard colleagues disparage LGBTQ patients, 52% had directly witnessed substandard care or denial of care to LGBT patients, and 14% had been victims of gay-bashing. Here are some of the comments that reflect the toxic nature of the climate in healthcare education and practice settings:

"I am a medical student and very in the closet as a bisexual woman. As a perceived straight woman, I hear the nasty comments. One of my residents supervising me in the 4th year in medicine spoke of a gay man with HIV in the ICU. He told me that he believed HIV was God's punishment for homosexuality, that he deserved to die, and that, in fact, all gay or lesbian people should be dead. I find it depressing and very angering that people like this man take care of gay and lesbian people."

"When I applied for residency as an out gay man, one of my interviewers asked me if I would have sex with my patients. I am sure no other candidate was asked this question."

A chief resident to a lesbian medical student: "I don't want to have gay patients because they'd all come in all the time for rectal exams."

"In the post-operative recovery room after my lover's operation for breast cancer, a nursing assistant saw me holding my lover's hand and heard me call her 'lover' and 'honey.' She walked by, shoved me a bit, and said, 'queer.' What is unsettling to me is that I work for this hospital." (all quotes from Schatz & O'Hanlan, 1994)

The Schatz and O'Hanlan (1994) study was repeated and extended in 2009 with a sample of 425 LGBTQ physicians drawn from three sources: the American Medical Association's database (a random sample), the GLMA membership (convenience sample), and via an invitation to GLMA members to share the link to the survey with their LGBTQ colleagues (a snowball sample). This resulted in a sample with an average

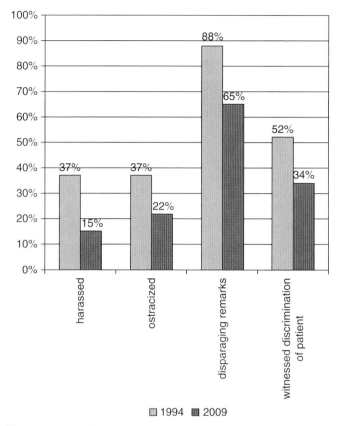

□ 1994 ■ 2009

Figure 12.1 – LGBTQ Physician Experiences in 1994 and 2009.

age of 47 and range of 25 to 92 (Eliason, Dibble, & Robertson, 2011). The sample was 70% male with only a handful of transgender respondents, and was 85% White. These demographic characteristics might indicate that women, people of color, and transgender physicians may still be reluctant to out themselves on a survey, and limits the findings to some extent. We know the most about gay men's experiences as healthcare professionals.

Figure 12.1 shows a few of the comparisons between the data collected in 1994 and 2009. Although conditions did improve in the intervening years, a significant number of physicians still experienced harassment and social ostracization in the workplace, and at least one in three had witnessed outright discrimination of LGBTQ patients. Fortunately, only 4% were denied a residency because of their sexual orientation or gender identity in the 2009 survey, compared to 11% in the 1990s.

Disclosure continues to be a sensitive issue for many LGBTQ doctors, and anxiety about the decision to disclose or not, may create a great deal of stress. Whereas much psychological literature finds that there are mental health benefits to disclosure, sometimes the environment is simply not perceived as safe for coming out. One study found that 95% of students applying for medical school did not disclose their sexuality for fear of discrimination, and 46% did not disclose when applying for a residency (Merchant, Jongco, & Woodward, 2005). A recent study finds similar rates of concealment. Mansh et al. (2015) surveyed medical students from all 176 medical schools in the United States, and Canada, obtaining nearly 600 respondents of whom 16% were sexual minorities, 1% were gender minorities, and a handful (*n* = 21) identified as both sexual and gender minority. Of the sexual minority respondents, overall 30% had not come out about their sexuality. There were major differences by sexual identity category, with lesbian and gay respondents the least likely to conceal their identities (15%), whereas rates of concealment were higher for those who identified as queer (22%), bisexual (54%), and questioning (92%). Of respondents who identified as gender minorities, 60% were not out in school. Racial ethnic minority respondents were somewhat less likely to be out (but not statistically significant except for East Asian students), and many reported fear of discrimination as a reason for not coming out (43% to 44%).

The following studies suggest that the fears of disclosure are valid. Brogan, Frank, Elon, Silvanesan, and O'Hanlan (1999) reported that 41% of lesbian physicians surveyed had experienced harassment in healthcare settings, and a later study reported that lesbian physicians weighed more and were more likely to have histories of depression than heterosexual female physicians, suggesting that added stress impacted the health of even these highly educated women (Brogan, O'Hanlan, Elon, & Frank, 2003). A study of first year medical students found that those who identified as LGB were more likely to have symptoms of depression and anxiety, 23% reported harassment, and 54% felt isolated (Przedworski et al., 2015). In another study, 25% of family practice program directors said that they would hesitate to match openly gay residents to their programs (Oriel, Madlon-Kay, Govaker, & Mersy, 1996).

Other data that supports the dangers of disclosure have examined coworkers and patients' attitudes. Regarding heterosexual doctors and medical student coworkers, one study of over 1,000 physicians in New Mexico (Ramos, Tellez, Palley, Umland, & Skipper, 1998) found that 11% would not refer a patient to an LGBTQ physician. Chapter 11 addressed the attitudes of heterosexual physicians toward LGBTQ people. Most of the studies focused on attitudes about patients, but doctors with negative attitudes about patients are likely to also have negative attitudes toward LGBTQ coworkers. In regards to patients' attitudes, a study of internists in Canada revealed that 30% had been subjected to homophobic remarks by patients on three or more occasions (Cook, Griffith, Cohen, Guyatt, & O'Brien, 1995). Another study in Canada showed that 12% of randomly selected adults said that they would refuse to see an LGB family physician (50% because they perceived the LGB physician would be incompetent); older respondents were more likely to refuse to see LGB physicians than younger respondents (Druzin, Shrier, Yacowar, & Rossignol, 1998).

No wonder healthcare professionals are hesitant to come out at work. In addition to facing potentially hostile or condescending coworkers and patients, there is little in the medical school curriculum to counter negative attitudes or foster disclosure. Tesar and Rovi (1998) found that over half of medical school curricula had no information about LGBT people, and Wallick, Cambre, and Townsend (1992) reported that for programs that do have LGBT content, there is less than

1 hour of content per year over the 4-year curriculum. McGarry, Clarke, Landau, and Cyr (2008) surveyed the program directors of U.S. internal medicine residency programs about their inclusion of vulnerable populations in the curriculum. Whereas 58% of schools covered health of racial/ethnic minorities, only 30% addressed health of gay men and 11% addressed the health of lesbians. Twenty-two percent devoted less than 1 hour to racial/ethnic populations compared to 37% for gay men's health and 73% for lesbian health topics. A study of 132 medical schools found that the median number of hours of LGBT content was 5 hours across the entire curriculum (Obedin-Maliver et al., 2011). Of the top five topics covered in the medical school curriculum, three of them were related to HIV and sexually transmitted infections. Another study found that even LGBTQ physicians experienced little content on sexual orientation or gender diversity in their medical school education: Average hours of content across the entire medical school experience was 1.4 hours for content about lesbian health; 2.3 hours on gay male health; 1.0 hours on bisexual health, and 0.9 hours on transgender health (Eliason, Dibble, et al., 2011). When the curriculum is inclusive and accepting, it provides an opening for LGBTQ students to come out. When the curriculum is silent on LGBTQ issues, or only discusses HIV/AIDS, students may be less likely to disclose. Curriculum inclusion (or not) sends a clear message to students about how the program perceives LGBTQ issues. The current lack of education reinforces heterosexism within the health professions, implying that LGBTQ issues are not important enough to be included in the curriculum.

In addition, the placement of the content, when it is so limited, becomes a critical factor in maintaining stereotypes. If the LGBTQ content is only found in a unit on human sexuality, where it is most often found if it exists at all in the curriculum, this reinforces a stereotype that sexual identities are all about sex and nothing else. If the LGBTQ content is found only in a unit on ethics, there is an implication that LGBTQ people are one of the populations that physicians "have to" care for whether they like it or not. Finally, if the LGBTQ content is only found in a unit on HIV/AIDS and/or other sexually transmitted infections, it implies that this is the only health problem in the LGBTQ community (and that being LGBTQ is all about sex).

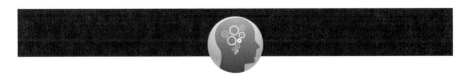

Think About It 12.1

In one university in the late 1980s, a 1-hour lecture on LGBT issues was imbedded in a summer unit called "Human Sexuality Week." But students called it "porn week" because each day included watching at least 2 hours of heterosexually oriented sexually explicit materials in an attempt to "desensitize" students to overt sexual images. The other content of human sexuality week focused on sexual dysfunctions. How do you think this placement of LGBT content might have affected the reception of heterosexual students? How might LGBTQ students have felt about this? Does this type of curricular placement reinforce stereotypes that being LGBTQ is only about sexual difference?

The lack of education for physicians interacts with the stigma of sexuality and internalization of shame and guilt on the part of some people, or as one gay man said,

> *"It's just a bad combination—there's shame on one side, and untrained professionals on the other. So [sexuality] doesn't get dealt with, and it's avoided. And when it comes up as an issue professionally, you're dealing with people who are really dealing with it on a personal level."* (Beehler, 2001, p. 138)

Some professional organizations within medicine are beginning to address LGBTQ issues. The American Medical Association has a GLBT Advisory Committee; the American Medical Student Association has an LGBT Action Committee, and their website contains information on starting local chapters as well as excellent educational resources. Many specialty associations also have LGBTQ interest groups or committees, such as the Society for Adolescent Medicine and American Psychiatric and Psychological Associations. There is a free-standing Association of Gay and Lesbian Psychiatrists (http://www.aglp.org/). These resources can be very helpful for LGBTQ physicians for support and help with dealing with hostile or benignly negligent workplaces. See Chapter 11 for other examples of advocacy and education efforts within medicine.

Nurses and Nursing Schools

> *"When I moved to ... begin nursing education, I was warned by heterosexual nurses and physicians...that an open lesbian could not be a nurse ... So after seven years of being out at work as a file clerk, I became a closeted nursing student. The sudden reversal to a double life was jolting, because it takes different sets of skills, compromises, and self-justifications to live either openly or in the closet ... After nursing school, I became more secretive again, because I was afraid of losing my new career. In each of my work settings, I saw gay and lesbian patients laughed at, mistreated, or denied. I was effectively intimidated by medical, nursing, and social work colleagues who challenged my tentative efforts at lesbian and gay patient advocacy."* (Deevey, 1993, p. 21)

The first articles about LGBTQ issues in nursing journals appeared in the 1960s and seem incredibly dated by today's standards. For example, Juzwiak (1964) recommended:

> *"The female nurse dealing with a homosexual patient ought to avoid behavior that, while potentially pleasing to a heterosexual male, might be irritating or seem threatening to the homosexual male. Specifically, she should avoid being flirtatious with him, or unduly pressuring ... The male nurse or attendant working with a male homosexual patient should bear in mind the possibility that normal friendly and solicitous behavior might be misinterpreted"* (p. 57) *... the degree to which she is able to view the homosexual person as a human being with a special problem rather than as an unspeakable and frightening 'pervert' will not only help her to work with such patients but will also beneficially influence the attitudes of other hospital personnel who come into contact with them"* (p. 118).

In the 1970s, the tone of articles began to change. Lawrence (1975) writing as an openly gay man, called for nurses to treat patients with respect and noted "to endure a hospital stay may be one of the most bitter and unpleasant of any of the oppressive experiences that homosexual persons are subject to daily" (p. 308). By the mid 1980s and early 1990s, studies began to appear about the nursing curriculum and attitudes of nurses and nursing students. Randall (1987) surveyed 100 midwestern nurse educators and found that 52% believed that lesbians are "unnatural," 34% thought lesbians "disgusting," and 23% considered lesbians "immoral." Four percent would refuse to care for a lesbian patient, and 13% said they would not allow a lesbian nurse to care for them. Over 50% of these educators had never addressed lesbian health issues in a clinical setting or the classroom, and 10% thought that lesbians should not be allowed to teach in schools of nursing.

Early studies of nursing students found similar attitudes. In one study, 26% of students said lesbians were unacceptable and that they would try to avoid any contact with one (Eliason & Randall, 1991), and a follow-up study of nearly 200 nursing students identified common stereotypes about lesbians. Nursing students worried that lesbian coworkers or patients would try to "hit on me" (38%) or "push their beliefs on me" (29%). About one-third of students thought that lesbians could be identified by their masculine appearance, and 13% objected to working with lesbians on the basis of their moral or religious beliefs. A more recent study of undergraduate nursing students and faculty (Dinkel, Patzel, McGuire, Rolfs, & Purcell, 2007) found relatively low homophobia scores, but the authors speculated that they might reflect neutrality and/ or heterosexist attitudes rather than acceptance. Blackwell (2006) conducted a random sample survey of Florida nurses and found that 22% had high scores on a homophobia scale, indicating overtly negative attitudes in about one in five nurses. Those in their 20s were the least homophobic, suggesting that there is hope for the future. Some studies have found higher rates of homophobia among heterosexual male nursing students and those with more conservative religious beliefs (Eliason, 1998; Eliason & Raheim, 2000). These studies did not address the issues of LGBTQ nurses in the workplace, but show that the general environment may be challenging.

Few studies have focused on the experiences of gay men in nursing, although the stereotype is that all men in nursing are gay. Nursing is constructed as "women's work" thus any man who enters the profession is suspect (Harding, 2007). Lesbian and bisexual women have a very different experience, stemming from the history of women in the workforce. Prior to the women's equality movements of the 1970s, many women only stayed in the workforce until they married and/or had children. Therefore, the leadership of nursing education and practice consisted primarily of "spinsters" and nuns. Both groups have historically included high numbers of sexual minority women. As nursing struggled to be seen as an autonomous profession, rather than merely being a physician's hand-maiden, lesbian and bisexual women were forced to be closeted to avoid tarnishing the reputation of nursing. This led to a dynamic of lesbian witch-hunts in many settings (Randall & Eliason, 2012). Many older lesbian nurses were forced to fake out-of-town boyfriends or live with "room-mates" rather than reveal the nature of their relationships with other women.

Giddings and Smith's (2001) research on the experience of lesbian nurses revealed seven themes in the stories of their experiences in nursing: closeting of lesbianism in nursing, isolating and hiding from self and others, living a double-life, self-loathing and shame, experiencing discrimination from others, keeping safe, and threatening other nurses who are closeted. They concluded that the experiences of the nurses they interviewed point to a double standard where nurses claim to embrace diversity but fail to respect the differences represented by lesbian experience. Men, because of stereotypes about nursing as women's work, were automatically assumed to be gay, therefore those who actually were, did not have conceal their identities. Less is known about the experiences of bisexual or transgender nurses, who face even greater negativity in society in general.

Any wonder that LGBTQ nurses might not always disclose their sexuality to coworkers? Rose (1993) surveyed 44 lesbian nurses, and found that 25% were not out to anyone at work. Half of those who were out said that it had been a very difficult process. Many had witnessed discriminatory behaviors by their nurse coworkers, including refusal to care for an LGB person (25%). One nurse in this study commented, "I have experienced other nurses/doctors refusing to give a gay man a painkilling suppository in case 'he enjoyed it'" (p. 51).

In 2004, GLMA: Health Professionals Advancing LGBT Equality, drafted an online survey for LGBTQ nurses (Eliason, DeJoseph, et al., 2011). It was distributed to all contacts in their membership and newsletter lists who indicated that they were nurses. Of the responding nurses (*n* = 264), 88% were currently practicing nurses and 21% were students; 54% were female, 44% were male, and three were transgender identified. By sexual identity, 44% were lesbians, 43% gay, 6% bisexual, and the rest noted "other." Figure 12.2 shows data for the percent of respondents who reported that they were out to all or most of these individuals in their lives—the vast majority of respondents were out to their friends and family but only a few were out to patients.

Most of the survey consisted of open-ended questions to elicit positive and negative experiences within the practice of nursing. When asked if the respondents worked in an "LGBT-friendly" environment, 78% said yes. The factors that appeared to make

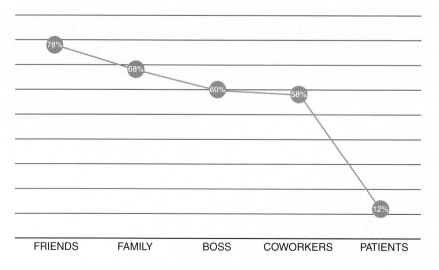

Figure 12.2 – Nurses' Degree of Disclosure: % "Out to All" (Based on **Eliason, DeJoseph, et al., 2011**).

an environment LGBT-friendly included having openly LGBTQ colleagues, having open-minded and accepting heterosexual colleagues, having institutional policies like nondiscrimination policies and domestic partner benefits, and working in LGBT-specific settings. Even though nearly 80% said their work environments were LGBT-friendly, their qualitative responses about what makes it friendly suggested that they may have had somewhat low expectations for what an LGBT-friendly environment was. For example, some responses indicated that the environment was tolerant, rather than accepting:

> *"I guess it's not that it's friendly so much as not hostile. For the most part, people just accept things and do the work that needs to be done."*

> *"Basic tolerance ... I would not go overboard in calling it friendly, however."*

> *"People know and are not hostile about it. Also, they know about my partner and include her in conversations. I am not sure that this makes it a friendly environment, but I am not threatened that others know."*

Most scholars suggest that tolerance is a rather condescending position to hold; it implies that one is superior to person with the tolerated identity. This does not make for a healthy work climate. Other respondents experienced a "don't ask, don't tell" environment:

> *"The question is hard to answer. Nobody disdains me, or anyone else. But it is not an open environment where it is discussed as easily as any other topic. For example, I have no idea who else is GLBT in the organization. It is just not talked about."*

> *"Yes and no, it's an environment of don't ask don't tell."*

Those who reported that the work environment was unfriendly had experiences that ranged from feeling they should remain silent about LGBTQ issues on the workplace, to hearing anti-gay comments, to experiencing harassment. Some examples include:

> *"I was told by colleagues when I wanted to do research on lesbian issues that I would 'be boiled in oil' and that I had a 'Jesus Christ complex,' critics may have been closeted themselves."*

> *"A resident doctor who made fun of an effeminate male nurse; when that guy tried to commit suicide, the resident merely said, 'He was a pansy.'"*

> *"The expectation that as a gay man in nursing, that I am only interested in sexual health issues."*

> *"Received email from nurse manager that included a 'you should repent' type of message."*

> *"I have a senior co-worker who has been here 20+ years who deems it necessary to harass me about my sexual identity. Particularly making sexual comments and then covering with, 'You know I'm kidding, right?'"*

Some respondents had experienced job loss because of their sexuality or gender identity:

"I lost my job after posting my wedding in the local paper, after over a decade at the same job. Never underestimate the power of a Catholic hospital."

"Being outed by a colleague at a faculty party. Although all of my evaluations had been excellent and I had just completed my Masters I did not have my contract renewed. I had been teaching in the program for 9 years. It may have had nothing to do with me being gay but it was awfully coincidental."

At this point in time, only one national nursing organization and a handful of state nursing organizations include sexual orientation and/or gender identity in their human rights statements, have committees, interest groups, or task forces for LGBTQ nurses, or acknowledge the presence of LGBTQ nurses in their documents or websites, even within discussions of diversity. The American Academy of Nursing established an LGBTQ Expert Panel in 2012, the first LGBTQ-related advocacy group in any nursing organization. In 2014, GLMA: Health Professionals Advancing LGBT Equality established a Nursing Section to help promote LGBT health concerns in nursing practice, education, research, and policy. The GLMA Nursing Section is one of the few places where LGBTQ nurses and their allies gather together to promote advocacy, workplace climate change, research, and educational reform for the discipline of nursing. Table 12.1 provides a list of LGBTQ policy statements that have begun to appear from major nursing organizations since 2012.

A few studies have considered the inclusion of LGBTQ topics in nursing school curricula. Lim, Johnson, and Eliason (2015) reported on a survey of over 1,200 nursing faculty across the United States. Many faculty reported a lack of awareness of LGBT health issues (37%), limited knowledge of LGBT health (43%), and they had rarely or never read any LGBT-related articles in professional journals in the past 2 years (70%). On the other hand, 70% said they were ready to teach these issues and only 25% were uncomfortable raising these topics. The mean amount of time devoted to LGBT topics

Table 12.1 – Examples of Policy Statements Issued by Nursing Organizations	
Organization	**Policy**
Oncology Nursing Society (https://www.ons.org/)	One of the first nursing organizations to include sexual orientation in their human rights statement; At one time, had an LGBT interest group.
American College of Nurse-Midwives (http://www.midwife.org/)	Position statement "Transgender/Transexual/Gender Variant Health Care" that affirms the right to quality nondiscriminatory care for all gender variant individuals and their families (November 2012).
American Academy of Nursing (http://www.aannet.org/)	• Position statement in support of Marriage Equality (July 11, 2012) • Position statement affirming quality health care for sexual minority and gender diverse populations (July 11, 2012) • Position statement opposing reparative therapy (January 2015) • Position statement supporting equal hospital visitation rights (January 2015)

for the entire nursing program was just over 2 hours. The two most commonly mentioned topics were homophobia (taught often or frequently by 19%) and HIV and other STIs (taught often or frequently by 18%). Not surprisingly, LGBTQ faculty members were more likely to report that they taught about LGBTQ issues than were heterosexual faculty members. Heterosexual men were the least likely to teach about LGBTQ issues. Sirota (2013) also found nurse educators to be willing, but unprepared to teach about LGBTQ patient care issues.

The lack of knowledge of LGBTQ topics among nurse educators is not surprising, given that the nursing research literature has only begun to seriously address LGBTQ topics (Eliason, DeJoseph, & Dibble, 2010). In an era of evidence-based practice, this is concerning, because if nursing research is not conducted on LGBTQ health topics, no evidence can accumulate to drive nursing practice, theory, or scholarship.

Other Healthcare Professions

More, Whitehead, and Gonthier (2004) sent surveys to student affairs administrators of all dental schools in the United States, and asked about LGBT student and staff issues. They obtained a response rate of 87%. They found that 62% of administrators reported that they had LGBT dental students, but 38% reported no LGBT students or faculty members in their programs. The majority did have nondiscrimination policies that included sexual orientation (75%), but most of the administrators were unaware of whether their school had LGBT support services, and only two schools had LGBT support groups in the dental school. Five administrators reported that they had experienced an incident of LGBT discrimination, 33% did not know if they treated LGBT patients, and the majority reported that the curriculum contained less than 2 hours of content on LGBT issues. There are no other articles related to sexuality or gender identity in the dental literature. The American Dental Association has a Gay-Straight Alliances Special Interest Group.

The American Public Health Association has had an LGBT Caucus since 1975, and The American Journal of Public Health did their first special issue on LGBTQ health in 2001. This does not mean that the curriculum of public health programs necessarily is more inclusive of LGBTQ issues than other health disciplines. Corliss, Shankle, and Moyer (2007) surveyed 102 faculty of 35 public health programs in the United States and Puerto Rico and found that most of the schools included sexual orientation in their nondiscrimination policies (71%), but fewer than half offered benefits to domestic partners (49%). Less than one-third (31%) had an LGBT student group within their program and about the same number reported that they had an out LGBT faculty member. When asked, "did your department offer a course in the past 2 years that covered LGBT health topics extending beyond HIV/AIDS," only 9% said yes. Nearly one-half (43%) of respondents felt that their curriculum inadequately addressed LGBT health issues.

A small body of research is emerging within the field of gerontology to examine knowledge and attitudes of elder care health workers, and this reveals much of the same concerns that are found in other healthcare settings (Hughes, Harold, & Boyer, 2011; Moone, Cagle, Croghan, & Smith, 2014; Porter & Krinsky, 2014). One difference, though, is that elders often feel much more vulnerable and may need caregivers in their homes who may potentially exploit, harass, or even harm them based on negative attitudes about LGBTQ people. Thus far, little is known about LGBTQ people who work as caregivers for older adults or in elder care settings.

Some other professions that might be found in healthcare settings, such as social work and psychology, have a longer history of having LGBT advocacy groups within their professional organizations, and have passed LGBTQ-affirmative policies and resolutions. For example, the American Psychological Association passed a resolution on the "normalcy" of homosexuality in 1975 (although it was slower to recognize bisexual and transgender issues). However, there continues to be significant numbers of professionals even in these professions that lack knowledge or hold negative attitudes (Division 44 Committee on LGB Concerns, 2000; Morrow & Messinger, 2006).

Finally, we know very little about the LGBTQ employees who work the service jobs: housekeeping, distributing meals, nursing assistants, technicians, and the hundreds of other jobs in healthcare settings. In general, these are low-paying jobs for people with less education, and the majority of studies of homophobia and transphobia find higher rates of negativity among those with lower education. These employees may feel the greatest degree of stress on the job, but have not been studied at all.

Improving the Climate for LGBTQ Healthcare Workers

The majority of LGBTQ healthcare professionals have experienced and/or witnessed discriminatory treatment in their own work environments. Ironically, having open LGBTQ role models in the health professions at educational programs and clinical sites could help to change the climate and change attitudes, however, many are afraid to be out at work. What will it take to improve this situation? In recent years, some healthcare professional organizations have taken small steps to become more inclusive of the LGBTQ workforce, and urged educational programs to consider greater curricular inclusion on these issues.

The Nursing Section of GLMA: Health Professionals Advancing LGBT Equality, has initiated a project to improve the workplace climate for LGBT employees. You can find a copy of this tool in Chapter 13 along with information about the Healthcare Equality Index, an assessment of workplace climate and policies/procedures that are LGBTQ inclusive. HEI is aimed at institutional assessment.

In the rest of this section, we propose three general sets of interventions to make the healthcare workplace safer for its LGBTQ workers; inclusive policies, training/education, and advocacy. These are discussed in more detail in Chapter 13.

1. Policies

Workplaces that had nondiscrimination policies including sexuality and gender, and that had domestic partner benefits were perceived as more LGBTQ-friendly in the GLMA physicians' survey (Eliason, Dibble, et al., 2011). Historically, the civil rights movement demonstrated that changing laws and policies is the first step in achieving equality—attitude change often follows. In health care as in the general population, there is a greater tendency to agree that LGBTQ people deserve equal rights than there is to agree that LGBTQ identities are a normal expression of human diversity. Sanchez, Rabatin, Sanchez, Hubbard, and Kalet (2006) found that the attitudes varied in medical

Table 12.2 – Medical Students' Endorsement of Statements about Lesbian and Gay Patients and Same-Sex Behaviors (Based on Sanchez et al., 2006)	
Statement	**Mean (range of 1–5[a])**
Lesbian and gay patients deserve the same quality of care from medical institutions as heterosexual patients.	4.9
I would be comfortable if I became known among my professional peers as a doctor that cares for LGBT patients.	4.3
Same-sex attraction is a natural expression of sexuality in humans.	3.8
Same-sex behavior is a natural expression of sexuality in humans.	3.6

[a]5 indicates strongly agree.

students in New York City, with a greater number of students agreeing that LGBT patients deserve quality care than those that agreed that same-sex behavior is "normal." Table 12.2 shows these data.

These findings suggest that appealing to heterosexual healthcare professionals' sense of social justice and civil rights might be an effective first step in changing the climate for LGBTQ healthcare professionals. Once the legal and policy protections for civil rights are in place, LGBTQ people can feel freer to be open and share their life experiences with coworkers, a strategy that may foster more personal attitude change.

Policies regarding workplace conduct are also important. Policies need to spell out what will happen if an employee acts in a discriminatory, hostile, or offensive manner with an LGBTQ coworker. Too often, harassing comments are ignored because supervisors have no clear policy to invoke, or cannot separate fact from stereotype themselves. The recent studies on implicit bias show that heterosexual healthcare providers may not be aware of their own bias.

2. Better training and education

Clearly there is a need to improve training programs for healthcare professionals to be more inclusive of LGBTQ people and their families. Ideally, this information should be integrated throughout the curriculum, although some students will want to specialize and may benefit from separate classes on LGBTQ health. Because the majority of healthcare education programs have not yet incorporated LGBTQ issues, there is a critical need for inservice and continuing education. Inservice education programs need to be sensitive to LGBTQ employees, by not assuming that everyone is heterosexual. The issues of content and placement of LGBTQ content in healthcare training curricula were addressed in Chapter 11, where we discussed how heterosexual healthcare providers need basic education. However, having this content in the curriculum is also a critical method of improving the climate for LGBTQ employees. Having LGBTQ content in healthcare training and education increases awareness that a subset of the population is "different," thus breaking the silence in health care that contributes to heterosexism and gender normativity. This content provides openings for LGBTQ employees or students to come out if they feel safe.

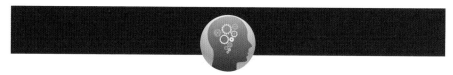

Think About It 12.2

James is a critical care nurse, and identifies as male, although a few years ago, he identified as female-to-male transgender. In his current setting, he is not out to any of his coworkers because of bad experiences in past jobs. The nurse manager announces in a staff meeting that they will be having an inservice the following week on transgender healthcare issues. James is happy they are doing this, but feels conflicted because he has not come out. He experiences much turmoil in the intervening week as he agonizes over whether to come out during the inservice, or wait and see how his coworkers react to the information. Either way, he knows that some of them will feel betrayed that he did not come out sooner.

If you were in James' shoes, what would you do (or not do!)? If James worked in the setting where you currently work or intern, how do you think your coworkers would react to the training and to James' coming out?

3. Support and advocacy

Finally, LGBTQ healthcare professionals need support in their local work environments and in their professional organizations. This can include support groups within hospitals and schools, LGBTQ committees or social/political groups, and recognition. For example, some hospitals have LGBTQ Pride Days in June when Pride celebrations occur in most communities, or celebrate Oct 11, National Coming Out Day. Professional organizations need to take a stand for social justice and pass resolutions, form interest groups or task forces, and change their policies to be inclusive. LGBTQ healthcare providers can find support and advocacy in organizations such as the GLMA, a national advocacy organization for all LGBTQ healthcare professionals and allies. We urge all healthcare professionals to pressure their mainstream professional organizations to be more inclusive, if they are not already.

For LGBTQ employees who are not at the "professional" rank, but occupy the vitally important support roles such as nursing assistant, technicians, unit clerks, and

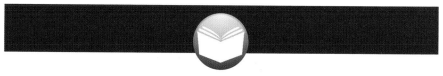

Read This 12.1

GLMA's White Paper is a comprehensive set of recommendations—authored by Shane Snowdon—that offer resources for making health professional schools more equitable, inclusive, and welcoming from an LGBTQ standpoint. Take the time to read this important paper for a comprehensive overview of important steps to create an inclusive climate for LGBTQ students and employees. https://goo.gl/PHHJzW

other jobs, labor unions can be important allies to forging LGBTQ inclusive policies and humane working conditions.

Conclusion

LGBTQ healthcare professionals are still largely invisible in their places of employment, and LGBTQ healthcare issues are absent or inadequate in the training of healthcare professionals. Minority stress stemming from fear of discrimination, harassment, or even loss of job may affect the health and well-being of employees and adversely affect their ability to be open and proud role models and resources in their work settings. LGBTQ employees are an untapped resource in healthcare agencies. This chapter has outlined some strategies for making the workplace and healthcare training more welcoming and inclusive of LGBTQ employees and patients.

References

Baumle, A. K., Compton, D., & Poston, D. L. (2009). *Same-sex partners: The social demography of sexual orientation.* New York: SUNY Press.

Beehler, G. P. (2001). Confronting the culture of medicine: gay men's experiences with primary care physicians. *Journal of the Gay and Lesbian Medical Association,* 5(4), 135–141.

Blackwell, C. (2006). Registered nurses' attitudes toward the protection of gay s and lesbians in the workplace: An examination of homophobia and discriminatory beliefs. In *Proceedings of the 2006 Annual Conference.* San Francisco, CA: GLMA: Health Professionals Advancing LGBT Equality.

Brogan, D. J., Frank, E., Elon, L., Silvanesan, S., & O'Hanlan, K. A. (1999). Harassment of lesbians as medical students and physician. *JAMA: The Journal of the American Medical Association,* 282, 1290–1292.

Brogan, D. J., O'Hanlan, K. A., Elon, L., & Frank, E. (2003). Health and professional characteristics of lesbian and heterosexual women physicians. *Journal of the American Medical Women's Association,* 58, 10–19.

Cook, D. J., Griffith, L. E., Cohen, M., Guyatt, G. H., & O'Brien, B. (1995). Discrimination and abuse experienced by general internists in Canada. *Journal of General Internal Medicine, 10,* 565–572. Retrieved from http://www.ncbi.nlm.nih.gov/pubmed/8576773

Corliss, H. L., Shankle, M. D., & Moyer, M. B. (2007). Research, curricula, and resources related to lesbian, gay, bisexual, and transgender health in US schools of public health. *American Journal of Public Health,* 97, 1023–1027. Retrieved from http://doi.org/10.2105/AJPH.2006.086157

Deevey, S. (1993). Lesbian self-disclosure: Strategies for success. *Journal of Psychosocial Nursing and Mental Health Services,* 31, 21–26.

Dinkel, S., Patzel, B., McGuire, M. J., Rolfs, E., & Purcell, K. (2007). Measures of homophobia among nursing students and faculty: A Midwestern perspective. *International Journal of Nursing Education Scholarship,* 4, Article 24. Retrieved from http://doi.org/10.2202/1548–923X.1491

Division 44 Committee on LGB Concerns. (2000). Guidelines for psychotherapy with LGB clients. Retrieved July 26, 2015, from http://www.apa.org/practice/guidelines/glbt.pdf

Druzin, P., Shrier, I., Yacowar, M., & Rossignol, M. (1998). Discrimination against gay, lesbian and bisexual family physicians by patient. *CMAJ: Canadian Medical Association Journal = Journal de l'Association Medicale Canadienne,* 158, 593–597.

Eliason, M. J. (1998). Correlates of prejudice in nursing students. *The Journal of Nursing Education,* 37, 27–29.

Eliason, M. J., DeJoseph, J., Dibble, S. L., Deevey, S., & Chinn, P. L. (2011). Lesbian, gay, bisexual, transgender and queer/questioning (LGBTQ) nurses' experiences in the workplace. *Journal of Professional Nursing: Official Journal of the American Association of Colleges of Nursing*, 27, 237–244.

Eliason, M. J., Dibble, S. L., & Dejoseph, J. (2010). Nursing's silence on lesbian, gay, bisexual, and transgender issues: The need for emancipatory efforts. *ANS. Advances in Nursing Science*, 33, 206–218. Retrieved from http://doi.org/10.1097/ANS.0b013e3181e63e4

Eliason, M. J., Dibble, S. L., & Robertson, P. A. (2011). Lesbian, gay, bisexual, and transgender (LGBT) physicians' experiences in the workplace. *Journal of Homosexuality*, 58(10), 1355–1371. Retrieved from http://doi.org/10.1080/00918369.2011.614902

Eliason, M. J., & Raheim, S. (2000). Experience and level of comfort with culturally diverse groups. *The Journal of Nursing Education*, 39, 161–165.

Eliason, M. J., & Randall, C. E. (1991). Lesbian phobia in nursing students. *Western Journal of Nursing Research*, 13, 363–374.

Fidas, D., Cooper, L., & Raspanti, J. (2014). The cost of the closet and the rewards of inclusion: Why the workplace environment for LGBT people matters to employers. Retrieved July 15, 2015, from http://hrc-assets.s3-website-us-east-1.amazonaws.com//files/assets/resources/Cost_of_the_Closet_May2014.pdf

Giddings, L. S., & Smith, M. C. (2001). Stories of lesbian in/visibility in nursing. *Nursing Outlook*, 49, 14–19. Retrieved from http://doi.org/10.1067/mno.2001.106906

Hanneman, T. (2014). Healthcare equality index 2014: Promoting equitable and inclusive care for lesbian, gay, bisexual and transgender patients and their families. Retrieved June 28, 2015, from http://www.hrc.org/campaigns/healthcare-equality-index

Harding, T. (2007). The construction of men who are nurses as gay. *Journal of Advanced Nursing*, 60(6), 636–644. Retrieved from http://doi.org/10.1111/j.1365–2648.2007.04447.x

Hughes, A. K., Harold, R. D., & Boyer, J. M. (2011). Awareness of LGBT aging issues among aging services network providers. *Journal of Gerontological Social Work*, 54(7), 659–677. Retrieved from http://doi.org/10.1080/01634372.2011.585392

Hughes, D. (2004). Disclosure of sexual preferences and lesbian, gay, and bisexual practitioners. *BMJ*, 328, 1211–1212. Retrieved from http://doi.org/10.1136/bmj.328.7450.1211

Juzwiak, M. (1964). Understanding the homosexual patient. *RN*, 27, 53–59.

Lawrence, J. C. (1975). Homosexuals, hospitalization, and the nurse. *Nursing Forum*, 14, 305–317.

Lim, F., Johnson, M., & Eliason, M. J. (2015). A national survey of faculty knowledge, experience, and readiness for teaching lesbian, gay, bisexual, and transgender health in baccalaureate nursing programs. *Nursing Education Perspectives*, 36(3), 144–152. Retrieved from http://doi.org/10.5480/14–1355

Mansh, M., White, W., Gee-Tong, L., Lunn, M. R., Obedin-Maliver, J., Stewart, L., … Garcia, G. (2015). Sexual and gender minority identity disclosure during undergraduate medical education: "In the closet" in medical school. *Academic Medicine: Journal of the Association of American Medical Colleges*, 90. Retrieved from http://doi.org/10.1097/ACM.0000000000000657

McGarry, K. A., Clarke, J. G., Landau, C., & Cyr, M. G. (2008). Caring for vulnerable populations: Curricula in U.S. internal medicine residencies. Journal of Homosexuality, 54, 225–232.

Merchant, R. C., Jongco, A. M., 3rd, & Woodward, L. (2005). Disclosure of sexual orientation by medical students and residency applicants. *Academic Medicine: Journal of the Association of American Medical Colleges*, 80, 786.

Moone, R. P., Cagle, J. G., Croghan, C. F., & Smith, J. (2014). Working with LGBT older adults: An assessment of employee training practices, needs, and preferences of senior service organizations in Minnesota. *Journal of Gerontological Social Work*, 57(2–4), 322–334. Retrieved from http://doi.org/10.1080/01634372.2013.843630

More, F. G., Whitehead, A. W., & Gonthier, M. (2004). Strategies for student services for lesbian, gay, bisexual, and transgender students in dental schools. *Journal of Dental Education*, 68, 623–632.

Morrow, D. F., & Messinger, L. (2006). *Sexual orientation and gender expression in social work practice: Working with gay, lesbian, bisexual, and transgender people*. New York: Columbia University Press.

Obedin-Maliver, J., Goldsmith, E. S., Stewart, L., White, W., Tran, E., Brenman, S., … Lunn, M. R. (2011). Lesbian, gay, bisexual, and transgender-related content in undergraduate medical education. *JAMA: The Journal of the American Medical Association*, 306(9), 971–977. Retrieved from http://doi.org/10.1001/jama.2011.1255

Oriel, K. A., Madlon-Kay, D. J., Govaker, D., & Mersy, D. J. (1996). Gay and lesbian physicians in training: Family practice program directors' attitudes and students' perceptions of bias. *Family Medicine*, 28, 720–725.

Porter, K. E., & Krinsky, L. (2014). Do LGBT aging trainings effectuate positive change in mainstream elder service providers? *Journal of Homosexuality*, 61(1), 197–216. Retrieved from http://doi.org/10.1080/00918369.2013.835618

Przedworski, J. M., Dovidio, J. F., Hardeman, R. R., Phelan, S. M., Burke, S. E., Ruben, M. A., … van Ryn, M. (2015). A comparison of the mental health and well-being of sexual minority and heterosexual first-year medical students: A report from the medical student CHANGE study. *Academic Medicine: Journal of the Association of American Medical Colleges*, 90(5), 652–659. Retrieved from http://doi.org/10.1097/ACM.0000000000000658

Ramos, M. M., Tellez, C. M., Palley, T. B., Umland, B. E., & Skipper, B. J. (1998). Attitudes of physicians practicing in New Mexico toward gay men and lesbians in the profession. *Academic Medicine: Journal of the Association of American -Medical Colleges*, 73, 436–438.

Randall, C. (1987). Lesbian-phobia: A survey of BSN educators. *Cassandra: Radical Feminist Nurses Newsjournal*, 5, 12–14.

Randall, C. E., & Eliason, M. J. (2012). Out lesbians in nursing: What would Florence say? *Journal of Lesbian Studies*, 16(1), 65–75. Retrieved from http://doi.org/10.1080/10894160.2011.557644

Risdon, C., Cook, D., & Willms, D. (2000). Gay and lesbian physicians in training: A qualitative study. *CMAJ: Canadian Medical Association Journal = Journal de l'Association Medicale Canadienne*, 162(3), 331–334.

Rose, P. (1993). Out in the open? Lesbianism. *Nursing Times*, 89, 50–52.

Sanchez, N. F., Rabatin, J., Sanchez, J. P., Hubbard, S., & Kalet, A. (2006). Medical students' ability to care for lesbian, gay, bisexual, and transgendered patients. Family Medicine, 38, 21–27.

Schatz, B., & O'Hanlan, K. A. (1994). Anti-gay discrimination in medicine: Results of a national survey of lesbian, gay, and bisexual physicians. *San Francisco, CA: American Association for Human Rights*.

Sirota, T. (2013). Attitudes among nurse educators toward homosexuality. *The Journal of Nursing Education*, 52(4), 219–227. Retrieved from http://doi.org/10.3928/01484834–20130320–01

Tesar, C. M., & Rovi, S. L. (1998). Survey of curriculum on homosexuality/bisexuality in departments of family medicine. *Family Medicine*, 30, 283–287.

Wallick, M. M., Cambre, K. M., & Townsend, M. H. (1992). How the topic of homosexuality is taught at U.S. medical schools. *Academic Medicine: Journal of the Association of American Medical Colleges*, 67, 601–603.

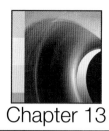

Chapter 13

Structural Barriers to Quality Care

"I had to dig through my bag to find this piece of paper that I carry around that confirms [I am my child's] legal guardian in health care, so she [the nurse] looks at it and the whole time she's looking at me like I've got six heads and then she goes, 'Well, that's not going to fit in my slot!'" (Respondent in Baker & Beagan, 2014, p. 586)

Mainstream healthcare settings are typically heterosexist, rendering LGBTQ people invisible or worse. Because of the stigma in society, LGBTQ people face more barriers to accessing health care and negotiating the healthcare system than do heterosexuals. The first section of this chapter reviews the components that make up the healthcare climate, the policies and procedures, including oral and written language, and describes how documents and agency policies can be made more inclusive. The second part of this chapter reviews some of the legal barriers to quality health care, including access to health insurance and the legal documents needed to protect relationships. Healthcare professionals need to be aware of the legal aspects that apply to their own settings.

Making Healthcare Settings Inclusive

Healthcare encounters begin even before a person walks in the door, and each part of these encounters can carry powerful messages that indicate if someone is welcome or not. For the most part, healthcare settings are overwhelming just by their physical traits—large, confusing, and intimidating buildings, reception desks behind protective windows, and people in uniforms that carry imposing nonverbal signals. A surprising number of these physical characteristics could and should be changed for the benefit of all consumers, but there are specific changes that are needed to send messages that are welcoming and inclusive of LGBTQ individuals and families. Table 13.1 shows the "Workplace Climate Scale" developed by the GLMA Nursing Section to promote inclusive environments for LGBTQ nurses, which in turn supports welcoming contexts for everyone, including patients.

The Website and Other Public Information

Some LGBTQ people will review the agency, institution, or clinic/office website prior to making an appointment to see if there is any sign that the healthcare setting is open and inclusive. Is there any wording on brochures, LGBTQ website links, or other public information that mark your agency as inclusive? If the agency is affiliated with a religious group, is there a statement that all religious/spiritual beliefs are welcome? Are there any links to community resources that are LGBTQ friendly?

Try This 13.1

Search the internet for patient pamphlets that focus on or incorporate LGBTQ issues that are relevant to your healthcare setting. Some relevant sites might include your professional organizations, LGBTQ community health center sites (e.g., Fenway Institute of Boston; Whitman-Walker Clinic in Washington, D.C.), or national LGBTQ organizations such as the GLMA, the Human Rights Campaign, the National Gay and Lesbian Task Force, and National LGBT Health Coalition. Check also the CDC, NIH, and SAMHSA for their dedicated pages to LGBTQ health.

Table 13.1 – Workplace Climate Scale—Self-Assessment Format (see http://glmanursing.org/workplace-climate/)	
Nurse Workplace Climate Scale[a]	**Score**
1. All recruitment and employment materials use prominent LGBT-inclusive language (sexual orientation and gender identity) and all forms provide opportunity for nurses to indicate sexual orientation, gender identity, preferred pronouns, and family affiliations in addition to other dimensions reflecting diversity.	
2. The workplace publishes policies that declare nondiscrimination in hiring, workload assignments, retention and promotion of nurses based on sexual orientation, gender identity, or family affiliation such as same-sex partners.	
3. The workplace openly recognizes and includes significant others, partners and spouses of LGBT nurses on all official records, as well as for all events where heterosexual partners are welcome.	
4. The workplace offers equal benefits to all domestic partners, spouses and children, regardless of sexual orientation or gender identity.	
5. There is a clear "zero tolerance" policy prohibiting workplace/event harassment of any kind toward nurses of diverse sexual orientations and gender identities.	
6. The workplace conducts accountability practices that require compliance with its policies prohibiting LGBT discrimination and harassment.	
7. The workplace has a defined and visible interest/support group that provides a safe space for LGBT nurses and allies to gather, network, and socialize.	
8. The workplace openly recognizes local and/or national events that celebrate and promote understanding of sexual orientation and gender diversity in equal measure with their acknowledgment of other kinds of "diversity" celebrations.	
9. There are ongoing employee educational programs, at least semiannually that are dedicated to promoting understanding of sexual and gender diversity.	
10. The workplace has documented relationships with stakeholders in the community that are devoted to serving the LGBT community.	

[a]Scoring: "Yes" = 1 point. "Working toward" = ½ point. "Not yet" = 0. "I/we do not know" = ?

The Waiting/Reception Area

The first entry into a hospital, clinic, or private practice is the waiting room or reception area. Several studies have found that LGBTQ patients scan the environment for clues that the setting might be safe (Eliason & Schope, 2001; Hitchcock & Wilson, 1992; Stevens, 1994). Visual clues that a healthcare setting is inclusive and welcoming to LGBTQ individuals can include, but are not limited to, the following:

- A nondiscrimination statement or patient rights policy that explicitly names sexual orientation and gender identity is prominently displayed at check-in or near admissions.
- Posters or art work that depict same-sex couples and gender variant people are displayed on the walls.
- There are magazines targeted to the LGBTQ community such as the Advocate, Curve, Genre, Out, Poz, Transgender Tapestry, or a local newspaper.
- If there is a rack of patient information, there are patient pamphlets that deal with LGBTQ issues.
- Local community LGBTQ newsletters or fliers about community social service agencies, health-related groups, or other resources are displayed.

The website for GLMA: Health Professionals Advancing LGBT Equality, has a pamphlet on creating a welcoming environment that may serve as a useful starting point for your work setting titled "Guidelines for Care of Lesbian, Gay, Bisexual and Transgender Patients" (available for download at http://glma.org/_data/n_0001/resources/live/GLMA%20guidelines%202006%20FINAL.pdf)

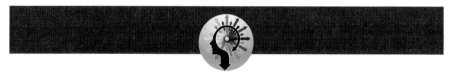

There Are No Dumb Questions 13.1

Question: If we display obvious LGBTQ magazines, pamphlets, and wall hangings, what about our patients/clients who have not yet come to understand that we need to do this, and who are offended and bothered by this? We can't afford to alienate them!

Answer: Unfortunately it is true that there are people who are negative or even hostile toward those who are LGBTQ. It is important that you and your colleagues who share a space have serious conversations about the kind of environment you want to create for your clients, and find ways to be inclusive of all, taking into account various racial/ethnic groups, religious and cultural affiliations, and socioeconomic status, and sexual/gender identities. Consider posting a prominent "What we believe ..." framed poster where everyone can see a statement that briefly summarizes your statement of inclusivity for all. Your statement might read: "We welcome people from all walks of life, from all religious and ethnic groups, and all sexual and gender identities."

Electronic Medical/Health Records

There are many structural factors that contribute to the institutionalization of healthcare disparities, but few are as powerful as the medical record. The institution of the electronic record makes the significance of the medical record all the more important because of the powerful ability to gather, analyze, and synthesize data. If medical records contain no indication of a person's sexual and gender identities, or worse yet, force everyone to conform to predetermined extremes such as male/female, married/single/divorced, the reality of LGBTQ people is invisible, and providers can completely ignore the particular issues that a person who is LGBTQ might be facing (Cahill & Makadon, 2013; Callahan, Hazarian, Yarborough, & Sanchez, 2014). In addition, to the extent that medical records include information related to intersecting factors such as race, socioeconomic status, relationship and family information, the potential exists to gain understanding of complex relationships between and among important social interactions. Statistical data provides a map that points the way to more in-depth understanding of complex relationships.

Thus far, most electronic medical record systems developed in the United States have not included questions on sexual orientation or gender identity. A concerted effort to be inclusive of all patients and their families has begun, prompted in part by the recommendations of the 2014 Institute of Medicine Committee on the Recommended Social and Behavioral Domains and Measures for Electronic Health Records. This report acknowledges lack of consensus on definitions, which hampers the development of standards for structured categories of data that are necessary for meaningful data analysis. Despite this barrier, the report strongly supports all efforts to begin to integrate data related to sexual and gender identity into medical records (Institute of Medicine, 2014, pp. 61–62).

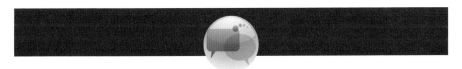

Talk About It 13.1

Get together with a group of colleagues and discuss the medical records you are now using. Examine them to determine the extent to which they are adequately gathering data related to sexual and gender identities and behaviors. You can download the IOM recommendations for electronic medical records here (https://goo.gl/Q2438B) and refer to page 61 for the section that highlights the importance of data related to sexual orientation.

Healthcare Intake Forms

"They take for granted that I'm heterosexual until I say that I'm not, and then everything comes to a halt. It's typical of the health care system … it's a very old-fashioned way to look at it." (Röndahl, Innala, & Carlsson, 2006, p. 376)

The language on the intake forms can put LGBTQ patients at ease or on the defensive. There is virtually no research on the impact of language on comfort levels of patients and clients, but we know anecdotally, and from qualitative studies, that these things matter. Inclusive language in intake forms is another clue that LGBTQ clients use to determine if they can trust a clinician with information about their sexual orientation, gender identity, and relationship status. There are no standardized ways for asking questions about sexuality and gender, as different information may be warranted in different healthcare settings. Some sample questions are listed below. We recommend asking questions about gender identity first, before sexual orientation. Some studies that have only had sexual orientation questions lead to people on the transgender or genderqueer spectrum selecting "other" or not define themselves because they were not given any option to acknowledge their gender first.

Gender Identity (this requires at least two questions):
- What was your sex assigned at birth? Male, female, another
- What is your current gender identification? Man, woman, transgender, another identification

Sexual Identity:

Do you identify as
- Straight, that is, not gay (some studies have found that many heterosexual people do not understand the term heterosexual, but define themselves in terms of not being gay)
- Gay or lesbian
- Bisexual
- Something else
- I do not use any sexual identity labels

Do you identify as
- Exclusively heterosexual, that is attracted to people of the other sex
- Mostly heterosexual
- Bisexual
- Mostly lesbian or gay
- Exclusively lesbian or gay, that is attracted to people of the same sex

Sexual Behavior:

In the past year, have your sexual relationships been with
- Only men
- Mostly men
- Equally men and women
- Mostly women
- Only women

If you work in a sexual health/STI setting, you may want to know more specifically about partners, and might ask:
- In the past year, how many of your sexual partners were men? ____
- How many were women? ____

For more information and recommendations related to inclusive language related to gender identity, refer to the "Best Practices" report from the Williams Institute at UCLA (Williams Institute & The GenIUSS Group, 2014). Think about the critical information you need to know in your healthcare setting and consider whether the questions you currently ask on written forms are inclusive and sensitive to LGBTQ patients.

Clinician Personal Interaction with the Client

When taking a history, if you use inclusive terms and language, you will vastly improve your relationships with all patients and increase the likelihood that you will elicit accurate information from anyone whose experience is different from cultural norms. Inclusive language does not make assumptions about a patient's sexual identity, sexual behavior, or gender identity (or race, social class, education, or other factors as well), particularly in situations where patients do not volunteer such information. Some examples of common questions that assume heterosexuality and gender normativity are:

- Are you married?
- Asking a patient you assume to be female: "Do you have a boyfriend?" or "Are you using birth control?"
- Asking a patient you assume to be male: "When did you first become interested in girls?"
- Asking a patient you assume to be male, "How about those … [insert the sports team]" or other gender-stereotypical statements.

Some examples of inclusive questions are:
- Are you dating anybody? Tell me about them.
- Do you have a partner or significant other?
- Is your partner male, female, or another identification?
- Are you currently in an intimate relationship?
- Are you sexually active with men, women, both, or neither?
- Who should be included in decisions about your health?
- Are you comfortable with your gender?
- What pronouns do you prefer to use?
- Is there anything related to your gender or sexuality that we should discuss on this visit?

Inclusive language conveys to LGBTQ patients that the interviewer is potentially open to hearing about their sexual identity, gender variation, and relationships. The accuracy and completeness of the information elicited will reflect the patient's level of comfort with the process. The goal of the interview is to work in the patient's best interest. The questions need to be tailored to the specific patient/client audience and setting. You may choose a different set of questions if you work in a reproductive health setting versus a psychiatric setting. For example, Garofalo and Bush (2008) proposed this introduction for interviewing adolescents:

> *"Some of my patients your age begin to find themselves attracted to other people. Have you been romantically or sexually attracted to boys, girls, or both" (p. 82) or "It is normal for young people to sometimes be confused about their feelings and experiences. Do you have any questions you'd like to ask me or things you would like to talk about?" (p. 83)*

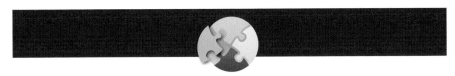

Try This 13.2

Set up a practice session with a colleague to role-play interviewing someone using only inclusive language. Consider working in a group of three, with one person being the interviewer, one person the patient, and the third an observer. After your first practice, stop to discuss the choices of language you used, and brainstorm better ways to ask questions. Rotate roles and repeat the process twice so that each person has an opportunity to be in each of the three roles. Keep practicing until you are comfortable with your new vocabulary.

Confidentiality

Confidentiality is the cornerstone of all clinician–patient relationships and assurances of confidentiality are crucial to taking a history. At the outset of the history, inform the patient that any information they provide will *not* be shared with others unless you are a mandatory reporter and are required to report something that could be a danger to self or others. In cases where complete confidentiality cannot be assured, a clinician should clarify the limits of confidentiality from the onset and respect patients' decision as to how much information about their sexuality or gender that they are willing to reveal to others. Details about patients' sexual orientation or gender variation should not be placed in the medical record without asking permission from the client. In these instances, it helps to create a code so that clinicians can remember the client's information without having the specific documentation in the record. Suggested ways to chart sexual identity without directly saying it include: "No need for birth control" (women in same-sex relationship); "has domestic partner"; or a special code. This is important because there is still considerable stigma attached to minority sexual and gender identifications. Some LGBTQ people will not want this information recorded on their medical files, but accept and appreciate that their provider knows this information without it having to be entered into a medical record. LGBTQ people still routinely lose jobs or promotions, lose custody of children, and lose the support of family, friends, and communities when they disclose their identities. In addition, many LGBTQ people have directly experienced poor quality of care, refusals of care, and/or unprofessional voyeurism or gossip in healthcare settings. While the medical record is supposed to be a confidential record, it is at the same time subject to review and inspection by any individual who gains access to it.

LGBTQ people have often experienced negative comments from healthcare providers. These types of comments are distressing at any time, but particularly when one is a patient and feeling vulnerable. As one respondent in Stevens and Hall's (1988) research said, "it's like putting your life in some one's hands who really hates you" (p. 72). Sometimes these inappropriate comments are violations of privacy, and sometimes they are in the form of malicious gossip or voyeurism, two forms of unprofessional practice, but that unfortunately still occurs. For example, one study found that nurses often reported that transgender patients were a source of gossip behind the patients' back:

"Not in front of the patient, but in particular like if it is a male to female and it is not that successful, people come back to the nurse's station and make a few comments like, 'Well, that's not working.'" (Carabez, Eliason, & Martinson, 2016).

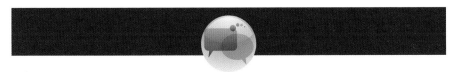

Talk About It 13.2

Talk with your colleagues about how you might deal with confidentiality issues and recording of information about sexuality and gender in patient records and in verbal communications among staff. Brainstorm special codes that might help you remember patients' information from one visit to another without revealing their sexuality or gender identifications in the medical record.

Special caution needs to be taken when working with children, adolescents, and young adults who may not have shared their concerns about sexual orientation or gender identity with their parents. Children and adolescents are particularly unlikely to share their intimate feelings unless their wishes and sensitivities are recognized. Special caution also needs to be taken when working with elders who may not have shared their sexual orientation or gender identity with their children or caregivers. Other situations where special caution needs to be taken include cases where revealing information may affect the outcome of a legal case such as child custody, divorce, or guardianship of an elderly dependent, or a patient who is at risk of losing employment if their identity is known. Once you have information about patients' sexuality and gender identity, remember the "A" in our model—always ASK the person who, if anyone, knows this information, and what they want to be included in their medical record.

Dignity and Safety Issues

Confidentiality of records and the Health Insurance Portability and Accountability Act (HIPAA) are legal mandates, but many LGBTQ people also report that their rights to privacy and dignity have been violated in healthcare encounters. Some have been asked voyeuristic questions, some have been exoticized, and others felt under undue scrutiny. Sometimes the questions are asked at inappropriate times that make patients feel unsafe. For example, one lesbian reported this story of what happened while she was having a pelvic examination:

"So he went to examine me, and halfway through the internal examination he said, 'Well, I don't really know much about these relationships. Can you tell me what your sexual practice is? What do you do?' ... and it was absolutely awful. I didn't know what to say, so I didn't say anything ... I decided I'd never go back to the GP ever again. When I got home I felt like I'd been abused ... I had to go and have a shower and I felt horrible." (Platzer & James, 2000, p. 196)

Making Referrals

Clinicians should not only be aware of the inclusivity of their own healthcare setting, but also of any referral sources that the healthcare agency uses for support services for their patients. This issue can be critical in settings where group treatments are the standard, such as substance abuse treatment settings—the LGBTQ client may have to face negative reactions or lack of understanding from counselors and other clients (Eliason, 2000). Another example might be referrals to clergy. Most clergy in healthcare settings are highly professional and provide client-centered services, but some may have negative attitudes about LGBTQ patients that hinder the healthcare experience. One gay man encountered physicians with anti-gay beliefs that were imposed on him:

> *"I have had a female doctor say she was fine with it and then try to coerce me into saying sexual identity is purely a choice. My worst experience, the doctor lectured me on the Bible and changed her diagnosis [when she discovered I was gay]"* (Respondent in Eliason & Schope, 2001, p. 130)

Policies in Healthcare Setting

Equitable policies and procedures help ensure that all patients/clients are treated fairly and help eliminate health disparities. Inequitable policies and procedures are one of the barriers for LGBTQ people in seeking healthcare, and as a result, many LGBTQ people wait until conditions are far advanced before seeking care. Once in the healthcare system, inequitable policies/procedures create greater levels of stress for the patient and family that compound the stress of the illness and its treatment.

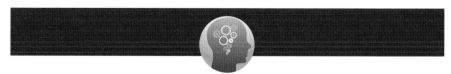

Think About It 13.1

Consider the two stories below, and the importance that legal relationships play in healthcare settings. Think about what needs to change in current healthcare systems to shift toward humane and sensitive treatment toward all LGBTQ patients and their families.

Situation #1: Bill Flanigan and his partner, Robert Daniel, were in the Washington DC area in 2000. Robert was admitted to a hospital due to complications from AIDS. Bill was not allowed to see Robert and the hospital staff would not give Bill any information about what was happening because he "wasn't family." The couple had durable power of attorney documents and were registered as domestic partners in the state of California. This information was disregarded, as was Bill's request not to insert a breathing tube, per Robert's wishes. Only when Robert's sister and mother arrived 4 hours later did Bill get to see his partner. By this time, Robert was no longer conscious, his eyes were taped shut, and a breathing tube had been inserted. The two men never had the chance to say goodbye before Robert died (for more information, see https://goo.gl/uo8Gw9).

Situation #2: In December of 2013, shortly after California reinstated same-sex marriage, three lesbian couples, all over the age of 65 who had been in their respective relationships

(continued)

for over 30 years, had a joint legal marriage ceremony to finally legalize and celebrate their long-standing commitments to one another. Two weeks later, just before the Christmas holiday, Joyce, Sue's partner (now wife) became violently ill and was rushed to the hospital. Sue remained with Joyce throughout the admission process. But when they rolled Joyce off to a hospital room, the admitting staff refused to let Sue accompany her. Sue protested, reminding the hospital folks who were involved, that she was Joyce's partner and wanted to remain with her. The hospital staff ignored her pleas and rolled Joyce down the hall. Finally Sue, in desperation, yelled loudly "but we are married and she is my wife!" The volunteer standing close by just stared at Sue, but finally ran after the person wheeling Joyce to the elevator, grabbed the chart, and sure enough, Sue's name was listed as the patient's spouse. Finally, just as the elevator arrived, they agreed that Sue could accompany them to the hospital room. Four days later, Joyce died, with Sue still by her side.

Healthcare Equality Index

In 2007, the Human Rights Campaign and GLMA: Health Professional Advancing LGBT Equality (formerly known as the Gay and Lesbian Medical Association) collaborated on a project called the Healthcare Equality Index (HEI), to rate whether U.S. hospitals have equitable policies and procedures for their LGBTQ patients and families. A questionnaire was sent out to hundreds of hospitals across the country, and the report provides information on 74 institutions that returned the questionnaire. While certainly not a scientific study, the report outlines equitable policies and procedures and the exercise of answering the questionnaire may prompt more hospitals to change their policies. Table 13.2 shows the questions on the survey, which can be accessed on the Human Rights Campaign web site (http://www.hrc.org/campaigns/healthcare-equality-index). The four core criteria in the Index are (1) patient nondiscrimination policies, (2) equal visitation, (3) training in LGBT patient-centered care, and (4) employment nondiscrimination.

Of the 74 hospitals initially surveyed in creating the Index,

- 58 (78%) had a written policy that prohibits discrimination on the basis of sexual orientation, and 47 (64%) prohibited discrimination on the basis of gender identity.
- 47 (64%) allowed LGBTQ domestic partners of patients the same access to visitation as spouses and next of kin.
- 39 (53%) allowed same-sex parents the same access to visitation as other-sex parents of minor children.
- 69 (93%) recognized advance healthcare directives such as durable power of attorney to give LGBTQ partners' rights over decision making for their incapacitated partners; but only 40 had a policy that allows same-sex parents the same rights for medical decision making as other-sex parents regarding their children.
- 57 (77%) provided diversity training to personnel that include issues related to LGBTQ people.
- 60 (81%) prohibited discrimination in employment on the basis of sexual orientation.
- 38 (51%) barred discrimination in employment based on gender identity or gender expression.
- 51 (69%) offered health insurance coverage to employees' domestic partners.

Table 13.2 – Sample Healthcare Equality Index Questions		
Question	Yes	No
Does your hospital have a nondiscrimination policy?		
If yes, does it include sexual identity/orientation?		
Does it include gender identity or gender expression?		
Does your hospital have a Patient Bill of Rights?		
If yes, does it have language on sexual identity/orientation and gender identity or expression?		
Does your hospital have a written definition of "family" or "immediate family?"		
Does your hospital have visitation policies that differentiate between friends, family, and/or immediate family? If yes, does the policy allow patients to designate their visitors?		
Does your hospital have any restrictions to its visitation policies, such as areas of the hospital or hours? Are these policies potentially discriminatory of LGBTQ families?		
Does your hospital have a written visitation policy that allows LGBTQ domestic partners the same access as spouses and next of kin?		
Does your hospital have a written policy that allows same-sex parents the same access as other-sex parents for visitation of their minor children?		
Does your hospital recognize advance healthcare directives such as durable powers of attorney for health care, healthcare proxies, or living wills in allowing LGBTQ domestic partners decision-making authority for their hospitalized domestic partner?		
Does your hospital counsel patients on their right to designate their domestic partner or someone else as medical decision maker when advising them of advance directive rights?		
Does your hospital provide any diversity or cultural competency training to personnel addressing the unique health issues related to LGBTQ patients and their families?		
Does your hospital specifically bar employment discrimination based on sexual orientation?		
Does your hospital specifically bar employment discrimination based on gender identity?		
Does your hospital have an LGBTQ staff association, affinity group, or network?		
Are the written forms inclusive of LGBTQ issues?		

Seven years after the first survey, while there is still a long way to go, the 2014 HEI Report shows considerable progress in achieving equitable and inclusive care for LGBT patients and families (Hanneman, 2014). The current Index is organized with four core criteria, with a total of 41 questions. The four core criteria are: (1) patient nondiscrimination policies, (2) visitation policies, (3) employment nondiscrimination policies, and (4) training in LGBT patient-centered care.

Active participation in using the Healthcare Equality Index is voluntary, but in addition to voluntary responses to the survey, the HRC staff research nonrespondent hospitals to estimate a broader understanding of the extent to which health care for LGBT patients and families is improving. A total of 507 healthcare facilities actively participated in the 2014 survey; an additional 997 nonrespondent and previous active participants were also evaluated by the HRC staff, for a total of 1,504 agencies in all 50 states. The contrast between the 507 active participants and the nonrespondent partic-ipants highlights the areas where there are major challenges. Ninety-seven percent of the participating hospitals had fully LGBT-inclusive patient nondiscrimination policies and 96% had fully LGBT-inclusive employment nondiscrimination policies, while only 51% of nonparticipating hospitals had fully inclusive LGBT patient policies and 50% had fully inclusive LGBT employment nondiscrimination policies.

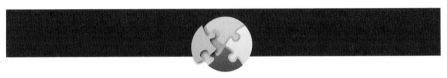

Try This 13.3

Review the information on the HRC web site at **https://goo.gl/Zi963g** explaining what is required to meet the first core criteria: patient nondiscrimination policies. Gather as much information as you can for an agency near you. Identify the agency's areas of strength, and what needs to happen to improve the agency's patient nondiscrimination policies.

Health Insurance

Compounding the problems in accessing health care that LGBTQ people face, securing medical insurance coverage for many LGBT people in the United States has been dif-ficult if not impossible because health care in the United States has not been universal. When the Affordable Care Act (ACA) reached full implementation in 2014, many of the barriers to healthcare coverage were removed. Specific changes that were particu-larly important for LGBT people and families included:

- The end of denial of coverage based on pre-existing conditions (particularly important for people with HIV/AIDS and for trans* people),
- The ability to obtain coverage regardless of employment status, and financial assistance for those who are not able to afford coverage,
- Improved coverage in most states for LGBT partners and children, depending on the state's definition of "family,"
- Mandatory coverage for preventive services and screening, mental health and for substance abuse issues, and
- Protection against discrimination based on sexual orientation and gender identity.

For more information and assistance in determining how to gain coverage under the new ACA plans, see the LGBT Guide to healthcare plans at http://strongfamilies-movement.org/assets/docs/where-to-start-what-to-ask.pdf (Strong Families, 2014)

Before the U.S. ACA, LGBTQ people were seriously disadvantaged in gaining access to health care, and some of those disadvantages persist, in part because people have yet to be informed about what is now available. The sudden legalization of marriage in the United States in June 2015 has the potential to open new possibilities for coverage for many, since marriage qualifies as a major life change, qualifying married partners to obtain coverage as soon as they marry. However, marriage is not an option or a choice that all want to make. Because of the gay rights movement, the workplace trend toward domestic-partner benefits is improving the lives of some committed couples, regardless of sexual orientation or marital status. Unfortunately, those in same-sex couples are less likely to be insured than heterosexual married couples. In fact, about 20% of same-sex couples (18.8% men and 21.4% women) had absolutely no health insurance in contrast to 11.5% of married couples (Ash & Bedgett, 2006). Even if health insurance were available for all same-sex partners, the federal government has determined that married couples have special rights. While the IRS allows the cost of health benefits for married spouses and dependents to be tax deductible, it has not yet given the same rights to unmarried same-sex couples. So the amount of money that the employer pays for health insurance for an unmarried partner and any children will be included as taxable income on W-2 of the employee. In addition the domestic partners must disclose their sexuality to an employer, which is not safe in some situations. Additionally, the federal Family and Medical Leave Act, which allows employees in larger companies to take paid or unpaid sick leave to care for a partner, child, or parent with a serious medical condition for up to 12 weeks out of a year, does not apply to most same-sex partners or to a partner's legal children, though some individual employers provide similar coverage.

Legal Issues

LGBTQ people have some unique legal challenges due to their inability to legally formalize their relationships in the state, national, or international arenas, which renders their families invisible and unprotected. Even though now all LGBTQ have been granted the right to marry in the United States and many other countries, some will choose not to marry and still need additional legal documents to protect their relationships and families. It is important for all healthcare providers to become aware of the extra legal documents required to protect LGBTQ patients and their families. Although many of these forms can be downloaded and completed without the assistance of a lawyer, an estate-planning specialist concentrating on LGBTQ issues is an excellent source of information and help. The following information has been adapted from NCLR and Rainbow Laws' websites: (http://www.nclrights.org/site/DocServer/NCLR_LIFELINES.pdf?docID=521 and http://rainbowlaw.com/)

Living Will/Medical Directive

In every state in the United States, and in most other western countries, people can sign documents describing their wishes concerning life-prolonging medical care. Depending upon the state, this document may be called by any one of several different names including: living will, medical directive, healthcare directive, directive to physicians, or declaration regarding health care. This document contains directions to healthcare professionals about what the person wishes when they are no longer capable of making or communicating choices regarding life-prolonging and other medical care.

Durable Power of Attorney for Health Care/Healthcare Proxy

A durable power of attorney for health care (which is also sometimes called a "healthcare proxy") allows a designated person to make medical decisions for another person in the event they are unable to do so. This is a very important document for LGBTQs, even if they are legally married, since agency personnel might ignore a legal marriage as equivalent to a heterosexual union, and turn to a biological family member instead as the person with the right to make healthcare decisions. A durable power of attorney is more likely to be universally recognized, and protects a person's right to have their designated person make healthcare decisions on their behalf, instead of someone from the biological family.

Hospital Visitation Authorization

A hospital visitation authorization allows the naming of specific individuals to visit them in the event individuals are no longer able to communicate their wishes.

Authorization for Consent to Medical Treatment of Minor

The medical treatment of a minor requires authorization by the legal parents. This form allows the legal parents to permit someone other than a child's legal parents to authorize a doctor or other healthcare professional to provide medical services to a minor child. In states that do not recognize both parents in a same-sex couple as legal parents, this form is critical so that all parents and appropriate grandparents are able to consent to emergency medical treatment for the child. For couples who are about to have children, it is very important to complete this document before the birth mother goes into the hospital. While this form may not be legally binding, hospitals will usually honor the authorization.

Durable Power of Attorney for Finances

A durable power of attorney for finances allows a designated person, the "agent," to take care of finances when a person is not able to do so. A general power of attorney for finances authorizes this designated agent to control a broad range of financial matters, including paying medical bills, cashing checks, or receiving benefits.

Wills

A will is a legal document that allows a person to designate who will receive their property when they die. When someone dies without a will, their property is distributed to their legal heirs. In locations where there is not yet marriage equality, a same-sex partner is NOT considered to be a legal heir and therefore is not legally entitled to inherit property when an individual dies without a will. This is true regardless of how long people have been with their partners and regardless of the quality of their relationship with their relatives.

Trusts

Another way to designate who and/or what charities will receive property upon death is through a revocable living trust. A living trust is similar to a will in that it allows one to say who should get what; it differs from a will in that property left by a will must go through the court probate process—which means that the will must be proven valid, and the person's debts must be paid before the property is distributed. The probate process often takes about a year. With a living trust, this process is avoided and the property goes directly to the people and/or charities named in the trust. In some circumstances, transferring the property through a living trust rather than a will also helps to reduce or avoid some estate taxes.

Nomination of Conservator or Guardian for a Minor

The care and custody of a child to another responsible adult in the event that the child's legal parent dies or becomes physically or psychologically unable to care for the child can be problematic if a guardian for the child(ren) has not been legally named. This is especially challenging for the child(ren) when the birth mother dies without providing for her children's future. Usually, a person who is appointed to be the child's guardian is given physical custody of the child and authority to manage the child's financial matters.

Elder Guardian/Conservator

LGBTQ elders are more likely to live alone and not have children. If the time comes when LGBTQ elders are unable to manage their affairs, who will handle these matters? If someone has not been named through a durable power of attorney, advanced medical directive, and/or a trust then someone will have to seek to qualify as a guardian and/or conservator. A petition will have to be filed in the Circuit Court of the city or county of residence asking the Judge to appoint an individual to serve as a guardian and/or conservator. A guardian is appointed to be responsible for the person, that is, to take care of physical needs, medical treatment, medication, and living arrangements. A conservator is appointed to attend to financial affairs, protect assets, pay bills, invest funds, and preserve resources of the LGBTQ elder. The best option is for LGBTQ elders to carefully plan for this eventuality and memorialize it in writing, yet hope that they can maintain control over their own environment and care.

Autopsy and Disposition of Remains

In the absence of written instructions, nearly every state gives biological relatives or relations by marriage the right to control the disposition of a body, including funeral arrangements, upon death. As is true for wills and power of attorney for health care, with the exception of married spouses this right to control disposition of remains is not provided automatically to a same-sex partner. But because there is still uneven acceptance of same-sex relationships even in locations where marriage equality exists, LGBTQ families should have written instructions regarding decisions after death of a loved one.

Tables 13.3 and 13.4 provide checklists that healthcare professionals can use with their LGBTQ clients to ensure that they are adequately protected. This information

Table 13.3 – Are You Legally Protected?

	Yes	No
Do you have a will or trust?		
If yes, do you regularly review it to insure that it still reflects your wishes?		
Have you named someone who you are confident will carry out wishes. Have you also named a back up?		
Do you have a "living will" detailing your healthcare wishes?		
Have you completed a medical power of attorney naming someone to make healthcare decisions for you if you cannot?		
Have you given a copy of your completed medical power of attorney to your doctors and communicated to them who should get information about your health?		
Have you completed a financial power of attorney naming someone to make financial decisions for you if you cannot?		
Have you made your wishes known about organ donation?		
Have you recorded information about your wishes regarding a funeral and disposition of your remains including financial limits?		
Have you discussed your wishes with those people you have named as power of attorney or executor?		
Have you stored all your important documents someplace where your executor/loved ones can access them (not in a bank safety deposit box)?		

Table 13.4 – Protection of Loved Ones Checkup: Is Your Family Protected?

	Yes	No
Do you have adequate life insurance?		
Have you named beneficiaries for bank accounts, investment accounts, and retirement plans so that the funds skip the probate process?		
Have you titled your assets so that they actually pass on as you intended?		
Have you named a guardian for your children in your will or trust?		
Have you signed up for disability insurance?		
Have you considered a living trust so that someone you have faith in, in the event of your incapacity, will manage your assets?		
If you have a living trust, have you titled all your assets in the name of the trust?		
If you own a business, do you have a succession plan or buyout agreements?		
Have you done everything you can to reduce your estate taxes?		

could be put into a pamphlet format and displayed in the waiting or reception area of a healthcare setting.

Conclusions

In other chapters, we have focused mostly on the individual level factors associated with stereotypes, stigma, discrimination, and differential treatment. Clearly, changes need to be made on the individual provider level, but these changes will not improve the quality of care that LGBTQ patients receive unless the system changes as well. Systems level factors such as policies, procedures, written forms, and the climate of the setting must be addressed simultaneously with provider education for real social change to occur.

For more information about achieving workplace equality for all LGBT employees, see the Human Rights Campaign Corporate Equality Index (http://www.hrc.org/campaigns/corporate-equality-index). Strategies for improving your climate may be found with TeamSTEPPS (http://teamstepps.ahrq.gov/).

References

Ash, M. A., & Bedgett, M. V. L. (2006). Separate and unequal: The effect of unequal access to employment-based health insurance on same-sex and unmarried different-sex couples. *Contemporary Economic Policy*, *24*, 582–599.

Baker, K., & Beagan, B. (2014). Making assumptions, making space: An anthropological critique of cultural competency and its relevance to queer patients. *Medical Anthropology Quarterly*, *28*(4), 578–598. Retrieved from http://doi.org/10.1111/maq.12129

Cahill, S., & Makadon, H. (2013). Sexual orientation and gender identity data collection in clinical settings and in electronic health records: A key to ending LGBT health disparities. *Journal of LGBT Health Research*, *1*, 1–8.

Callahan, E. J., Hazarian, S., Yarborough, M., & Sanchez, J. P. (2014). Eliminating LGBTIQQ health disparities: The associated roles of electronic health records and institutional culture. *The Hastings Center Report*, *44*(Suppl 4), S48–S52. Retrieved from http://doi.org/10.1002/hast.371

Carabez, R., Eliason, M. J., & Martinson, M. (2016). Nurses' knowledge about transgender patient care: A qualitative study. *ANS. Advances in Nursing Science*, *39*(3), 257–271.

Eliason, M. J. (2000). Substance abuse counselor's attitudes regarding lesbian, gay, bisexual, and transgendered clients. *Journal of Substance Abuse*, *12*(4), 311–328. Retrieved from http://doi.org/10.1016/S0899–3289(01)00055–4

Eliason, M. J., & Schope, R. (2001). Does "Don't Ask, Don't Tell" apply to health care? Lesbian, gay, and bisexual people's disclosure to health care providers. *Journal of the Gay and Lesbian Medical Association*, *5*, 125–134.

Garofalo, R., & Bush, S. (2008). Addressing LGBTQ youth in the clinical setting. In H. J. Makadon, K. H. Mayer, J. Potter, & H. Goldhammer (Eds.), *The Fenway guide to lesbian, gay, bisexual, and transgender health* (pp. 75–100). Philadelphia, PA: American College of Physicians Press.

Hanneman, T. (2014). *Healthcare equality index 2014: promoting equitable and inclusive care for lesbian, gay, bisexual and transgender patients and their families*. Retrieved June 28, 2015, from http://www.hrc.org/campaigns/healthcare-equality-index

Hitchcock, J. M., & Wilson, H. S. (1992). Personal risking: Lesbian self-disclosure of sexual orientation to professional health care providers. *Nursing Research*, *41*(3), 178–183.

Institute of Medicine. (2014). *Capturing social and behavioral domains and measures in electronic health records: Phase 2*. Washington, DC: The National Academies Press. Retrieved from http://www.nap.edu/download.php?record_id=18951

Platzer, H., & James, T. (2000). Lesbians' experiences of healthcare. *Nursing Times Research*, 5(3), 194–202. Retrieved from http://doi.org/10.1177/136140960000500305

Röndahl, G., Innala, S., & Carlsson, M. (2006). Heterosexual assumptions in verbal and non-verbal communication in nursing. *Journal of Advanced Nursing*, 56(4), 373–381. Retrieved from http://doi.org/10.1111/j.1365–2648.2006.04018.x

Stevens, P. E. (1994). Protective strategies of lesbian clients in health care environments. *Research in Nursing & Health*, 17(3), 217–229.

Stevens, P. E., & Hall, J. M. (1988). Stigma, health beliefs and experiences with health care in lesbian women. *Image–The- Journal of Nursing Scholarship*, 20(2), 69–73.

Strong Families. (2014). *Where to start, what to ask: A guide for LGBT people choosing healthcare plans*. Retrieved June 28, 2015, from http://strongfamiliesmovement.org/assets/docs/where-to-start-what-to-ask.pdf

Williams Institute, & The GenIUSS Group. (2014). *Best practices for asking questions to identify transgender and other gender minority respondents on population-based surveys*. Retrieved July 26, 2015, from http://williamsinstitute.law.ucla.edu/wp-content/uploads/geniuss-report-sep-2014.pdf

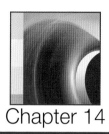

Chapter 14

Conclusions and A Call to Action

"It doesn't make much sense, but today in America, millions of our fellow citizens wake up and go to work with the awareness that they could lose their job, not because of anything they do or fail to do, but because of who they are – lesbian, gay, bisexual, transgender. And that's wrong. We're here to do what we can to make it right – to bend that arc of justice just a little bit in a better direction." (President Obama on July 21, 2014, on signing an executive order to ban workplace discrimination against LGBT people)

This book has summarized some of the important terms and concepts related to sexuality and gender identifications and outlined the potential role of minority stress in affecting access to health care, quality of health care, and development of physical and mental health problems. We have emphasized the structural issues that are at the root of these health problems. The book offers a starting point for understanding the health disparities experienced by many LGBTQ people, as well as describing the unwelcoming environment of many healthcare settings. The hostile climate in society as a whole and healthcare institutions in particular, stem from historic prejudices that became embedded in the very fabric of society, permeating the legal system, religion, education, medicine and healthcare policy and systems, and politics. Changing this environment means that dedicated people of all identities must work together to change these systems, not just educate people about LGBTQ healthcare issues. The first section of this final chapter outlines the different levels of interventions needed to create a welcoming and inclusive environment.

A Levels Approach to Change

One way to consider how to implement the action steps needed to improve healthcare access and quality is to examine the interventions that need to be undertaken at different levels of the system, from the individual to the larger societal level. An ecological approach to LGBTQ health care would include the individual person (with their attitudes, knowledge, identities, experiences, and education), interpersonal dynamics (communication and interactions between two or more people), the community (both LGBTQ and other components that make up local communities), the institutional level (the systems that exist in communities, such as law enforcement, healthcare agencies, schools, churches, and government), and the larger societal level (the state and national laws and policies, national politics, media, religious discourses, and so on). Some ideas for change at each level are outlined briefly below. Creating the kinds of changes that are needed may seem daunting, because change is sometimes difficult and slow. But each of us as individuals can contribute to creating change at each and every one of these levels. We expand on the individual level interventions in the final section of this chapter, ending with ten recommendations for change that readers can begin immediately.

Individual Level

- Seek out continuing education/inclusive education about LGBTQ health care.
- Get experienced (ask your patients/clients about how their sexual and gender identities have affected their lives, and their health).
- Use inclusive language.
- Study your own body language and evaluate your attitudes.
- Examine the beliefs that you have carried over from youth into your adulthood. Where did they come from (family, religion, media, etc)? Do they serve you well now? What beliefs can be discarded as stereotypes, and which ones help you to provide quality care to all of your patients/clients?

Interpersonal Level

- Get to know your LGBTQ coworkers if you don't already know them.
- Talk to LGBTQ community members and find out what issues affect your own region.
- Practice using inclusive language in your work and daily life.
- Be a role model for inclusion in your family.

Institutional Level

- Evaluate the institution where you work or get your own health care: Is it inclusive and welcoming?
- Encourage/initiate changes in policies and procedures, such as nondiscrimination policies, visiting hours, and definitions of family and relationships.
- Demand staff training at all levels that covers all types of diversity.
- Support having an LGBTQ task force, committee, or work group to consider what changes in climate are needed: Volunteer for such a group.

Community Level

- Support education and dialogue about sexuality and gender in your larger community through social and political practices, such as urging your faith communities to be open and accepting, making your neighborhoods safe for LGBTQ people to live in, and fostering social justice in all aspects of community life.
- If you have children, find out what they learn about LGBTQ people at school and other settings. Advocate for comprehensive sexuality education that includes LGBTQ issues. By doing this, you are positively impacting the future for all.

Societal Level

- Vote for politicians who support civil rights for LGBTQ (and all) people.
- Learn about legislation and national issues related to LGBTQ people.

- Join social justice movements or coalitions.
- Encourage state and national professional organizations to which you belong to be inclusive of LGBTQ people if they are not already.

Social justice change requires working at all of these levels. It may be helpful to assess your own healthcare setting in terms of a continuum from very rejecting and actively negative about LGBTQ people to one that embraces sexual and gender difference. Figure 14.1 outlines a continuum with five levels of environments. Which one best describes your workplace? Which one best describes the setting where you receive health care? The final section will outline the steps that you as an individual can take to move your agency or institution up the continuum to welcoming and inclusive.

The Ten Things Healthcare Professionals Can Do

We end this book with our top ten list of things that healthcare professionals can do to improve the quality of care for their LGBTQ patients/clients. These ten things are in no particular order. We offer them for readers who are ready to take action for social justice.

In spite of the lack of research in many areas and the gaps in knowledge that we have pointed out throughout the book, we know enough to start making changes in healthcare systems and in individual healthcare professionals that begin the process of improving the quality of health care. We know about concepts of equity, respect, social justice, and human dignity and can build on those values that are already central to healthcare practice. In this book, we presented a useful cultural model that focuses on awareness, sensitivity, and knowledge

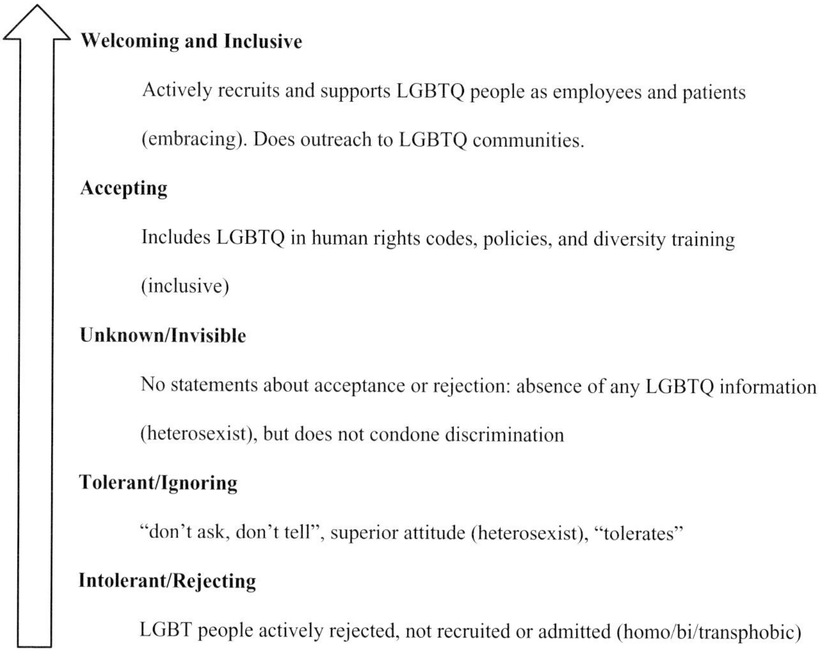

Welcoming and Inclusive

Actively recruits and supports LGBTQ people as employees and patients

(embracing). Does outreach to LGBTQ communities.

Accepting

Includes LGBTQ in human rights codes, policies, and diversity training

(inclusive)

Unknown/Invisible

No statements about acceptance or rejection: absence of any LGBTQ information

(heterosexist), but does not condone discrimination

Tolerant/Ignoring

"don't ask, don't tell", superior attitude (heterosexist), "tolerates"

Intolerant/Rejecting

LGBT people actively rejected, not recruited or admitted (homo/bi/transphobic)

Figure 14.1 – Levels of Acceptance in Healthcare Environments.

(Lipson & Dibble, 2005). Building on the knowledge and skills presented in this book, we offer an action plan, based on the top ten things that healthcare providers can do to be culturally appropriate with their LGBTQ clients/patients and coworkers.

Number 10: Understand the Far-Reaching Effects of Social Stigma on LGBTQ People, Families, and Communities

If nothing else, the content of this book should have resulted in greater awareness of the myriad ways that stigma impacts LGBTQ people, from lack of validation of relationships and families to employment discrimination to experiencing harassment and violence in public to being ignored or humiliated in healthcare settings. Stigma has affected access to health care because same-sex relationships were not legal in most locales until 2015, resulting in many partners not being covered by health insurance. In addition, many LGBTQ people experience discrimination, harassment, and invisibility in healthcare systems, and these experiences may lead them to delay or avoid mainstream healthcare services, such as preventive screenings. Stigma has also created minority stress, which contributes to the onset and maintenance of a wide variety of physical and mental health problems, such as depression, anxiety disorders, substance abuse, and asthma. Stigma impacts the ways that healthcare professionals interact with LGBTQ clients and the likelihood that LGBTQ patients will feel safe to disclose their sexuality or gender identities. To reduce stigma, we first must make it visible and healthcare systems need to acknowledge it.

- *Action Steps*
  1. Share this knowledge with others—coworkers, fellow students, family members, your children, etc. In other words, break the silence about sexuality and gender. You can start by saying, "I just read this book about LGBTQ health care and learned … Did you know that?"
  2. Examine your own practice—do you unwittingly allow invisibility, harassment, or discrimination to occur un-remarked? When you see the effects of stigma at work, name it as such. If you hear an anti-LGBTQ joke, tell others it is offensive. When you see an LGBTQ coworker ignored or treated differently, speak up. When you treat LGBTQ patients who experience shame and guilt, help them to see that the stigma is not their fault. Show compassion to all of your patients in every way you can.

Number 9: Know Inclusive Language and Use It in Written and Oral Communications

Most of the forms and assessments used in healthcare settings render LGBTQ people invisible. Words have a great deal of power and being rendered invisible is alienating. In fact, it is one form of microaggression. Take a look at the language used in your setting, and also examine how comfortable you are with the language. Can you say "lesbian, gay, bisexual, and transgender" without feeling discomfort or being self-conscious? Are you comfortable asking patients/clients about their sexual identities and discussing their concerns about sexuality and gender? How comfortable are you speaking with a patient who is early in a gender transition process? It may take practice for some healthcare professionals to include sexual and gender histories as a natural part of the history-taking process. For those who are direct care providers, was it easy to ask about bowel habits at first? Most of what we do as healthcare professionals takes practice before we are comfortable and competent at it. Becoming comfortable talking to patients about sexuality and gender will benefit all of your patients or clients and could improve communications within your own family and intimate relationships as well.

- *Action Steps*
1. Point out to administrators or coworkers if your forms are not inclusive, but do not wait for the forms to change—you can change your own language and oral communication immediately.
2. Volunteer to be on a committee or task force to recommend changes in official documents and forms.
3. Request training on LGBTQ issues, and sexual and gender history-taking for all staff.
4. Make changes in your own individual history-taking or intake process to be inclusive if you are not already (e.g., use terms like partner, ask about sexuality and gender).

Number 8: Develop Written Policies That Are Inclusive of LGBTQ People and Their Families

As we have seen, many LGBTQ relationships and families are not always protected by existing laws, and LGBTQ families are often invisible in hospital and clinic policies and procedures. Examine your own work setting and determine if there is equality for LGBTQ patients, clients, and staff members. The policies to examine include human rights or nondiscrimination policies, patient rights statements, definitions of family, visiting policies, and policies governing staff conduct such as sexual harassment policies. Employee partner benefits and staff training policies are also important.

- *Action Steps*
1. Point out to administrators or coworkers if your policies are not inclusive.
2. Volunteer to be on a committee or task force to recommend changes.
3. Learn about the laws in your own state and local region that address LGBTQ people, such as same-sex marriage, domestic partner registries, civil unions, adoption laws, employment nondiscrimination, and hate crimes. Remember that some of these policies may include sexual orientation but not gender identity. Policies need to include both sexuality and gender to be truly inclusive.

Number 7: Recognize the Broad Diversity and Creativity of LGBT Family Structures

Examine how family is defined where you work, live, or receive your own health care. Why do we focus on legal relationships or blood to define family? Shouldn't family be the people we care most about and want around us in the times of stress? The people who support us in making important decisions about our health? Examine the rationale for current policies, for example, why do so many settings limit visitors in emergency departments or intensive care units to legal spouses or blood relatives? Aren't there many heterosexual individuals who rely on people other than those sanctioned individuals for their support? Inclusive policies could benefit more than just LGBTQ people.

- **Action Steps**
  1. Advocate for the broadest possible definitions of family that allow patients/ clients to choose who gets to be involved in healthcare decision-making and who gets to visit and support them while hospitalized.
  2. Respect and include families, whatever form they take, in the care of patients/ clients.
  3. Make sure that agency/institution documents, posters, flyers, brochures, and other written materials reflect the diversity of the families that the institution serves.

Number 6: Develop Policies and Procedures for How to Deal with Confidentiality Issues and Recording of Information about Sexuality and Gender in Patient Records, and for Dealing with Inappropriate Comments in Verbal Communications Among Staff

We know that some LGBTQ people are afraid to disclose their sexual/gender identities to healthcare professionals, and why this might be the case. Are those fears valid in your work setting? What happens now when a patient is known to be LGBTQ? Is it recorded on their records without their consent? Do staff members gossip about the sexuality or gender identities of patients? If so, how do we convey to staff a professional procedure to protect client/patient confidentiality and to maintain patient's dignity? What are the sanctions for unprofessional behavior?

- **Action Steps**
  1. Make it policy to ask permission from patients to record sexual or gender identity on medical records.
  2. Develop a code that allows you to remember this information from one visit to another for patients/clients who do not want the information on their records. Respect patients' reasons for not disclosing whether you think the reason is valid or not. They are the only ones who can determine what is safe for them.
  3. Develop employee policies that contain sanctions for breaking patient confidentiality.
  4. Set a tone of professional conduct among staff members—be a role model for respecting the privacy and dignity of patients/clients. Gossip about patients is unprofessional.

Number 5: Recognize The Legal Issues: Have Forms or Information Available for LGBTQ Families for Release of Information, Power of Attorney for Health Care, Guardianship, etc.

Because of the lack of legislation that protects LGBTQ relationships in many parts of the world, other legal documents are needed. Many LGBTQ people are unaware of these legal protections, or do not know how to go about accessing the forms. All healthcare settings should provide information about the legal documents needed to protect families without recourse to the benefits of marriage, in the same way that information is provided about living wills and organ donation. In some cases, LGBTQ people have produced legal documents such as power of attorney and they have not been honored. Staff members need training about these documents, and healthcare settings need a mechanism for recording that such documents exist. Finally, they must be honored in emergency situations. Chapter 13 contained detailed information about these legal issues.

- *Action Steps*
  1. Inform yourself about the state and local laws related to power of attorney and guardianship in your region.
  2. Keep copies of the relevant forms, or information about how to get these forms available and ask every patient/client if they need this information.
  3. Have a designated place to keep copies of these documents or record that they have such documents.

Number 4: Know the Potential Consequences of Stress Related to Stigma: Assess for Substance Abuse, Including Tobacco Dependence, Mental Health Problems, Body Image and Weight Issues, Unsafe Sexual Practices, and Domestic Violence as Well as Physical Health Problems

We know that there are higher rates of many physical and mental health disorders in LGBTQ people, at least of the disorders that are influenced by stress. Stigma has enormous impact on individual's lives. As a healthcare professional, you can educate your patients/clients about their risk factors. Many LGBTQ people do not recognize the impact of stress on their health—they have lived with the stress for so long that it has become "normal." You can help them name the stress, learn more positive coping strategies, and recognize the role of minority stress to relieve individual self-blaming.

- *Action Steps*
  1. Recognize that the higher rates of illness are due to stigma, not one's sexual or gender identity.
  2. Help clients/patients understand this fact as well, so they do not blame themselves. Help them reduce internalized oppression if they suffer from it by treating them as worthy, unique individuals.
  3. Share the information you learned in this book with coworkers, so they do not "blame the victim" and assume that health problems in LGBTQ people are because of their "lifestyles."

Number 3: Celebrate the Diversity of LGBTQ Communities, Based on Differences in Age, Racial/Ethnic Identities, Geography, Immigration Status, Language, Socioeconomic Class, and Education

LGBTQ people are as diverse in every way as any other client/patient. Some of their other identities may influence health as much or more than their sexual or gender identities, because minority stress can stem from the oppression based on race/ethnicity, social class, age, and other human differences as well as from sexuality and gender variations. All healthcare professionals need reminders to resist stereotypical thinking based on any of these characteristics, and examine social justice issues that occur in the workplace. **Diversity is a good thing, both in employees and in patients/clients, and adds to the richness of our culture.**

- *Action Steps*
  1. Treat every patient/client as a unique individual and do not assume that you know anything about them based on some visible presenting characteristic.
  2. Make sure that assessments take into account the patient/client's understandings of the role of their diverse identities in their illness or treatment needs. Listening to patient's own cultural understandings of health and illness will lead to better treatment planning.
  3. Seek out diversity training that considers the intersections of multiple oppressed identities rather than viewing each one separately.
  4. Examine the power dynamics in your own workplace. Who has power and authority and who does not?

Number 2: Understand the Effects of Homophobia/Biphobia/ Transphobia in the Healthcare Workplace Setting for LGBTQ Employees

We have described the far-reaching effects of stigma on patients and clients, but also on LGBTQ healthcare professionals. As we have seen, many LGBTQ healthcare professionals are afraid to be "out" in their workplaces. They fear how they will be treated by coworkers and by patients/clients. How does oppression play out in your work setting? How ironic is it that settings that are supposed to be about "caring" and "healing" are so often among the most hostile and uncaring places where LGBTQ people may work? What is the climate of the workplace where you work for LGBTQ staff members?

- *Action Steps*
  1. Examine employee policies. Do they prohibit discrimination on the basis of sexual orientation? How about gender identity? If they do not, advocate for policy change.
  2. What about sexual harassment policies? Do they include sexual and gender identities?
  3. What happens if someone does harass or mistreat an employee on the basis of sexual identity and gender identity? Are there any sanctions? If not, propose that there be consequences for acting in a discriminatory way.
  4. Consider the overall climate. Even when inclusive policies are in place, are LGBTQ employees expected to be invisible? Are they treated differently? How could this climate be changed? You can start the change process by being a role model of acceptance and inclusivity.

Number 1: Reflect on What It Might Be Like to Be an LGBTQ Patient in Your Healthcare Setting—Do You Have Realistic Concerns about How an LGBTQ Person Might Be Treated? If They Are Not Realistic, How Can You Convey to Patients that Your Environment Is Safe?

This recommendation requires that you put yourself in the shoes of an LGBTQ patient in your work setting. How would you feel about the waiting or reception area, the pamphlets and patient education materials, the posters on the wall, and the forms and policies? Several of the action steps above have focused on the policies and language in the written forms. What about the physical environment? Is it friendly and inclusive in the types of magazines, the patient education brochures or pamphlets, or the artwork on the walls? What about the staff members that a patient/client first encounters? Have they had diversity training? How can you make it feel safe and welcoming to as many patients/clients as possible? Your healthcare setting exists within a larger community, and many communities have some LGBTQ resources that healthcare agencies have not utilized. What resources does the local community have for LGBTQ people? Are there LGBTQ social service or political organizations and social outlets? Are there community activists who could help your setting become more inclusive and welcoming? Sometimes healthcare institutions have "bad" reputations in LGBTQ communities and do not even know it. The reputation could stem from one incident years earlier, and could be improved by even a small outreach to the LGBTQ community.

- **Action Steps**
1. If it is hard for you to put yourself in the place of an LGBTQ patient, ask someone from the LGBTQ community to do a "walk through" or review policies, procedures, and climate issues with you and your coworkers. Even if you are LGBTQ yourself, it may be hard to see your own workplace objectively.
2. Conduct a needs assessment of the local LGBTQ community to find out the reputation of your setting and identify strengths and weaknesses of your setting.
3. Identify LGBTQ specific materials to place strategically in the setting—these could include local or national LGBTQ newsletters or magazines, health education pamphlets, and/or books that depict LGBTQ families.
4. Advertise job openings and your agency's services in LGBTQ community newspapers or at LGBTQ centers or social institutions.

Conclusions

We hope that this book has been helpful to you personally and will serve as a resource to you and your coworkers. We have tried to balance information with thought-provoking questions and real life stories to facilitate the learning. Knowledge and attitudes are one component of change, but real change also requires action. This final chapter, in particular, has outlined a number of steps that you can take as an individual to improve the climate in healthcare settings and society as a whole, for LGBTQ people. There are numerous other resources that you can access to continue the process of being an inclusive and welcoming provider of healthcare services, including books, websites, and organizations. We invite you to continue on this path of social justice and leave you with these final words.

> *"Never doubt that a small group of thoughtful, committed citizens can change the world.*
>
> *Indeed, it is the only thing that ever has."*
>
> *Margaret Mead*

Reference

Lipson, J., & Dibble, S. L. (2005). Providing culturally appropriate health care. In *Culture and critical care*. San Francisco, CA: UCSF Nursing Press.

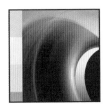

Index